Learning Strategies for Allied Health Students

Learning Strategies for Allied Health Students

Susan Marcus Palau, MA
Learning Specialist
Private Practice
Westchester, NY

Marilyn Meltzer, MA
Hunter College
New York, NY

W.B. SAUNDERS COMPANY
A Division of Harcourt Brace & Company
Philadelphia   London   Toronto
Montreal   Sydney   Tokyo

W.B. SAUNDERS COMPANY
A Division of Harcourt Brace & Company

The Curtis Center
Independence Square West
Philadelphia, PA 19106

Library of Congress Cataloging-in-Publication Data

Palau, Susan Marcus.
    Learning strategies for allied health students / Susan Marcus Palau, Marilyn Meltzer. — 1st ed.
      p.   cm.
   ISBN 0-7216-5603-X
    1. Paramedical education.   2. Study skills.   3. Allied health personnel.   I. Meltzer, Marilyn.   II. Title.
R847.P35   1996
610.73'7'0711—dc20   95-901

LEARNING STRATEGIES FOR ALLIED HEALTH STUDENTS   ISBN 0-7216-5603-X

Copyright © 1996 by W.B. Saunders Company

All rights reserved. No part of this publication may be reproduced or transmitted in any form or by any means, electronic or mechanical, including photocopy, recording, or any information storage and retrieval system, without permission in writing from the publisher.

Printed in the United States of America

Last digit is the print number: 9 8 7 6 5 4 3 2 1

To my Mother
and the memory of my Father
SMP

In memory of my Mother,
Esther Cohen Astalos
MM

Preface

Learning Strategies for Health Care Students is intended for those health care students who need additional help in reading the textbook, writing school and work-related reports, solving math problems, and studying. The purpose of this book is to provide these students with the learning strategies that will enable them to successfully finish their health care programs and to function well in the workplace. With this book, health care students can practice basic reading, writing, math, and study skills on materials taken from currently used health care textbooks in a wide variety of fields.

Organization

Unit I, Reading Strategies, will teach students better techniques for understanding what they read. They will learn ways of organizing the vast amount of information they will be getting from their texts and ways of learning the new terminology they will be exposed to as students in health care.

Unit II, Writing Strategies, will present students with the procedures for writing reports for classroom and work purposes. Students will be shown the various processes for getting started, producing the first copy, editing for errors, and writing the final copy.

Unit III, Mathematics Strategies, will introduce students to the basic concepts of health care mathematics. These strategies should help them overcome any anxiety or resistance they may have to math.

Unit IV, Study Strategies, will provide the student with all the strategies they will need to perform well in class and on examinations.

Unit V, Reading Selections, contains 15 reading selections taken from health care textbooks and will allow the students to practice all the major strategies they learned in the other units.

Each chapter in Units I through IV contains the following:

- Learning objectives
- Vocabulary words
- Vocabulary check
- Strategies presentations
- Examples
- Exercises
- Chapter summary

Unit V, Reading Selections, gives students the chance to practice the following strategies they learned in the previous four units:

- Previewing
- Developing vocabulary
- Reading
- Writing
- Answering objective questions
- Solving word problems

Using the Textbook

Since this textbook contains 15 chapters, it is intended to be used in one semester with the students doing one chapter weekly. Unit V, Reading Selections, can be used at the same time the students are working on the chapters or when the students have finished Chapter 15.

Learning Strategies for Health Care Students can be used in one of three ways:

1. It can be used in the traditional classroom setting with an instructor explaining and modeling the strategies to be learned.
2. Students can use this text for self-study, since the strategies are clearly explained and abundant examples are given for each strategy.
3. Students can form small groups to use this book, with an instructor acting as a consultant to these groups.

Setting Up the Course

Learning Strategies for Health Care Students can be used by students who may have had difficulties with entrance examinations or standardized reading tests. The course can be a requirement for all incoming freshman students. This book is especially helpful for older adult students returning to school after a long time. Instructors will find this text useful for introducing all students to a higher level of academic work.

If *Learning Strategies for Health Care Students* is used in a traditional class setting, the instructor should provide guided practice — working closely with students initially and then gradually allowing the student to work independently. If students are using this text individually or in small groups, they are encouraged to do each chapter in the given order. However, the first four units are independent of each other and can be done in any order. The instructor can be responsible for grading and assessing the students' progress or the students can assess their own progress individually or in small groups. Finally, an answer key at the end of the book will make doing this task easier.

Motivating the Students

The strategies in *Learning Strategies for Health Care Students* are presented in a straightforward manner so that students will be successful using this book. Once they have had ample time to use these strategies in the classroom and workplace and get positive results, motivational problems for the students should be resolved.

Acknowledgments

We would like to extend a hearty thanks to Lisa Biello, Editor-in-Chief Health-Related Professions, for her good sense and great laugh. In addition, we would like to thank Margaret M. Biblis for first taking on this project. We also would like to thank Sara Meltzer and Michael Meltzer for their extraordinary word processing skills, and Mary Espenschied and Jeanne Gulledge of CRACOM Corporation who helped us in the production process.

Susan Marcus Palau
Marilyn Meltzer

Contents

Unit I	**Reading Strategies**		**1**
	1	Identifying the Three Levels of Understanding	3
	2	Recognizing Details	16
	3	Developing Vocabulary	38
	4	Monitoring and Improving Comprehension	53
	5	Reading the Textbook	65
Unit II	**Writing Strategies**		**93**
	6	Organizing Ideas	95
	7	Writing the First Draft	106
	8	Rewriting the Final Draft	114
Unit III	**Mathematics Strategies**		**131**
	9	Learning Computation Skills	133
	10	Understanding Algebra, Geometry, and the Metric System	150
	11	Solving Word Problems	172
Unit IV	**Study Strategies**		**187**
	12	Managing Time	189
	13	Learning Active Listening Skills	198
	14	Taking Notes	204
	15	Improving Test Scores	223
Unit V	**Reading Selections**		**245**
References			**324**
Glossary			**325**
Answer Key			**329**
Index			**347**

UNIT 1

READING STRATEGIES

As a student of the allied health professions, one of your first responsibilities will be to grapple with a great amount of reading. In many instances, this will be the first time that you will have been exposed to medical vocabulary and concepts. Because your time is so precious, it will be necessary that you get the meaning of what you are reading as efficiently as possible. You will have to recognize and understand important facts and details and apply them to real-life situations. You will have to develop a new vocabulary for your future career and learn ways of becoming aware of when you do not understand these new words and ideas from your textbook. Lastly, you will have to familiarize yourself with the layout of a textbook so that you can learn the strategies for being an active reader.

Chapter 1, Identifying the Three Levels of Understanding, will teach you how to read for a purpose. You will also be taught the strategies for reading and interpreting factual information, and for applying these new ideas to real life situations. Chapter 2, Recognizing Details, will teach you the organization of the many facts in a passage so that your comprehension will improve. Chapter 3, Developing Vocabulary, will offer you strategies for improving your medical and general vocabulary. Chapter 4, Monitoring and Improving Comprehension, will suggest ways in which you can become aware of when you are not understanding what you are reading and strategies to correct this. Finally, Chapter 5, Reading the Textbook, will explain the layout of textbooks and give you strategies for becoming an active reader of your health care texts.

Once you have completed the exercises in Unit 1, Reading Strategies, you should be better equipped to meet the first big challenge of your health care program, reading and comprehending your reading assignments as effectively as you can.

BUTTON TO MONITOR COMPREHENSION

To improve your comprehension, you must first become aware of when you are not understanding. You do this by asking yourself frequently if you are understanding what you are reading. To help you get used to monitoring your comprehension, the following button will appear throughout the text:

This button will act as a reminder to monitor your comprehension by asking yourself if you are comprehending what you are reading.

Chapter 1

Identifying the Three Levels of Understanding

LEARNING OBJECTIVES
VOCABULARY WORDS
VOCABULARY CHECK
READING WITH A PURPOSE
INTRODUCING THE THREE LEVELS OF UNDERSTANDING
    Literal Understanding
        Identifying the Topic of a Passage
        Identifying the Main Idea
    Interpretive Understanding
        Details as Clues
    Applied Understanding
REVIEWING THE LEARNING STRATEGIES

LEARNING OBJECTIVES

In this chapter you will learn how to
- Improve your reading comprehension by reading for a purpose
- Identify the appropriate level of understanding that fits your purpose for reading
- Use strategies for reading at the literal, interpretive, and applied levels

VOCABULARY WORDS

The following vocabulary words are important to your understanding of the ideas in this chapter. These vocabulary words are underscored the first time they are used in the chapter. Read the list of words and definitions. Then check your understanding of these words before you read the chapter.

asepsis freedom from infection (Miller-Keane, p. 141).
autocratic pertaining to one who has total power.
conclusions outcomes or results.
document informational paper.
efficiently pertaining to being productive without any waste.
hemostasis stopping blood flow by natural and artificial means.
lymph a transparent, usually slightly yellow, often opalescent liquid found within the lymphatic vessels (Miller-Keane, p. 867).
neurologist a specialist in the branch of health science that deals with the nervous system (Miller-Keane, p. 1021).
supine lying with the face upward (Miller-Keane, p. 1438).
topical pertaining to a particular area (Miller-Keane, p. 1506).

VOCABULARY CHECK

Directions: Choose the vocabulary word that best fits into the sentence.

1. The unit coordinator prided himself on working as _____ as possible.
2. In the operating room, the principles of _____ are applied.
3. One of the major fluids in the human body is the _____.
4. The pharmacist sold me over-the-counter _____ medicine to put on my sunburn.
5. I saw a _____ after I had a severe headache for over a month.
6. Before surgery, the orderly placed the patient on the operating table in the _____ position.
7. Her _____ personality in the classroom made her young students dislike her.
8. In order to manage the patient during the operation, the technician maintained the _____.
9. He typed a copy of the _____ on the computer.
10. The two mystery stories with the same name ended with different _____.

READING WITH A PURPOSE

As students in the health care professions, you quickly discover the great amount of reading that you are required to complete. It is necessary that you accomplish these reading tasks as <u>efficiently</u> as possible. This means that you get as much understanding as you can during each of your study sessions. You cannot afford to waste time by performing at less than your best each time you sit at your desk and read. An excellent strategy that guarantees that each reading session will be successful is to read with a purpose. When you read with a purpose, you create a goal that you wish to accomplish each time you read. Having a goal to reach will keep you focused and involved in your reading. Your comprehension will be improved by reading with a purpose.

INTRODUCING THE THREE LEVELS OF UNDERSTANDING

There is more than one way to understand what you are reading in your textbook. The goal or purpose you set for yourself as you read will determine the level of understanding required for comprehension of the reading material.

- The first level of understanding is called **literal understanding.** This level of understanding requires that you know what the subject of your reading is and the most important points being made about the subject. For example, when you need to learn important terms, names and functions of different parts of the body, or steps in a procedure from your textbook, you use literal understanding.
- The second level of understanding is called **interpretive understanding.** This level of understanding requires that you draw <u>conclusions</u> about what you are reading by examining the facts that are presented. For example, when you are reading to learn how to schedule patients according to the seriousness of their complaints, reading to learn how to decide on the proper medical insurance forms to fill out for a patient, or reading to learn how to examine stained smears for the presence of certain microorganisms, you use interpretive understanding.
- The third level of understanding is called **applied understanding.** This level of understanding requires that you see how ideas are similar so that you can use ideas from one situation in another related situation. For example, when you are asked to read a chapter about focusing the microscope and then you use one correctly in the laboratory or when you memorize from your text the proper handwashing technique and then use it when you handle patients, you use applied understanding.

Again, your goal or purpose for reading will determine which level of understanding you need to use when reading your textbook.

EXERCISE 1–1

Directions: Your instructor gives you assignments to learn different types of information. These assignments are listed below. If the assignment requires literal understanding, write "L" in the blank next to the assignment. If the assignment requires interpretive understanding, write "I" in the blank next to the assignment. If the assignment requires applied understanding, write "A" in the blank next to the assignment.

Assignment 1: You are asked to memorize the names of the important parts of the human brain. ____
Assignment 2: You are asked to make up a patient chart following a model chart that the instructor has created. ____
Assignment 3: The instructor asks you to retype a document that has been corrected and marked with proofreading symbols. ____
Assignment 4: You are asked to figure out what the different tail positions of a cat mean. ____
Assignment 5: You are given a chart of the components of blood and are asked to label the different parts. ____
Assignment 6: The instructor hands you a study sheet describing the different plural endings of medical terms. You are asked to use the plural endings for every medical term in a report you are writing. ____
Assignment 7: After successfully completing Chapter 9 in your textbook, you are expected to be able to fill a syringe. ____
Assignment 8: You are expected to spell all the important words in the first chapter of your health care textbook. ____
Assignment 9: You are asked to list the four major food groups. ____
Assignment 10: You need to determine whether a patient's diet includes all the proper food groups. ____

Let us now take a closer look at each of the different levels of understanding and see how each level suggests a strategy for improving reading comprehension.

Literal Understanding

When you read for literal understanding, you are reading for facts and information. You are trying to determine what the passage is saying in a basic, straightforward way. The strategy to use for literal understanding is to identify the topic and main idea of the selection you are reading. Finding the topic and main idea of a passage will give you a purpose for reading and will help you to concentrate on the essential points in the selection that you need to learn.

Identifying the Topic of a Passage

The topic is the key subject of the passage. To find the topic, you ask:

- What is this passage mostly about?

The answer will be the topic or subject of the passage and should be stated as briefly as possible.

Example 1-1

Following is a selection from Solomon (p. 183). Read the passage and notice how one reader identified the topic of the passage by asking, What is this passage mostly about?

When filtering and destroying bacteria from the <u>lymph</u>, the lymph nodes help prevent the spread of infection. When bacteria are present, lymph nodes may increase in size and become tender. You may have experienced the swollen cervical lymph nodes that often accompany a sore throat. An infection in almost any part of the body may result in swelling and tenderness of the lymph nodes that drain that area.

- Question: What is this passage mostly about?
- Answer: lymph nodes = Topic.

Notice also that the term *lymph nodes* appears many times in the selection. A repeated word is also a clue that the topic of the passage is "lymph nodes."

EXERCISE 1-2

Directions: Read the following selections. In the space provided, write the topic of each selection. Remember to use the strategy of asking yourself, What is this passage mostly about? Be as brief as possible with your answer. Check to see if the word or words you choose appear frequently in the selection.

1. The health unit coordinator has access to a great deal of confidential information. By the very nature of your job, you are exposed to information that is considered confidential, such as surgical procedures, diagnostic results, and other medical reports. This information should be treated with absolute confidentiality—that is, secrecy—by all health personnel (LaFleur-Brooks, p. 53).

Topic: _____

2. The surgical assistant is often responsible for maintaining <u>hemostasis</u> during surgery. Hemostasis is needed both to limit the volume of blood loss and to obtain adequate visibility in the incision. Hemostasis can be obtained by a variety of methods with which the surgical assistant should be familiar (McCurnin, p. 310).

Topic: _____

3. It is always advisable to carefully check all references and to follow through on any leads for information. It is best to use the telephone in checking references because people are sometimes less than <u>candid</u> in a letter; furthermore, letter writing is time-consuming, and you may not get a reply (Kinn, Woods, and Derge, p. 365).

Topic: _____

4. The cat has been used increasingly in psychotherapy sessions to stimulate communication, provide an object for affection, and allow the patient's mastery of a situation. Cats also have been prescribed for home therapy, working 24 hours a day to draw individuals into an awareness of their surroundings or to provide affection and emotional security where they might be lacking. Therapy in institutional settings for the emotionally disturbed and the mentally retarded also has received a big boost when cats are part of the settings because the animals increase the effect of the professional staff and provide continuity during staff turnovers (Beaver, p. 7).

Topic: _____

5. Appointment scheduling is the process that determines which patients will be seen by the physician, how soon they will be seen, and how much time will be allotted to each patient on the basis of his or her complaint and the physician's availability. A vital step in efficient time management is to realize that there will always be unforeseen interruptions and delays. Most providers of medical care find that efficient scheduling of appointments is one of the most important factors in the success of the practice. However, some providers do no scheduling. They conduct their practices with open office hours.

Topic: _____

Identifying the Main Idea

The main idea of a passage is what the passage is all about. The strategy to use to identify the main idea is to ask,

- What is the most important point being made about the topic?

The answer will be the main idea and should be stated in sentence form.

Example 1–2

Read the following excerpt from a health care textbook and pay attention to how the reader found the main idea by identifying the topic and then asking the question, What is the most important point being made about the topic?

Good business writing depends on clarity. If the basic element used to convey meaning—the sentence—is unclear, the entire message may be difficult to understand. Good sentence structure requires the application of all the rules of English grammar and the avoidance of certain particularly common errors (Diehl and Fordney, p. 304).

- What is this passage mostly about? Good writing = Topic.
- What is the most important point being made about good writing? Good writing depends on clear sentences = Main idea.

Notice that the first sentence in the paragraph, "Good business writing depends on clarity," contains the main idea of the selection. In this example the main idea was the first sentence. In other cases, however, the main idea may be in the last sentence, in the middle sentence, or in both the first and last sentences. In some instances, you may not be able to find a main idea sentence. In such cases, you will need to create you own main idea sentence. The strategy will be the same as you used for finding a given main idea sentence. You determine the topic and then ask the main idea question: What is the most important point being made about the topic? As long as you use this strategy, your answer should lead you to the main idea, regardless of where it is located. As long as you create and answer the main idea question, you should be able to make up your own main idea if one cannot be found in the passage.

EXERCISE 1-3

Directions: Read the following passages taken from health care textbooks. In the space provided, write in the topic and underline the main idea sentence. If the main idea is not stated, create your own in the space provided. In either case, don't forget to use the strategy of asking yourself the two questions:

- What is this passage mostly about? = Topic
- What is the most important point being made about the topic = Main idea

Don't forget that the main idea sentence can appear anywhere in the passage, or not at all.

1. The **cell** is the basic unit of all life. The human body is made up of millions of cells. Cells perform specific functions, and their size and shape vary according to function. Bones, muscles, skin and blood are each made up of different kinds of cells. The cell was discovered by Robert Hooke over 300 years ago. Body cells are microscopic; approximately 2000 are needed to make an inch (LaFleur-Brooks, p. 358).

Topic: _____

(Unstated main idea: _____)

2. Three types of connective tissue fibers are collagen fibers, reticular fibers, and elastic fibers. **Collagen fibers** are the most numerous. Collagen fibers contain the protein **collagen,** the most abundant protein in the body. Collagen is a very tough substance, and collagen fibers give great strength to body structures (Solomon, pp. 35–36).

Topic: _____

(Unstated main idea: _____)

3. Liquid <u>topical</u> anesthetic agents are in the form of a thick liquid containing a flavoring agent. They are applied by having the patient swish a small amount of the solution around in the mouth.

    In patients who have an excessive gag reflex, liquid topical anesthetics are used to numb the surfaces of the oral tissues just prior to taking impressions or making intra-oral radiographs.

    They also may be used to provide temporary relief from the pain of ulcers, wounds, and other injured areas in the mouth (Ehrlich and Torres, p. 319).

Topic: _____

(Unstated main idea: _____)

4. One type of computer service is based on a telephone-linked terminal on a time-share basis with other users. Another is the batch type, in which the information is picked up at the office and taken to a computer center for processing. Whether to use computer services and the selection of what service to use are highly individualized decisions that require study and analysis of the practice. It is important to choose a service

that will explain what can be expected from the computer and that will provide all the instruction and supervision necessary to ensure success in using it (Kinn, Woods, Dirge, p. 265).

Topic: _____

(Unstated main idea: _____)

5. On the day of surgery, the surgical site is prepared after the animal is anesthetized. If the hair was not previously clipped, it is done at this time (No. 40 clipper blade in small animals, No. 10 in large animals). The hair should be closely clipped for an area extending at least 7 cm in all directions from the site of the proposed skin incision. Long hair that originates outside this area, but droops into the field, should also be clipped. If an open wound is present, it should be packed with a sterile, water-soluble lubricant prior to clipping the hair. The lubricant traps hair and debris, allowing it to be flushed away during skin preparation. Areas with obvious signs of infection should be clipped last so that the clippers will not spread infective fluids and debris toward the intended incision site. A chemical depilatory (hair remover) is occasionally used to remove hard-to-clip residual hair (after clipping). Several antiseptic soaps are available for skin preparation (Betadine, Purdue-Frederick Co.; Nolvasan, Fort Dodge; Hibiclens, Stuart Pharmaceuticals). Several effective methods for preparing the surgical site are available. Initial skin preparation should be done in the preparation room. The skin is initially washed to remove gross contamination. Some modifications of the scrubbing technique may be necessary, depending upon the surgical scrub used. The surgical site is scrubbed at least three separate times. It is extremely important to begin the scrub in the center of the clipped area, over the proposed incision site, and scrub toward the periphery, *never* going back to the center of the area with the same gauze sponge. The animal is carefully moved to the operating table and positioned. If contamination occurs during transit, the animal is rescrubbed. Many veterinarians prefer to have the surgery site scrubbed after the animal is positioned on the operating table. This method is acceptable but does result in increased contamination of the surgery room (McCurnin, p. 270).

Topic: _____

(Unstated main idea: _____)

Interpretive Understanding

When you read for interpretive understanding, you are reading to figure out something unstated in the passage. The strategy you use for interpretive understanding is to examine the facts or details in the passage and to use your own experience and background knowledge to draw a conclusion about the meaning of the passage. Drawing the correct conclusions about what you are reading will allow you to understand better what the writer really means and will allow you to function better in your workplace.

Details as Clues

When you use interpretive understanding, you need to go beyond the literal meaning of the passage and reason out in what direction the facts or details are leading. This requires that you infer or make a judgment about the meaning of the details. In other words, your responsibility when using interpretive understanding is to examine the details and use them as clues to help you form your own logical conclusions. In addition, you need to rely on information you have learned from your other classes and from you own life in order to come to the right explanation of the passage.

Example 1–3

Read the following description of a medical assistant's boss from Kinn, Woods, and Derge (p. 73). Then read how the medical assistant interpreted this behavior and drew the conclusion on the best way to behave with this boss. Notice that she uses facts describing the boss and her own experience to interpret the situation.

An <u>autocratic</u> supervisor is a leader. This person dictates procedure, policy, and tasks. This individual tells you how to do a task and when to do it. An autocratic person may feel uncomfortable in delegating authority. He or she seldom accepts employees who have traits such as initiative, creativity, and assertiveness.

MEDICAL ASSISTANT'S INTERPRETIVE UNDERSTANDING:

I see that the boss is a leader. That means that he must need followers. I guess that means that I must carefully follow whatever orders he gives me. I see that he likes to tell you how and when to do things. My dad is like that and, boy, does he get angry when I take that responsibility on myself. I'd better wait and let the boss show me how to do things around here and let him decide on my schedule. I also understand that he likes to do everything himself. I remember reading about that type of personality in my psych class. It will be in my best interest not to seem too bossy. It seems that, to get along with this guy, I must follow all his directions and stick to the rules of the office.

Note that the medical assistant used both the details or facts describing the boss and her own personal knowledge and experience to determine what type of behavior would be best with the autocratic type of boss.

EXERCISE 1–4

Directions: Below are a series of situations taken from health care textbooks. Following each is an interpretive understanding question. Read the question and choose the best answer by circling the letter of the best choice. Remember to use facts from the passages and your own personal experience and knowledge to help you choose the correct answer.

1. When you are ushered into the interviewer's room, wait to be seated until you are invited to do so. Let the interviewer lead the conversation. Be prepared to answer such questions as "Tell me about yourself" and "Why do you want to work here?" (Kinn, Woods, and Derge, p. 88).

You can conclude that the reason the interviewer starts the interview in this way is to

    a. see if you are made nervous easily
    b. have a chance to get acquainted
    c. check how well you memorized your résumé
    d. determine whether you think and talk like the interviewer

2. All patients, when initially seen, need to give the physician a complete history of their problems and be examined. How many questions they are asked, the types of questions, and body area emphasized are determined both by the patient's problem and by the medical specialty involved (Diehl and Fordney, p. 245).

You can conclude from this that
   a. A patient with headaches will have a <u>neurologist</u> pay more attention to his head than his other body systems to some extent.
   b. The neurologist would not be interested in the fact that the patient hit his head 2 months ago.
   c. The neurologist would ask for a medical history only after she has examined the patient thoroughly.
   d. A general practitioner would make an automatic referral to a neurologist for this patient before examining him.

3. Respiratory care is the department within the hospital that performs treatments ordered by the doctor that are related to respiratory function. The task of the health unit coordinator is to communicate these orders to the respiratory care department. The treatments are performed at the patient's bedside by a respiratory technician or therapist. If the doctor orders medication as a part of the treatment, it may be the health unit coordinator's task to order medication from the pharmacy (LaFleur-Brooks, p. 266).

Which of the following questions does the passage answer?
   a. Who is responsible for writing in the patient's chart?
   b. What respiratory treatments are the best?
   c. What medications did the doctor order?
   d. Who is responsible for communicating with the respiratory department?

4. Urine is an excellent growth medium for many bacteria because it contains electrolytes, water-soluble vitamins, residual amounts of glucose, and various nitrogenous compounds (McCurnin, p. 110).

You can conclude that
   a. The proper collection and handling of urine for culture is important.
   b. You should collect urine only by catheterization.
   c. Because there is bacteria in urine, it does not need refrigeration.
   d. All of the above.

5. For vision to occur, light must pass through the eye and form an image on the retina. Light passes through the transparent cornea, the aqueous humor, the lens, and the vitreous body before reaching the retina. After the image is formed on the retina, nerve impulses must be transmitted to the visual areas of the cerebral cortex (Solomon, p. 121).

Which of the following statements can be concluded from the passage?
   a. The only organ involved with seeing is the eye.
   b. The retina does not have nerve endings.
   c. Light is crucial to seeing.
   d. The retina is the first part of the eye that light reaches.

EXERCISE 1-5

Read the following excerpt on minimizing waiting time for a patient on the telephone (Kinn, Woods, and Derge, pp. 143–144). Using your background knowledge and experience and details from the passage, write the best responses in the spaces provided.

When a call cannot be put through immediately, ask,

_____.

If the caller elects to wait, remember that waiting with a silent telephone can be irritating. The waiting time, no matter how brief, always seems long. Let no more than 1 minute pass without breaking in with some reassuring comment, for instance,

_____.

If the wait is longer than expected, the caller may wish to reconsider and call back at another time or have the call returned, but he or she needs to communicate this to you. By going back on the line at frequent intervals, you give the caller an opportunity to express such concerns. In fact, you may ask the caller if he or she wishes to continue waiting. Say something like,

_____.

Try to give the caller some estimate of when he or she may expect the return call. In any event, irritation can be lessened by your consideration in saying:

_____.

When it is necessary for you to leave the telephone to obtain information, ask the caller:

_____,

and then wait for a reply. When you return to the telephone, thank the caller for waiting.

Applied Understanding

When you read for applied understanding, you are reading to learn ideas from your textbook so you can use these ideas in school or in the workplace. The strategies you will use for applied understanding include the strategies you use for literal and interpretive understanding.

- In order to apply information, you must first learn the facts. This will require that you learn and remember ideas literally. Finding the topic and the main idea will help you focus on what is important.
- In order to apply information, you must be able to interpret what you are reading. This will require that you have some background knowledge of the subject and of the situation to which you will be applying the information.
- Finally, in order to apply information, you must use good judgment. You must be able to recognize the similarities and differences between the facts you read and the situations in which you will be applying these facts. You must be able to judge when and where it is appropriate and correct to apply these facts. This judgment requires that you know your facts and have experience. Following is an example from Ehrlich and Torres (p. 137) of how one dental assistant student thought through an emergency situation and successfully used applied understanding in the workplace.

14 READING STRATEGIES

Example 1-4

Today was my third day of clinical placement and I was working with Dr. Pepper and his patients. The night before, I had finished reading Chapter 9 in my textbook, and one part of the chapter stuck in my mind—the procedure for responding to the patient who feels faint. I remember it said the following:

1. *Immediately reposition the patient in the <u>supine</u> position.*
2. *After a few minutes, slowly return the patient to an upright position.*
3. *If the patient still feels dizzy and faint, immediately lower him to the supine position once again.*
4. *Administer oxygen if necessary.*

Was I glad that I learned this because Mrs. Klein, who must be about 6 months pregnant, appeared to faint as I raised the back of her chair. My first responsibility was to judge whether or not she had actually fainted. I called her name and she responded that she felt faint. At this point I buzzed for Dr. Pepper, while I slowly lowered the back of the chair. After a few minutes I raised the chair slowly and by this time Dr. Pepper had arrived and started to give Mrs. Klein some oxygen. Dr. Pepper praised me for acting so calmly and using good judgment in an emergency situation. I was glad I knew my facts also so I was able to do the right thing.

EXERCISE 1-6

Directions: In the left-hand column are titles of chapters from a textbook by Kinn, Woods, and Derge. In the right-hand column are tasks taken from Kinn, Woods, and Derge that you should be able to complete after reading and learning the correct chapter. In the blank space next to the task, write in the letter of the chapter you would need to learn in order to perform the task. The first one has been done for you.

A. Basic Concepts of <u>Asepsis</u> (Ch. 23)   <u>I</u>   Explain the difference between "good" and "bad" cholesterol (p. 691)

B. Banking Services and Procedures (Ch. 17)   ___   Obtain a patient's height and weight within $\frac{1}{4}$ inch and $\frac{1}{4}$ pound of your evaluator's measurements (p. 467)

C. Patient Reception (Ch. 9)   ___   Address envelopes using the guidelines for optical scanning (p. 184)

D. Correspondence and Mail Processing (Ch. 12)   ___   Perform a 2-minute medical handwash according to medical aseptic principles without missing a step or incorrectly performing a step (p. 407)

E. Dictation and Transcription (Ch. 13)   ___   List at least 10 items that should be completed on a patient's registration form (p. 119)

F. Management Responsibilities (Ch. 22)   ___   Correctly type numbers in a dictated report (p. 204)

G. Vital Signs and Anthropometric Measurements (Ch. 26)

H. Microbiology in the Physician's Office (Ch. 31)

I. Nutrition and Diet Modification (Ch. 34)

J. Assisting With Minor Surgery (Ch. 36)

K. Medical Emergencies (Ch. 40)

___ Collect a throat culture and prepare it for immediate examination (p. 596)

___ Discuss the advantage of using checks for the transfer of funds (p 285)

___ Prepare an outline of contents for a basic office manual (p. 389)

___ Recognize the major symptoms of a heart attack (p. 877)

___ Put on a pair of sterile gloves without contaminating them (p. 756)

REVIEWING THE LEARNING STRATEGIES

TO LEARN — **USE THIS STRATEGY**

Literal understanding — Identify the topic of the passage by asking What is this passage mostly about?
Identify the main idea of the passage by asking, What is the most important point being made about the topic?

Interpretive understanding — Examine the facts and details.
Use your own experiences and background knowledge to draw conclusions.

Applied understanding — Learn the facts for literal understanding.
Use experience and background knowledge to interpret situation.
Use your best judgment to determine when it is appropriate to apply facts to a new situation.

Chapter 2

Recognizing Details

LEARNING OBJECTIVES
VOCABULARY WORDS
VOCABULARY CHECK
LOCATING SUPPORTING DETAILS
DISTINGUISHING BETWEEN MAIN IDEA AND SUPPORTING DETAILS
MAPPING DETAILS
VERIFYING FACTS FROM THE TEXT
RECOGNIZING LOGICAL RELATIONSHIPS
FOLLOWING THE ORDER OF DETAILS
    Sequence
    Classification
    Examples and Illustrations
    Comparison and Contrast
    Cause and Effect
REVIEWING RECOGNIZING DETAILS

LEARNING OBJECTIVES

In this chapter you will learn how to
- Locate details
- Distinguish between the main idea and important details
- Verify facts from the text
- Recognize logical relationships

VOCABULARY WORDS

The following vocabulary words are important to your understanding of the ideas in this chapter. These vocabulary words are underscored the first time they are used in the chapter. Read the list of words and definitions. Then check your understanding of these words before you read the chapter.

accredited credentialed.
aneurysm a sac formed by the localized dilation of the wall of an artery, a vein, or the heart.
aneurysmectomy surgical removal of an aneurysm.
apprenticeship the practical experience of training under skilled workers.
beneficence kindness.
disclosure something made known.
pancreas a large gland located behind the stomach.
quadrant one of four parts.
sodium salt.
veracity truthfulness.

VOCABULARY CHECK

Directions: Choose the vocabulary word that best fits into the sentence.

1. He learned his trade as a carpenter by serving as an _____.
2. Her _____ toward others made everyone love her.
3. Is the school that you are attending an _____ institution?
4. Although hearing the truth was difficult, I appreciate the doctor's _____.
5. The _____ of health records is unethical without the patient's permission.
6. You should be on a low _____ diet.
7. Will you measure one of the _____ of the circle?
8. The _____ in his heart was fatal.
9. The _____ is the surgery that saved his life.
10. The _____ is an organ of the digestive system.

LOCATING SUPPORTING DETAILS

When you are learning information in the health care fields, it is essential that you learn to locate the important details that explain, illustrate, or prove the main idea. These important details are the facts that help you to understand the main point of the reading material. These facts explain how things work, how things are made, what they are, and why things happen. Locating the supporting details and understanding how these details relate to the main idea is key to your understanding your textbooks.

DISTINGUISHING BETWEEN MAIN IDEA AND SUPPORTING DETAILS

As you read your textbooks, you concentrate on identifying the main idea. In the health care fields, understanding the important details and following the way these details develop the main idea are necessary tools to help you learn the information in your textbooks. As you read your assignments, it is important for you to be able to distinguish the main idea from the important details. Remember that the main idea is a general statement and that the details are specific facts.

MAPPING DETAILS

Details are facts and examples that give you a better understanding of the most important point of a paragraph. Details, then, will relate to or support the main idea.

There are two kinds of details—**important details** and **less important details.** **Important details** relate directly to the main idea. They describe and tell you more about the important point of a paragraph. The relationship between important details and the main idea would look like this diagram or map:

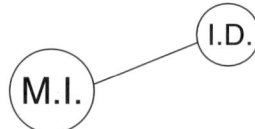

Most paragraphs from your health care textbooks will be filled with many important details. A mapping of the details would look more like this:

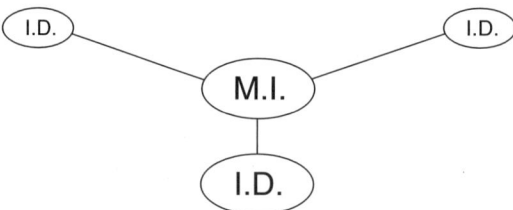

Less important details are details that relate directly to important details. They describe and tell you more about these important details. The relationship among less important details, important details, and the main idea would look like this map:

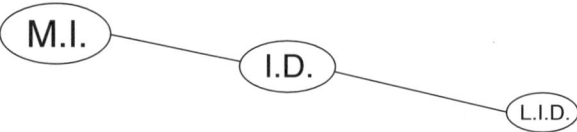

Again, paragraphs from your health care textbooks will be more complex than this. A mapping of both types of details would look more like this:

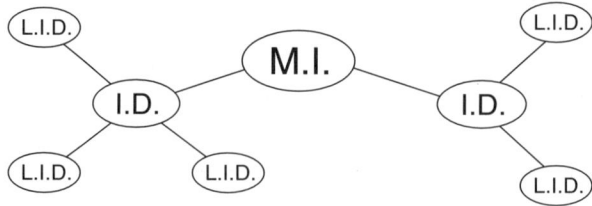

Mapping the main ideas and details will help you visualize, or see, the relationship of the important and less important details to the main idea. This will enable you to better understand what you are reading. It makes sense, especially when you are having trouble understanding a paragraph, to try this strategy. Sometimes seeing how the details relate to each other and the main idea will make the reading clear.

Example 2-1

Below is a selection from the Kim, Woods, and Derge health care textbook *The Medical Assistant: Administrative and Clinical* (p. 95). Following the passage is an example of how to map the main ideas, important details, and less important details.

The medical faculty that uses a batch system sends information daily, by mail or messenger, to a central location; at this location, the data is entered into a main-frame computer. The service bureau then prepares statements, insurance forms, and reports and returns them to the physician by mail or messenger. One of the major problems with this system is the time lag between the sending and the receiving of information; however, it is the simplest and the least expensive way to use a service bureau.

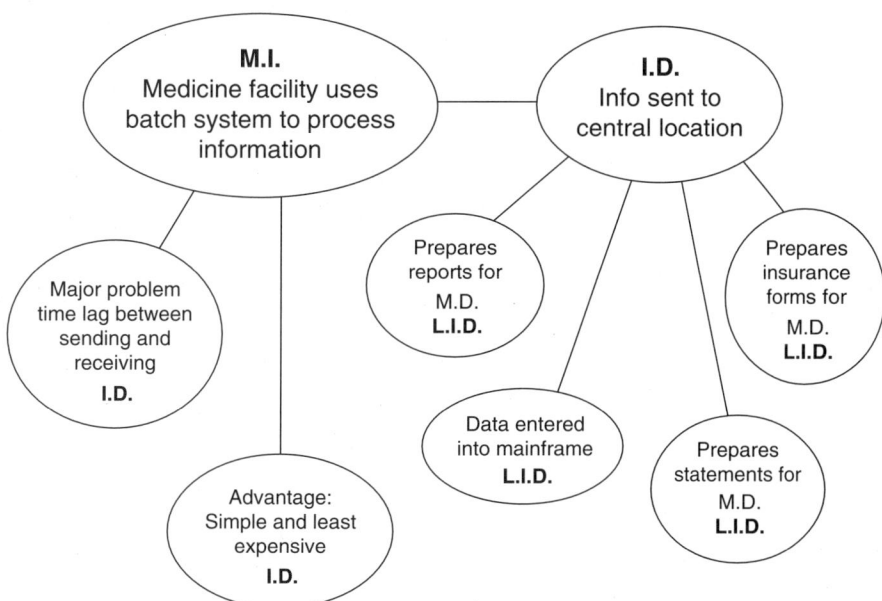

EXERCISE 2-1

Directions: Read the following selection from the Ehrlich and Torres health care textbook *Essentials of Dental Assisting* (p. 24). In the space provided at the top of page 20, draw a details map showing the relationship of the main idea to the important details and less important details.

Well-groomed hair is an important part of your professional appearance. A suitable hairstyle is one that is neat, clean, easily controlled, and not falling over the face (either yours or the patient's).

It is impossible to maintain a clean or clear operating field if the chairside assistant must keep fussing with her hair. Therefore, a hairstyle must also be manageable. This means that it does not require constant fussing, touching, or pushing back into place. If the chairside assistant's hair is long, it must be secured effectively throughout the hours of employment.

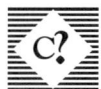

VERIFYING FACTS FROM THE TEXT

When reading your textbooks, your purpose is to learn the information in the assigned chapters. You will most likely have to answer questions following the reading. These questions may be at the end of the chapter or on a study guide provided by the instructor. When you are answering these questions, you want to be able to verify, or prove, that your answers are correct by scanning back to the pages you have read in the text. Scanning for facts is an essential reading strategy that will help you use your textbook more efficiently. Focus on key words in the question to help you find the information you need in the text.

Example 2–2

Directions: Read the following excerpt from a health care textbook (Torres and Ehrlich, p. 13). Answer the multiple-choice questions based on the selection. Then read the explanation of the answers.

THE DENTAL LABORATORY TECHNICIAN

The dental laboratory technician may legally perform only the mechanical, technically skilled tasks specified by the written prescription of the dentist.

Many dental laboratory technicians maintain their own laboratories, providing services for many dentists. Others are employed by individual dentists, larger laboratories, or the military services.

Dental laboratory technicians receive their training through apprenticeship, commercial schools, or accredited programs. The **Certified Dental Technician** (CDT) program was established in 1958 by the National Association of Dental Laboratories in cooperation with the ADA.

Programs approved by the ADA are 2 academic years in length and preferably are conducted in an accredited 2- or 4-year college or post-high school institution.

1. The dental laboratory technician may legally perform
    a. all the mechanical tasks of the dentist.
    b. the written information prescribed by the dental laboratory.
    c. the mechanical tasks specified by the written prescription of the dentist.
    d. none of the technical skilled tasks required by the dentist.

2. Dental laboratory technicians are employed by
   a. the military.
   b. self-employed.
   c. large laboratories.
   d. all of the above.

3. Dental laboratory technicians must be in training programs which are
   a. two calendar years.
   b. two academic years.
   c. four college years.
   d. four high school years.

The answer to question 1 is c. The key word in the question—*legally*—helps you to scan back to the first sentence of the passage. Read this sentence carefully, and you will be able to prove that you have chosen the correct answers. The word *all* in choice a makes that answer incorrect. Choice b is incorrect because a careful reading reveals that the information is prescribed by the *dentist*, not by the dental laboratory. Choice d is incorrect because the word *none* is too exclusive.

The answer to question 2 is d. *Employed* is the key word in the question. Use the key word to scan paragraph 2. All of the choices are correct; therefore choice d is the answer.

The answer to question 3 is b. The key word in question 3 is *training*. Scan the selection to find information about training in the third paragraph. A careful reading of the details will reveal that the information in answer choices a, c, and d are factually incorrect based on the information in the text.

EXERCISE 2–2

Directions: Read the following excerpt from a health care textbook (Torres and Ehrlich, p. 17). Answer the multiple-choice questions based on the selection. Use key words in the question to scan back to the passage to locate the correct answer. On the line next to the question, fill in the paragraph and line number of your answer choice.

THE DUTY OF CARE

The duty of care owed by a dentist to a patient includes the following: The dentist (1) is licensed; (2) uses reasonable skill, care, and judgment; and (3) uses standard drugs, materials, and techniques.

The dentist may refuse to treat a patient; however, this action must *not* be based on the patient's race, color, or creed. Under the Americans with Disabilities Act, patients with an infectious disease such as HIV disease cannot be refused treatment because of their infection.

In rare cases in which the dentist refuses treatment—for example, if the necessary equipment for such treatment is not in the office, or if the patient requires extensive emergency treatment or general anesthesia—the dentist should refer the patient to a facility where he could receive treatment.

22 READING STRATEGIES

Once a dentist undertakes to render dental care, he or she is expected to charge a reasonable fee and to continue that treatment to completion within a reasonable length of time (usually within two years). Otherwise, the dentist may be held liable for abandonment (discontinuation of care after treatment has commenced but before it has been completed).

Also, instructions to the patient must be reasonable and be given in a manner and language that the patient can understand. The dentist may not dismiss or abandon the patient without giving written notification of termination. After notification, care must continue for a reasonable length of time (usually 30 days) to allow the patient to secure another dentist's services.

As for the duties of the patient to the dentist, the patient is legally required to pay a reasonable and agreed-upon fee for services rendered, to cooperate, and to follow instructions.

1. A reasonable length of time for dental treatment is
   a. more than 2 years.   par#____
   b. within 2 years.   line#____
   c. 30 days.
   d. within 30 days.

2. The patient is required to pay the dentist's fee, when the fee is
   a. set by the dentist's overhead.   par#____
   b. based on insurance payments.   line#____
   c. what the patient can afford to pay.
   d. agreed upon by the patient and the dentist.

3. The dentist can dismiss a patient
   a. any time.   par#____
   b. after 2 years.   line#____
   c. after giving written notice.
   d. after finding another dentist to continue the patient's treatment.

4. If a dentist refuses treatment, the dentist
   a. must find another dentist to treat the patient.   par#____
   b. should direct the patient to a dental clinic.   line#____
   c. could lose his license.
   d. should indicate to the patient where treatment might be received.

5. The drugs that a dentist uses on his patient must be
   a. standard.   par#____
   b. prescription.   line#____
   c. over-the-counter.
   d. nonaddictive.

RECOGNIZING LOGICAL RELATIONSHIPS

When reading health care textbooks, you must pay close attention to details. As you read, you should think about these facts and how they are organized. Details in your textbook are grouped so that you can easily identify the relationship between the main idea and details. These organizational patterns make it easier for you to remember information.

TYPES OF PATTERNS

There are patterns of organization that are often found in textbooks. Both single paragraphs and longer selections are structured in these patterns and in combinations of these patterns. When you learn to recognize these organizational patterns, you will be able to closely follow the ideas in your texts.

FOLLOWING THE ORDER OF DETAILS

When you are reading, it is important to follow the order of details. Following the order of details is important when you are studying for exams or following written directions on the job.

Correctly following the order, or steps, is necessary if you are to do your work correctly. If you confuse the order of the directions, you could make a serious mistake. To avoid these errors, pay attention to the order of details. Your first step in reading is to identify the topic and the main idea of the reading material. Details in a reading passage are put together so that readers can better understand the main idea. All the details relate to the main idea and help the reader understand the main idea.

There are words that signal you to be aware of the correct order of details. Some of these directional words are

- First
- Second
- Last
- Finally
- When
- In conclusion
- Then
- Before
- Next
- After
- During
- Following

Just as traffic signals help you to follow the correct road when you travel, directional words help you to stay on track and follow the correct order of the details. Paying attention to the order of details helps you to understand and remember what you are reading.

Example 2-3

Read the following example from the Bonewit-West health care textbook *Computer Concepts and Applications for the Medical Office* (p. 71) and pay attention to the boldface directional words. Focus on the order of the information presented. Count the number of steps in the procedure.

FLOPPY DISK

Loading an application program stored on a floppy disk into the computer memory involves the following **steps:** The program disk is **first** inserted into the disk drive, and the drive is activated. Activation of the disk drive is accomplished by either a cold start or a warm start procedure. The *cold start method* is used **when** the computer has not been previously turned on, whereas the *warm start method* is used **when** the computer is currently in use. **During** activation, a copy of the program is retrieved from the disk and loaded into the computer's memory. The computer is **then** able to perform the functions specified by the application program.

EXERCISE 2-3

Directions: Read the following selection from a health care textbook (Bonewit-West, p. 59). Then answer the questions that follow.

Because 5.25-inch disks are enclosed in a vinyl rather than a hard plastic jacket they are more susceptible to harm, and some additional precautions must be followed as listed below.

1. Always complete the label before attaching it to the disk jacket. If information needs to be modified on an affixed label, a felt tip pen must be used. Using a ball point pen or pencil causes pressure on the disk surface which could damage it. (*Note:* Because of their hard plastic jacket, a ball point pen or pencil can be used to write on an affixed label of a 3.5-inch disk.)
2. Each 5.25-inch disk comes with a paper or cardboard envelope. The disk envelope must be removed before the disk is inserted into the disk drive. Always return the disk to its envelope *immediately* after use to protect it from dust and dirt. Leaving an unprotected disk lying out is courting disaster.
3. Handle the disk so that the data access area does not come in contact with anything other than the disk drive head. Touching this exposed area may cause body oils to be transferred to it resulting in dust particles sticking to its mylar surface. Dust particles can scratch the surface of the disk when the read/write head moves over them leading to a loss of data. The proper method for holding a 5.25-inch disk is to place the thumb of the right hand on the top of the label with two fingers supporting the underside of the disk directly below the label.
4. Do not bend or fold the disk. The disk is able to withstand a certain amount of flexing, however, excessive bending or flexing could cause the magnetic material coating the disk to flake off resulting in loss of data.
5. Do not use rubber bands or paper clips on the disk.

1. The selection is mainly about_____.

2. How many steps must be followed to complete the directions?
_____

3. List the directional words that lead you to each step. _____
_____

4. Look at this scrambled list of steps from the reading selection. Rearrange the steps in the correct order. Number the steps in their proper order.

____ Complete the label before attaching it to the disk jacket.

____ Do not bend or fold the disk.

____ Do not use rubber bands or paper clips on the disk.

____ Hold the disk properly so that the data access area does not come in contact with anything other than the disk drive head.

____ Remove the disk envelope before you insert the disk into the disk drive.

Sequence

The sequence pattern helps you to understand a process when you read your health care textbook. Sequence helps you to answer these questions about any procedure: What does it do? How does it work? You answer these questions by following an order or sequence. This helps you to organize the information into a system. Some signal words that help you to follow a sequence pattern are *steps, when, then, first, last, stages*. Following a sequence helps you understand each step of any procedure described in your textbook.

Example 2–4

Read the following example of a **sequence** pattern of organization from the Chabner textbook *The Language of Medicine* (p. 371). Notice how the signal words *first* and *next* help you to follow the process of digital subtraction angiography (DSA).

Video equipment and a computer are used to produce x-ray pictures of blood vessels. First, an x-ray is taken of the area to be studied, and the results are stored in a computer. Next, contrast material is injected into a vein, and a second image is produced that is also recorded in the computer. The computer then compares the two images and subtracts the first image from the second (removing parts not being studied such as bone, muscle, and fat), leaving nothing but an image of the contrast medium and vessels.

EXERCISE 2–4

Directions: Read the following excerpt from a health care textbook (Torres and Ehrlich, pp. 468 and 469). Follow the pattern of organization. Answer the questions following the selection.

PREPARATION OF SYRINGE-TYPE MATERIAL

1. Dispense approximiately 11/4 to 2 inches of the syringe-type base material onto a clean papaer pad. Wipe the tube opening clean with a gauze sponge and recap immediately.
   ☐ *RATIONALE*: Cleaning the top of the tube and the threads prevents a messy cap, which may stick closed.
2. Dispense an equal length of syringe-type accelerator onto the pad near, but not touching the base material. Wipe the tupe opening clean and recap immediately.
3. Place the blade of the spatula into the catalyst so both sides are coated. Then incorporate the catalyst into the base paste.
   ☐ *RATIONALE*: Having this catalyst on the spatula makes cleanup easier because the catalyst causes the base material to set so it does not stick to the spatula.

26 RECOGNIZING DETAILS

4. Spatulate smoothly (wiping back and forth) to produce a homogeneous, streak-free mix withing 45 to 60 seconds.
   ☐ *RATIONALE*: This material is mixed most effectively by spreading it over a wide area of the pad.
5. Load and complete assembly of the syringe in less than 30 seconds, and pass the prepared syringe to the dentist.

PREPARATION OF TRAY-TYPE MATERIAL

1. Use a clean mixing pad and clean spatula.
2. Extrude the trya-type base material to the appropriate length (2 to 3 inches). Wipe the tube opening clean and recap immediately.
3. Extrude an equal length of tray-type catalyst. This is placed on the pad about an inch from the base paste. Wipe the tube opening clean and recap immediately.
4. Place the blade of spatula into catalyst on the mixing pad so that both sides of the blade are covered.
   ☐ *RATIONALE*: Coating the spatula with catalyst makes cleanup easier because it is not as sticky as the base material.
5. Use the edge of the spatula to scrape the remaining catalyst into the base.
6. Use a flat spreading motion with the spatula to spread the mix in crosswise strokes on the pad.
   ☐ *RATIONALE*: This material is mixed most effecively by spreading it over a wide area of the pad.
7. Continue to scrape up the mix and spread it smoothly on the pad in even crosswise strokes, to incorporate all material.
   ☐ *RATIONALE*: The mix must be homogeneous and should appear creamy, of even texture and color, and free of streaks.
8. Complete a homogeneous mix within the time recommended by the manufacturer. (This is usually 45 seconds to 1 minute.)
   ☐ *RATIONALE*: If the mix is not completed within the recommended working time, the quality of the imipression will be compromised.
9. Pick up the bulk of the tray mix with the spatula and load the material into the tray. The mass should flow into the tray.
10. Spread the material until the tray is evenly loaded.
11. Receive the used syringe from the dentist, and pass the loaded tray.

1. What is the pattern of organization? _____

2. What is the topic? _____

3. How many steps are in the procedure? _____

4. Number these steps in the order in which they take place in the procedure.

   ____ Place the blade of the spatula into the catalyst..

   ____ Dispense syringe-type material onto a clean paper pad.

   ____ Load and complete assembly of syringe in less than 30 seconds.

   ____ Dispense syringe-type accelerator onto the pad.

   ____ Spatulate smoothly.

Classification

The classification pattern is used to group and subgroup the different facts in your text. Classification helps you to understand structure. By following classification patterns, you will be able to understand **how things are organized, how things are made,** and **what things are.** Classification is also used to describe things. Charts are often used to illustrate this pattern. Some signal words that are clues to recognizing this pattern are *breaks down, parts, components, group, heading,* and *subheading.* When you recognize and follow the classification pattern in your health care texts, you will be able to find the more important and less important details. Therefore, you will be able to understand the content of your reading assignment.

Example 2-5

Read the following example of a **classification** pattern from Chabner (pp. 497–498). Follow the organization of details. See how the relationship between the six parts and the whole (facial bones) help you to understand the content. Examine how labeling the parts of the diagram will help you to understand and remember the information in the selection.

FACIAL BONES

All the facial bones, except one, are joined together by sutures, so that they are immovable. The mandible (lower jaw bone) is the only facial bone capable of movement. This ability is necessary for activities such as mastication (chewing) and speaking.

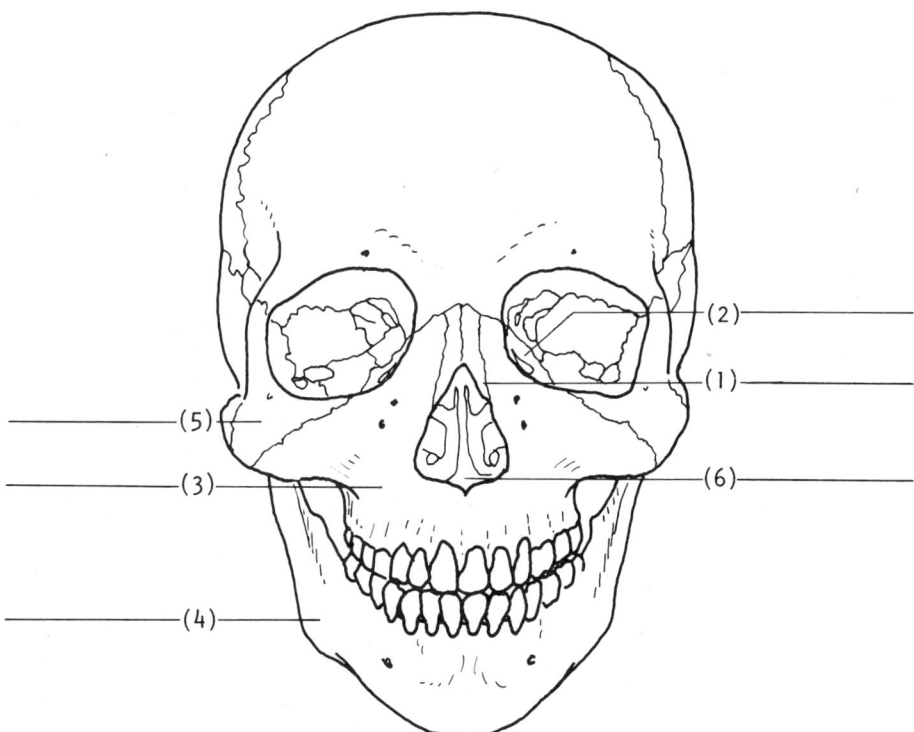

FIGURE 2-1 Facial bones. (From Chabner D-E: The Language of Medicine, 4th ed. Philadelphia, WB Saunders, 1991, p. 498.)

Figure 2–1 shows the facial bones; label it as you read the following descriptions of the facial bones:

(1) **Nasal bones**—two slender nasal (nas/o means nose) bones support the bridge of the nose. They join with the frontal bone superiorly and form part of the nasal septum.

(2) **Lacrimal bones**—two paired lacrimal (lacrim/o means tear) bones are located one at the corner of each eye. These thin, small bones contain fossae for the lacrimal gland (tear gland) and canals for the passage of the lacrimal duct.

(3) **Maxillary bones**—two large bones compose the massive upper jaw bones (maxillae). They are joined by a suture in the median plane. If the two bones do not come together normally before birth, the condition know as cleft palate results.

(4) **Mandibular bone**—this is the lower jaw bone (mandible). Both the maxilla and the mandible contain the sockets called alveoli in which the teeth are embedded. The mandible joins the skull at the region of the temporal bone, forming the temporomandibular joint (TMJ) on either side of the skull.

(5) **Zygomatic bones**—two bones, one on each side of the face, form the high portion of the cheek.

(6) **Vomer**—this thin, single, flat bone forms the lower portion of the nasal septum.

EXERCISE 2–5

Directions: Read the following textbook selection (Chabner, p. 44). Answer the questions based on the selection. Identify the pattern of organization. Use this pattern to help you understand the passage.

QUADRANTS

The abdominopelvic area can be divided into four quadrants by drawing two imaginary lines—one horizontally and one vertically through the body. Figure 2–2 shows these quadrants. You add the proper abbreviation under each label on the diagram.

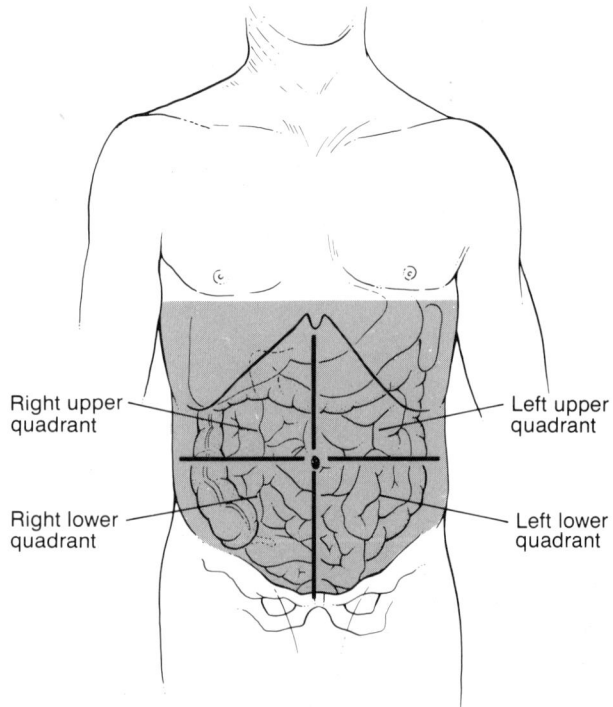

FIGURE 2–2 Quadrants of the abdomen. (From Swartz MH: Textbook of Physical Diagnosis: History and Examination. Philadelphia, WB Saunders, 1994, p. 303.)

Right upper quadrant, RUQ: contains the liver (right lobe), gallbladder, part of the <u>pancreas</u>, parts of the small and large intestines.
Left upper quadrant, LUQ: contains the liver (left lobe), stomach, spleen, part of the pancreas, parts of the small and large intestines.
Right lower quadrant, RLQ: contains parts of the small and large intestines, right ovary, right uterine (fallopian) tube, appendix, right ureter.
Left lower quadrant, LLQ: contains parts of the small and large intestines, left ovary, left uterine tube, left ureter.

1. What is the pattern of organization? _____

2. Did you add the abbreviations under each label?
   Yes ____
   No ____

3. What is the main topic? _____

4. How many parts are there? _____

5. List the parts: _____
   _____

6. Which part contains the gallbladder? _____

EXERCISE 2–6

Directions: Read the following excerpt from a health care textbook (Chabner, pp. 45–46). Follow the pattern of organization. Answer the questions following the selection.

DIVISIONS OF THE BACK (SPINAL COLUMN)

The back is separated into divisions corresponding to regions of the spinal column. The spinal column is composed of a series of bones extending from the neck downward to the tailbone. Each bone is called a **vertebra** (plural: **vertebrae**).

Label the divisions of the back on Figure 2–3 as you study the following:

DIVISION OF THE BACK	ABBREVIATION	LOCATION
(1) Cervical	C	Neck region. There are 7 cervical vertebrae (C1–C7).
(2) Thoracic	T or D (D = dorsal)	Chest region. There are 12 thoracic vertebrae (T1–T12). Each bone is joined to a rib.
(3) Lumbar	L	Loin (waist) or flank region (between the ribs and the hip bone). There are 5 lumbar vertebrae (L1–L5).
(4) Sacral	S	Five bones (S1–S5) are fused to form one bone, the sacrum.
(5) Coccygeal		The coccyx (tailbone) is a small bone composed of 4 fused pieces.

30 RECOGNIZING DETAILS

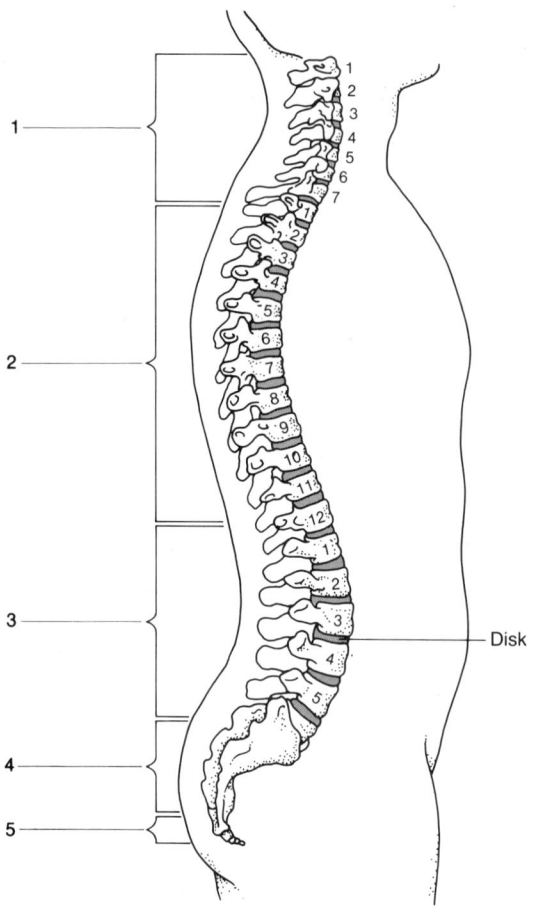

FIGURE 2–3 Anatomical divisions of the back (spinal column). Disks are shown in color. (From Chabner D-E: Medical Terminology: A Short Course. Philadelphia, WB Saunders, 1990.)

1. What is the pattern of organization? _____
2. Did you label each part?
   Yes ____   No ____
3. What is the main topic? _____
4. Write the number of the part that contains the neck region. _____
5. Write the number of the part that contains the chest region. _____

Examples and Illustrations

When you read health care textbooks, the author may give examples or illustrations as the details to back up his main ideas. Signal words that are a clue to this pattern are *for example, shows, explains, kinds of*. Following these examples will help you to understand the ideas in your text.

Example 2–6

Read the following example of an **examples or illustrations** pattern (Torres and Ehrlich, p. 437). The signal words, *types of*, gives you a clue to follow examples. Read and follow these types of dental cement. Look at the figure to see how these types of dental cement are used.

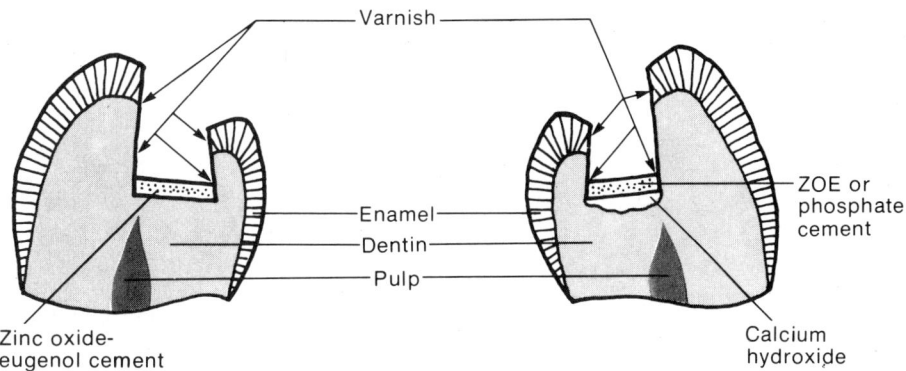

FIGURE 2-4 The use of dental cements as pulpal protective material and sedative base in cavity preparation. (From Torres HO, Ehrlich A: Modern Dental Assisting, 5th ed. Philadelphia, WB Saunders, 1994, p. 522.)

BASES

Different types of cements are used to form specialized types of bases under restorative materials (Fig. 2-4).

Protective Bases. After a tooth has been prepared, it is necessary to protect the pulp before the restoration is placed. Without this protection, there may be post operative sensitivity and possible damage to the pulp.

Calcium hydroxide is most commonly used for this purpose because it soothes the pulp and promotes the formation of reparative dentin. It is placed directly over the pulpal floor of the preparation. (**Reparative dentin**, also known as *tertiary dentin*, is a protective layer of dentin formed by the tooth over the pulpal area in response to irritation or injury.)

Insulating Bases. When the cavity is deep, it is necessary to place an insulating base under the restoration to protect the tooth from thermal shock. This base is placed *over* the protective base.

The thermal qualities of metal allow it to conduct hot and cold more quickly than does dentin. For this reason, an insulating base is particularly important under a metal restoration.

Sedative Bases. Sometimes a sedative base, of a material such as zinc oxide-eugenol cement, is placed to soothe the pulp. When a sedative base is used, it is placed directly over the pulpal area of the tooth.

EXERCISE 2-7

Directions: Read the following excerpt from a health care textbook (Chabner, p. 367). Follow the pattern of organization. Answer the questions following the selection.

An <u>aneurysm</u> may occur anywhere in the body but most commonly occurs in the aorta. A frequent site is just inferior to the origin of the renal arteries. The danger of an aneurysm is that as the wall of the artery pushes outward it becomes progressively thinner and may eventually rupture. Figure 2-5 shows an aneurysm of the aorta. An <u>aneurysmectomy</u> is surgical removal of an aneurysm. After removal of a large aortic aneurysm in the abdomen, a synthetic graft is stitched to the aorta at one end and the two iliac arteries at the other end (Fig. 2-5).

High Blood Pressure in Arteries

There are two kinds of arterial hypertension: essential and secondary. In essential hypertension, the cause of the increased pressure is idiopathic. In secondary hypertension, there is always some associated lesion, such as glomerulonephritis, pyelonephritis, or disease of the adrenal glands, that is responsible for the elevated blood pressure.

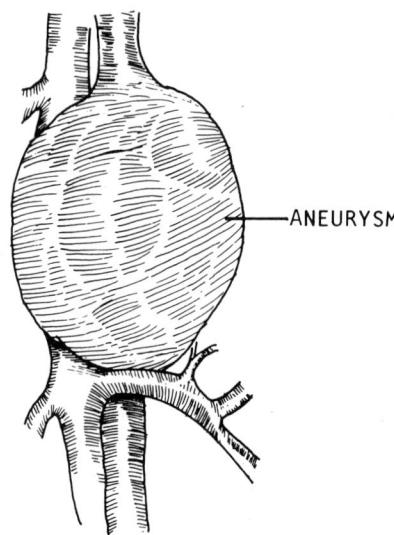

Figure 2-5 Aneurysm of the aorta. (From Chabner D-E: The Language of Medicine, 4th ed. Philadelphia, WB Saunders, 1991, p. 367.)

In adults, a blood pressure equal to or greater than 140/90 mm Hg is considered high. Diuretics, beta-blockers, and other drugs are used as treatment for essential hypertension. Losing weight, limiting sodium (salt) intake, stopping smoking, and reducing fat in the diet are also important in therapy.

1. What is the pattern of organization? _____
2. What is the topic? _____
3. What was given as an example of high blood pressure in adults? _____
4. What are treatments for hypertension? _____
5. What are the two kinds of hypertension? _____

Comparison and Contrast Pattern

Writers often organize details to compare or contrast information. Some signal words that help you to make comparisons are *alike, some, similar,* or *compare*. Some signal words that help you to contrast details are *different, unlike*. Comparison-contrast patterns help you to organize information so that you will remember which details are the same and which are different.

Example 2-7

Read the following example of a comparison-contrast pattern from Bonewit-West (p. 114). The word *difference* is a signal to a contrast in the organization of the details. Read about the difference between a manual and a computerized office. Use comparison and contrast to help you determine which system you prefer.

The main difference between a manual and computerized office, however, is that all the data that you enter into your computer becomes part of the database, not just the patient records. In other words, the database for a medical practice consists of patient records, patient transactions, diagnosis codes, procedure codes, insurance carriers, and so on (refer to Fig. 2–6). This information is stored on a hard disk for later retrieval and use as needed. A database also provides the ability to add new information, to modify existing information, and to delete unneeded information. When you need to look up something that has been stored in the database, it is displayed on the same screen that was used for entering the data. In addition, this information can be printed out, as needed, in hardcopy form.

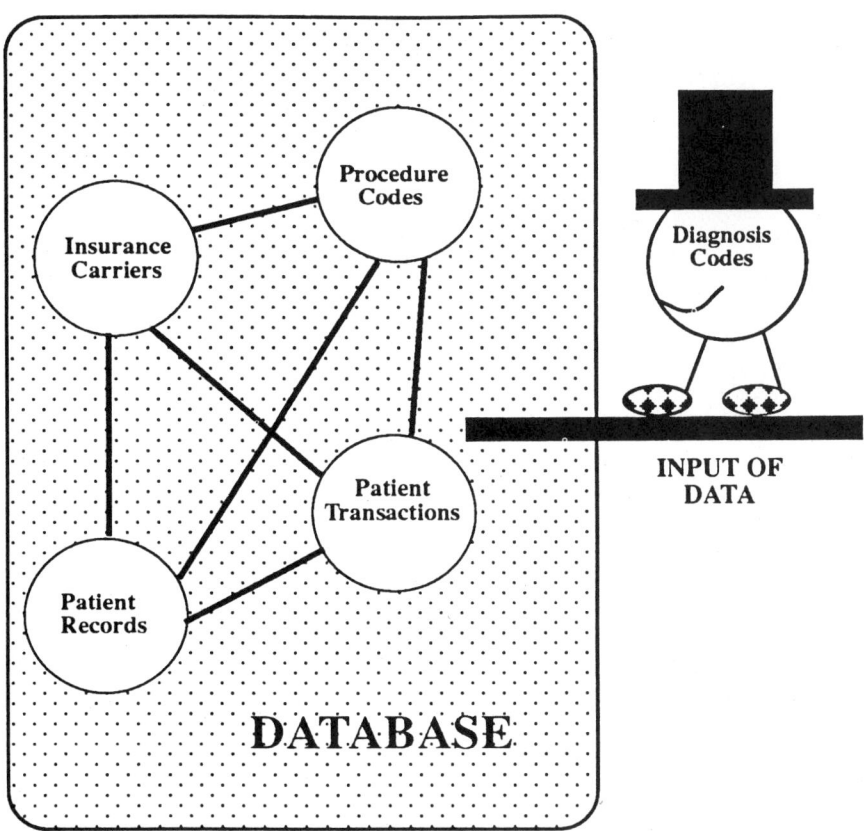

FIGURE 2–6 All of the data entered into the computer becomes part of the database. A database is a large "pool" of information that can be accessed in a multitude of ways according to the task being performed. (From Bonewit-West K: Computer Concepts and Applications for the Medical Office. Philadelphia, WB Saunders, 1993, p. 114.)

EXERCISE 2-8

Directions: Read the following excerpt from the Purtilo health care textbook *Ethical Dimensions in the Health Professions* (pp. 109–111). Follow the pattern of organization. Answer the questions following the selections.

AN ARGUMENT AGAINST DISCLOSURE

The main argument advanced against disclosure of "bad news" is that the health professional's role is to maintain the patient's hope, and hope may be shattered by bad news. Do you agree that this is an important function you will have to assume?

yes _____

no _____

Throughout most of the history of Western health care, the patient has been defined as the one who needs to be cared for, who has little knowledge of medical science, who suffers passively from a disease, and who brings her- or himself to the health care system much in the same way that a car is brought to an automobile mechanic. As Edward said to Dr. Reilly in T. S. Eliot's *The Cocktail Party*,

> I can no longer act for myself
> Coming to see you—That's the last decision
> I was capable of making. I am in your hands.
> I cannot take any further responsibility.

The patient's choice has been whether or not to follow the strong recommendations of the physician. In this view, a benevolent disposition has been regarded as more important than an honest one, although both are extremely important. You can also think about which duties are involved in this situation. They are

_____ or _____
and
_____

If you answered "beneficence or nonmaleficence" and "veracity" you have correctly identified the duties that are consistent with being a "benevolent" and "truthful" or "honest" person.

As you may recall from our earlier discussions about duties, sometimes the idea of acting beneficently means acting independently in the patient's best wishes. Such a way of acting is called _____ or _____. (The answer: paternalistic or parentalistic.)

The arguments against disclosure of information have been based on paternalistic thinking. The physician is privy to the awful truth of the inexorable progress of most diseases, and decides what patients ought to be told, based on an assessment of their welfare. Of course, such perceptions are heavily influenced by the physician's own concept of his or her role in the system and attitudes about sickness and death.

This portrays a relationship that is unequal and paternalistic, but well-intentioned. In order to maintain a patient's trust it is believed that honesty may have to be sacrificed to benevolence.

ARGUMENTS FAVORING DISCLOSURE

Today, there is mounting pressure on the health professions from within their own ranks (as well as from lay people) to be more candid or "honest" with patients, especially concerning the health professional's own limitations. In the 1960s Elisabeth Kübler-Ross, a physician, spearheaded a revolutionary movement in the health care world by clarifying simple concepts about the dying process and making suggestions for the better care of the dying. She was convinced that patients with fatal illnesses could handle the truth about that awesome knowledge, and therefore that knowledge ought not to be swept under the rug delicately but rather dealt with honestly, carefully, and realistically. She cited many cases of people having come to terms with the meanings of death and dying for themselves and their loved ones because they knew the truth about their own condition and its prognosis. Today, thanks to Kübler-Ross and others like her, the topics of dying and death are not as taboo as they were a few years ago. In the wake of this new openness, the idea that patients can handle difficult news, and may even benefit from knowing, has taken the health professionals down a new stream of thought: the truth, rather than being a barrier to hope, may set the patient free. The specter of AIDS has again raised truth telling questions and concerns to the forefront of health professionals' consciousness.

In this interpretation, an honest disposition is at least as important as, and is not necessarily in conflict with, a benevolent one. Acting truthfully is consistent with acting beneficiently. What is "best" for the patient cannot be discerned by the health professional who is acting independently on behalf of the patient. Caring entails sharing pertinent information: The best way to maintain trust is to share relevant information with patients, but do so in ways that will be supportive of them. The health professional is learned, but approaches the patient on more equal footing where matters of the patient's life and health are at stake.

Truth telling involves a relationship between people, so that the issue of "to tell or not to tell" is merely a juncture in an ongoing personal and professional relationship with the one who asks the questions. Underlying the bias towards greater disclosure of information is the conviction that if the health professional, both verbally and through his or her actions, conveys the message that he or she still cares, and has the intention and ability to comfort, then it is possible to tell the truth and still maintain the patient's trust and hope. Benevolence is expressed *through* honesty, rather than played off *against* it. Do you find these arguments compelling?

1. What is the pattern of organization? _____
2. What is the topic? _____
3. List the three details for disclosure. _____
4. List the three details against disclosure. _____
5. Which point of view do you agree with? _____ Why? _____

Cause-effect

Cause-effect patterns of detail help you to answer the questions: *Why does it happen? How does it happen? How does it work?* Some signal words that help you to recognize cause-effect patterns are *because, in order to, why, result, effect, reasons, factors*. When following cause-effect patterns, remember that the cause takes place first; the effect happens after the cause.

Example 2–8

Read the following example of a **cause-effect** pattern of organization from Chabner (p. 365). Following this pattern will help you to understand **why** high blood pressure affects the heart.

HIGH BLOOD PRESSURE AFFECTING THE HEART

This condition is caused by the contraction of arterioles of the body leading to increased pressure in arteries. The heart itself is affected because it has to pump more vigorously to overcome the increased resistance in the arteries. The vessels lose their elasticity, become like solid pipes, and place increased burden on the heart to pump blood through the body.

EXERCISE 2–9

Directions: Read the following excerpt from a health care textbook (Chabner, p. 363). Follow the pattern of organization. Answer the questions following the selection.

The heart is unable to pump its required amount of blood (more blood enters the heart from the veins than leaves through the arteries).

Blood accumulates in the lungs (left-sided heart failure) causing pulmonary edema (fluid seeps out of capillaries into the tiny air sacs of the lungs). Damming back of blood resulting from right-sided heart failure results in accumulation of fluid in the abdominal organs (liver and spleen) and subcutaneous tissue of the legs. Congestive heart failure often develops gradually over several years, although it can be acute. It is treated with drugs, such as digitalis, to strengthen the heart and diuretics to promote loss of fluid.

1. What is the pattern of organization? _____
2. What is the topic? _____
3. What is the reason for pulmonary edema? _____
4. What gets into the lungs? _____
5. Why is there a damming back of blood? _____

REVIEWING RECOGNIZING DETAILS

TO LEARN	USE THIS STRATEGY
To locate details	Locate the facts that give you a better understanding of the main idea
To distinguish between the main idea and important details	Remember that the main idea is a general statement and the details are specific facts
To map details	Recognize that there are important details which describe the main idea and less important details which describe the important details
To verify facts from the text	Scan for facts by focusing on key words to help you find the information you are looking for in the text
To recognize logical relationships	Recognize that main ideas and details are organized into types of patterns. Look for the following patterns in your textbook: • Sequence • Classification • Examples and illustrations • Comparison and contrast • Cause and effect

Chapter 3

Developing Vocabulary

LEARNING OBJECTIVES
VOCABULARY WORDS
VOCABULARY CHECK
THE NEED FOR A GOOD VOCABULARY
CONTEXT CLUES
    Locating Context Clues
WORD PARTS
    What Are Word Parts?
THE DICTIONARY, GLOSSARY, AND THESAURUS
    The Dictionary
        Reading a Dictionary Entry
    The Glossary
    The Thesaurus
        Reading a Thesaurus Entry
REMEMBERING NEW WORDS
    Word Cards
REVIEWING THE LEARNING STRATEGIES

LEARNING OBJECTIVES

In this chapter you will learn how to
- Improve your general and medical vocabulary by learning strategies for using context clues, word parts, dictionaries, glossaries, and thesauruses
- Remember the meanings of new vocabulary terms by creating word cards

VOCABULARY WORDS

The following vocabulary words are important to your understanding of the ideas in this chapter. These vocabulary words are underscored the first time they are used in the chapter. Read the list of words and definitions. Then check your understanding of these words before you read the chapter.

analyzing breaking down a whole into its parts.
context the words around an unknown word that are used to figure out the meaning of the unknown word.
hormones chemical transmitter substance produced by cells of the body and transported by the bloodstream to the cells and organs on which it has a specific regulatory effect (Miller-Keane, p. 702).
inadequate not good enough.
microorganisms organisms that are too small to be seen with the unaided eye.
ovum egg.
pathogenic having the ability to cause disease.
syllables parts of a word that contain at least one consonant and one vowel.
vague not clearly stated.
veterinary relating to the diagnosis and cure of disease in animals.

VOCABULARY CHECK

Directions: Choose the vocabulary word that best fits into the sentence.

1. The student figured out the meaning of "defibrillation" by looking at the _____ clue.

2. He did not understand what to do because her instructions were _____.

3. _____ the parts of the plant was easy for the botany student.

4. Because of a _____ imbalance, she was gaining much weight.

5. The small child was learning to read quickly by breaking up big words into _____.

6. The doctor received an _____ supply of the much needed drug.

7. The _____ surgeon operated on the dog.

8. In the laboratory, the scientists were looking at a human _____ in a test tube.

9. A _____ substance was released into the air causing thousands of people untold misery.

10. It is amazing that so many _____ can be seen on the laboratory slide.

THE NEED FOR A GOOD VOCABULARY

Having chosen to become health care students, you have entered an environment where you will be exposed to new and unfamiliar words. You will come across these words in your textbooks, lectures, and conversations with instructors and fellow students. A great deal of your school success will depend on how many of these words you understand and on the strategies that you use to learn and remember words you do not know.

You will be expected to know two types of vocabulary words. The first type, general terminology, includes the words you hear around you every day or words that you see in newspapers, magazines, and books that you read for pleasure. The second type, medical terminology, includes the specific words that relate to your studies in the health care field. Different strategies are required to learn and remember these two types of vocabulary words. When you read or hear a general vocabulary term that you do not understand, it is sometimes okay not to know the exact or precise definition of the word. If you have a close enough understanding of the word, that may be good enough. It is important in some instances not to stop the flow of your reading or quit taking class notes to look up an unknown word. However, this is not the case for learning and remembering medical terminology. When you read or hear new medical terms in your textbook and lectures, it is very important to get the precise definitions of these words. Therefore, it is necessary not only to learn new words but also to choose the right strategies for learning general vocabulary and medical vocabulary words.

CONTEXT CLUES

An excellent strategy for learning both general and medical vocabulary words is using context clues. When you use context clues, you try to figure out the meaning of the unknown word by reading the surrounding words in the sentence or paragraph.

EXERCISE 3–1

Directions: Look at the following exercise from a passage in *Clinical Textbook for Veterinary Technicians* by McCurnin (p. 1). Notice that some of the words have been left out. See if you can determine what words belong in the blanks by reading the surrounding words in the passage.

Most _____ who enter the field of veterinary medicine have had experience in handling _____, and some are even expert in handling and training certain species (e.g., dogs or horses). There is a tendency to think that if one has developed a good rapport with one species of animal the same knowledge can be transferred directly to another _____. Unfortunately, handling techniques may have little transferability among different animals; sometimes the _____ are merely inefficient, and sometimes they are _____ when applied to other animals.

After reading the entire passage you should have filled in "people," "animals," "species," "techniques," and "dangerous." What you have just done is use the surrounding and familiar words to figure out the unknown words. In other words, you have used context clues to fill in the blank spaces. The advantage to this strategy is that you do not have to stop reading to look up a word in the dictionary. Nor do you need to stop taking notes in a lecture class to get the definition of an unknown word. Using context clues, or the surrounding words, to figure out the meaning of an unknown word is a fine strategy for learning both general and medical vocabulary. However, some context clues will give you only a <u>vague</u> definition that may be acceptable for general vocabulary words and other context clues may give a precise definition that will work well with unknown medical words. It is your responsibility to be aware of when context clues are meeting your vocabulary needs, and when they are not you must use another strategy to learn the definition of the unknown word.

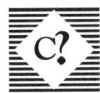

Locating Context Clues

To use context clues, you must be able to locate or recognize which words in the sentence or paragraph are suggesting the definition of the unknown word. Sometimes, the context clue will be right next to the unknown word, separated from it by a comma or a dash. Read the following example from *Health Unit Coordinating* by LaFleur-Brooks (p. 27).

Example 3-1

A **radiologist,** qualified in the use of x-ray and other imaging devices, is in charge of this department.

Note that in this example, the definition "qualified in the use of x-ray and other imaging devices" is separated from the unknown medical term *radiologist* by commas. This context clue gives us a precise definition of the word *radiologist*.

EXERCISE 3-2

Directions: Read the following sentences and circle the context clue for the **boldfaced** word in each sentence.

1. The use of a **radiopaque catheter** (a catheter coated with a substance that does not permit the passage of x-rays) allows the catheter to be followed on a television screen (LaFleur-Brooks, p. 250).
2. **Sebaceous glands** (see-bay' shus), also known as oil glands, are generally attached to hair follicles (Solomon, p. 43).
3. The **ventral coccygeal vein** ("tail vein") can be used for the administration of small quantities of nonirritating medications (see discussion of bovine venipuncture procedures) (McCurnin, p. 173).
4. **Disposable** thermometers (those that are used only once) are also available for obtaining body temperatures (Kinn, Woods, and Derge, p. 433).
5. A portable file, often referred to as the **kardex,** is maintained by each nursing unit (LaFleur-Brooks, p. 127).

Sometimes the context clue can be found in the same sentence as the unknown word. In this case, the context clue will appear as an exact definition of the unknown word. This type of context clue is frequently found in your health care textbooks. Look at this example of a context clue that appears in the same sentence as the unknown word.

Example 3-2

An **ectopic pregnancy** is a pregnancy in which the fertilized ovum is planted outside of the uterus; over 90% implant in the fallopian tubes (LaFleur-Brooks, p. 454).

In this example, the words *"the fertilized ovum is planted outside of the uterus"* provide a clear and precise definition for the unknown medical term *ectopic pregnancy*.

EXERCISE 3-3

Directions: In the space provided, write a definition context clue for each of the following medical terms. Consult a dictionary if necessary but use your own words for writing the sentences. The first one has been done for you.

1. Crown: <u>The crown of the tooth is above the gumline.</u>
2. Insomnia: _____
3. Nausea: _____
4. Tonsillectomy: _____
5. Iris: _____
6. Estrogen: _____

In some instances, however, you may have to read an entire paragraph or a longer passage to find the context clues that suggest the meaning of an unknown word. This may be the case for both general and medical terms. Read the following selection from LaFleur-Brooks (pp. 86–87). Notice that the italicized context clues for "imprinter card" are found in the sentences following the boldfaced word **imprinter card.**

Example 3-3

When a patient is admitted to the hospital, an **imprinter card** is prepared in the admissions department. The card, *which may be of plastic or metal, is used to imprint the patient's chart forms and the requisitions needed to obtain services.*

Information on the imprinter card *consists of the patient's name, sex, age, health records number, account number, and attending physician's name.*

EXERCISE 3-4

Directions: Read the following passage from *The Medical Assistant; Administrative and Clinical* by Kinn, Woods, and Derge (p. 74). Underline all the words that are context clues that help you figure out the meaning of the phrase *subtle discrimination*.

Discrimination that is not entirely defined by law may be just as harmful as the discrimination that is defined. This type of discrimination is often referred to as *subtle discrimination*. Subtle discrimination is not obvious and seldom expressed openly. It includes discrimination based on a person's appearance, values, or lifestyle or on some other personal factor.

Much of the discrimination that occurs in medical facilities falls into this category. Examples include discrimination against overweight people, divorced people, gay people, people receiving public assistance, and people with sexually transmitted diseases. Often, you may not even be aware that your words or actions reflect subtle discrimination against another.

WORD PARTS

Another good strategy for learning unknown words is analyzing the meaning of the word parts that make up the structure of the word. This strategy can be used for general vocabulary, but it is particularly effective for medical terms as long as these words have word parts. By learning and remembering a relatively small number of word parts, you will be able to discover the meanings of thousands of unknown words.

What Are Word Parts?

Many medical and general words in English are made up of two or more of the following word parts:

A **prefix** is a word part that is found in the beginning of the word. It changes the meaning of the main part of the word. For example, when you add the prefix *un* to the main part of the word *happy*, the meaning changes from "glad" to "not being glad."

A **root** is a word part that is the main part of the word and gives the basic meaning to the word. For example, in the word *review*, *view* is the root and means "to see." When you add the prefix *re*, the meaning of the root changes and the word now means "to see again."

A **suffix** is a word part that is found at the end of the word. It has two purposes. The first purpose is to change the meaning of the root. The second purpose is to change the part of speech. For example, in the medical word *endocrinologist*, the suffix *ologist* means "a person who studies." This suffix changes the meaning of the root *crin* ("to give off") to "one who studies that which is given off." The suffix changes the root from a verb (action word) to a noun (person, place, or thing). When you add the prefix *endo* ("within"), you now see that the word *endocrinologist* means "one who studies that which gives off from within." This refers to the various glands that secrete, or give off, hormones. Thus an endocrinologist is a person who specializes in the study of the function and disorders of the glands that give off hormones.

You can see from this example that when you know the meanings of some prefixes, roots, and suffixes you will be able to use your knowledge to analyze word parts to determine the meanings of many unknown words. However, you must be aware that in some cases a word may seem to have a word part but that word part may really be the root and cannot be used to figure out the meaning of the word. For example, the word *reptile* may appear to begin with the prefix *re*, but that is just a part of the root. Thus when you try to use the word part strategy, be sure that the word part is indeed a word part. To do this, familiarize yourself with some of the word parts and their meanings in Table 3–1.

TABLE 3-1   Prefixes, Roots, Suffixes

	DEFINITION	EXAMPLE	DEFINITION OF EXAMPLE	YOUR EXAMPLE
Prefix				
anti	against	anti-inflamatory		
*dys	bad, difficult	dyslexia		
*exo	outside	exoskeleton		
*hem, hemato	relating to the blood	hemodiagnosis		
*hyper	over, above, beyond	hyperkinesia		
inter	between	intersession		
mal	poor, bad	maladjusted		
*peri	around, near	perigastric		
semi	half	semisweet		
tele	distant, far	telescope		
Root				
*arthro, arthr	joint	arthritis		
bio	life	biology		
*cardi, cardio	heart	cardiopathy		
*derm, dermo	skin	dermatitis		
fac, fact	make, do	factory		
*path	disease	pathologist		
port	carry	portable		
*psych	mind	psychiatry		
spec, spect	to look at	spectator		
vers	turn	reversible		
Suffix				
able, ible	capable of	trainable		
ation	act of	sanitation		
*ectomy	excision	hysterectomy		
ful	full of	hateful		
*itis	inflammation of	bursitis		
ology	study	psychology		
*oma	tumor	hematoma		
*osis	condition	nephrosis		
*phobia	fear	xenophobia		
scope	see	periscope		

*Word parts with a medical use.

EXERCISE 3-5

Directions: In Table 3-1 in the column headed "Definition of Example," write the meanings of the example words for prefixes, roots, and suffixes. Check with a dictionary or glossary if necessary.

EXERCISE 3-6

Directions: In the column headed "Your Example," write your own example word for each prefix, root, and suffix. If necessary, use a dictionary, glossary, or thesaurus.

EXERCISE 3-7

Directions: Make up your own chart similar to the one in Table 3-1. Write in any prefixes, roots, and suffixes you see in your textbook and would like to learn.

THE DICTIONARY, GLOSSARY, AND THESAURUS

In this chapter, you have learned vocabulary development strategies that allow you to continue reading your textbook if you see a word you do not understand. However, you may discover that not all sentences and paragraphs contain context clues and not all words are made up of word parts. In that case, you will have to stop the flow of your reading and consult with a reference that will give you the definition. Also, when you are working with medical terminology, it is important to know the precise definition of the word. Then, again, it will be necessary to consult a dictionary, glossary, or thesaurus for help in finding the meaning of the unknown word.

The Dictionary

As a health care student, it will be necessary for you to own two types of dictionaries; a **collegiate** dictionary for learning general vocabulary and a **medical** dictionary for learning medical terms. You may find it convenient to own two versions of a collegiate dictionary—a hard-cover version to keep at home by your study area and a soft-cover version to carry to school.

Many students do not realize that a dictionary contains more than just definitions. A good dictionary will show you how to pronounce a word, the origin of the word, how to break the word into syllables, and other words that mean the same or the opposite of the word you are looking up.

Reading a Dictionary Entry

To be able to use the dictionary well, you must be familiar with the various parts of the entry. Following is an entry taken from *Miller-Keane's Encyclopedia & Dictionary of Medicine, Nursing, & Allied Health* (p. 913). The different parts of the entry have been numbered.

        1.   2.   3.   4.   5.

metastasis (me-tas´tah-sis), pl. *metas´tases* [Gr.] 1. the transfer of disease from one organ or part to another not directly connected with it. It may be due either to the transfer of patho-genic microorganisms (e.g., tubercle bacilli) or to the transfer of cells, as in malignant tumors. 2. a growth of pathogenic microorganisms or of abnormal cells distant from the site primarily
                                                     6.   7.
involved by the morbid process. adj., **meta-stat´ic.** (See also CANCER.)

Let us look closer at the different numbered parts of the entry:

1. The **main entry** or **headword** is printed in boldface type. This is the word you are looking up.
2. The **pronunciation** is found next to the headword and is enclosed in parentheses ( ). The headword is broken into syllables using dashes and written with accent marks to help you pronounce the word.
3. The **plural** form of the headword is given if it is not a standard English plural.
4. The **derivation** or **origin** of the word is given if the word comes from a foreign country. The derivation is abbreviated, and the meaning of the abbreviation can be found in the beginning of the dictionary.
5. The **definitions** or **meanings** of the headword follow and are printed in regular type. If there is more than one meaning for the word, the definitions will be numbered. When you are looking up an unknown word, it is important that you choose the definition that fits into the context of what you are reading.
6. The **adjective form** of the headword is also provided, if there is one. It is printed in boldface and broken up into its pronunciation.
7. **Synonyms** (other words that mean the same as the headword) end the entry, and you may be encouraged to look up the synonyms with the words "See also . . . ." Synonyms will appear in parentheses and are printed in capital letters.

EXERCISE 3–8

Directions: Reread the dictionary entry at the top of this page and answer the following questions in the space provided.

1. The headword is _____.
2. How is the headword printed? _____
3. How many syllables are in the headword? _____
4. The headword comes from what foreign country? _____
5. If you were reading about a cancerous tumor spreading from the breast to the brain, which numbered definition would be best? _____
6. Into what other part of speech can the headword be changed? _____
7. What is a synonym for the headword? _____

The Glossary

The glossary is a listing of key words found in the back of some of your textbooks. A glossary is like a dictionary because it gives you the definitions of words. However, the entries in a glossary are much briefer than dictionary entries. A glossary entry usually omits pronunciation, plural form, derivation, adjective form, and synonyms. It is generally just a collection of important words from the textbook and their definitions.

The advantage of the glossary is its convenience. You do not need to put down your textbook and start searching for a dictionary. The words are found in the back of the text you are reading. The disadvantage of the glossary is its limited number of words. You may discover that a needed word is not listed in the glossary. Only words that the author believes are important are included in the glossary. A word that you believe is important or do not know may not be included. Also, the glossary entry, as mentioned earlier, is much briefer than an entry in the dictionary, so you will not learn all you can about an unknown word. In any case, if you need to know the exact definition of a medical term, the glossary can be the first place you look. If the information is <u>inadequate</u>, use your medical dictionary.

EXERCISE 3-9

Directions: The first page of a glossary taken from the Solomon health-care textbook *Introduction to Human Anatomy and Physiology* (p. 271) is shown on p. 48. Study the page and then answer the following questions in the space provided.

1. How many glands make up the adrenal glands? _____
2. The Adam's apple is enlarged by which hormone? _____
3. The Achilles' tendon is attached to which bone? _____
4. AIDS is an abbreviation for _____.
5. The area of the body between the diaphragm and the pelvis is the

   _____.

The Thesaurus

A thesaurus is a listing of words and their synonyms (different words that have the same meaning). In addition, some thesauruses will give words that mean the opposite of the headword (antonyms). Most thesauruses resemble a dictionary; you look up the entry the same way you would look up an entry in your dictionary. However, instead of giving pronunciations, origins, and definitions, a thesaurus lists only the words that can be used to substitute for the headword.

The thesaurus is most useful for good writing. When you are writing a paper, you may see that you are using the same word repeatedly. If this is so, look up the word in

GLOSSARY

abdomen (ab-doe-men) The region of the body between the diaphragm and the pelvis.

abdominal cavity (ab-dom-ih-nal) The superior part of the abdominopelvic cavity containing the liver, gallbladder, spleen, stomach, pancreas, and small intestine and part of the large intestine.

abdominopelvic cavity (ab-*dom*-ih-no-pel-vic) The lower part of the ventral body cavity below the thoracic cavity.

abduction (ab-duk-shun) A movement whereby a body part is drawn away from the main body axis or the axis of a limb.

ABO blood types A system of categorizing blood, based on the presence or absence of specific surface antigens.

abortion (ah-bor-shun) Expulsion of an embryo or fetus before it is capable of surviving outside the uterus.

absorption (ab-sorp-shun) The passage of material into or through a cell or tissue, as in the movement of digested nutrients from the GI tract into the blood or lymph.

acetylcholine (*as*-ee-til-koe-leen) A neurotransmitter released by cholinergic nerves, such as those stimulating skeletal muscle contraction.

Achilles' tendon (ah-kil-eez) The tendon of the gastrocnemius and soleus muscle that inserts upon the calcaneus (heel bone).

acid (as-id) A proton donor or compound that dissociates in solution to produce hydrogen ions and some type of anion.

acquired immune deficiency syndrome (AIDS) A disease caused by the HIV virus in which a deficiency develops in helper T cells. Symptoms include fever, night sweats, sore throat, coughing, enlarged lymph nodes, body aches, fatigue, and weight loss. No cure is presently known.

acromegaly (*ak*-roe-meg-ah-lee) A condition resulting from a hypersecretion of growth hormone in the adult. It is characterized by enlarged bones in the extremities and face along with the enlargement of other tissues.

actin (ak-tin) A contractile protein of the thin filaments within a muscle cell.

action potential The electrical activity developed in a muscle or nerve cell during activity; also called a nerve or muscle impulse.

active immunity An acquired immunity resulting from the production of antibodies in response to exposure to antigens.

active transport The movement of substances through cell membranes against concentration gradients. Active transport requires energy expenditure.

acute (a-kyout) Having a short and relatively severe course; not chronic.

Adam's apple The thyroid cartilage of the larynx. In males, it is pronounced because of enlargement caused by testosterone.

adduction (ad-duk-shun) A movement whereby a body part is drawn toward the main body axis or the axis of a limb.

adenosine triphosphate (ATP) (a-den-oh-seen try-fos-fate) The energy currency of the cell; a chemical compound used to transfer energy from those biochemical reactions that yield energy to those that require it.

adipose tissue A type of connective tissue characterized by the presence of many fat cells.

adrenal cortex (ah-dree-nal kore-tekz) The outer part of the adrenal gland. It has three zones, each producing different hormones.

adrenal glands (ah-dree-nal) The two glands located superior to the kidneys. They are also known as the suprarenal glands.

adrenal medulla (ah-dree-nal meh-dul-ah) The inner part of the adrenal gland that secretes catecholamines (epinephrine and norepinephrine) in response to sympathetic stimulation.

adrenocorticotropic hormone (ACTH) (ad-*ree*-no-kore-ti-kow-trope-ik) A hormone produced and released by the anterior pituitary that causes the production and release of hormones of the adrenal cortex.

adventitia (*ad*-ven-tish-eah) The outermost layer or covering of an organ or structure.

271

---

the thesaurus and choose a different word with the same meaning. Or else, you may want to use a word that has a different meaning than the word you have written. Again, consult the thesaurus. Once you become familiar with the thesaurus and use it regularly, you should notice a big improvement in your writing.

Reading a Thesaurus Entry

Following is an entry taken from *Roget's New Pocket Thesaurus in Dictionary Form* (p. 309). The different parts of the entry have been numbered.

    1.   2.   3.   4.
physician, n. general practitioner, doctor (MEDICAL SCIENCE)

1. The **main entry** or **headword** is the word you are looking up in order to find a synonym for it.
2. A letter **abbreviation** tells you **the part of speech** of the headword. An explanation of the abbreviations is usually given in the front of the thesaurus. Headwords may have more than one part of speech. Make sure that the part of speech matches the way the word appears in your text.
3. The **synonyms** are given following the part of speech.
4. Suggestions for **other words to look up** that relate to the word you want to change are written in capital letters, enclosed in parentheses, and end the entry.

EXERCISE 3-10

Page 192 from *Roget's New Pocket Thesaurus* is shown on p. 50. Read the following passage with words in boldface print. After reviewing the thesaurus page, choose a better word for each of the boldface words and write it above the boldface term. Make sure the part of speech of the synonym matches the part of speech of the word you want to change.

The **healer** wished to **heal** the patient with the bad heart. It was a **heartbreaking** situation because the patient came from a **heartless** family who did not care if she became **healthy** or not. They were very **headstrong** in their feelings. The family's attitude make the healer **heartsick.** If she could convince them that a change of heart would allow the patient to **heal** quicker, then she would feel **heartened** by the patient's improved ability to get **healthy.**

REMEMBERING NEW WORDS

In this chapter, you have learned different strategies for finding the meanings of unknown general and medical terms. However, seeing the definition of the unknown word is not the same as remembering the definition of the unknown word. You must have a strategy for memorizing the meaning of the word so you do not have to relearn the word every time you see it.

> **HEADING**   192   **HEAT**
>
> mer (*slang*), derby, bowler (*Brit.*); castor, busby, cocked hat, coonskin hat, pith helmet, shako, sombrero, southwester *or* sou'wester, tricorn; bonnet, capote, sunbonnet, calash, breton, cloche, picture hat, pillbox, sailor, toque.
>   **cap**, beanie, beret, biretta *or* barret (*R. C. Ch.*), coif, fez, tarboosh, garrison cap, overseas cap, kepi, mobcap, mob (*hist.*), mortarboard, nightcap, bedcap, skullcap, tam-o'-shanter, tam, tuque; cap and bells, fool's cap, dunce cap.
>   **high hat**, beaver, crush hat, opera hat, plug hat (*slang*), silk hat, stovepipe hat (*colloq.*), top hat, topper (*colloq.*).
>   helmet, headpiece, crest, casque (*poetic*); visor, beaver.
>   See also CLOTHING, CLOTHING WORKER, COVERING, HEAD, ORNAMENT. *Antonyms*—See FOOTWEAR.
>
> ---
>
> **heading**, *n.* caption, rubric, inscription (TITLE).
> **headland**, *n.* promontory, cape, head (LAND).
> **headline**, *n.* banner, streamer, heading (TITLE).
> **headlong**, *adv.* full-tilt, posthaste, pell-mell (SPEED); violently, headfirst, precipitately (VIOLENCE).
> **headstrong**, *adj.* self-willed, obstinate, willful (STUBBORNNESS, WILL, UNRULINESS); ungovernable, uncontrollable, unruly (VIOLENCE).
> **headway**, *n.* headroom, elbowroom, leeway, seaway (SPACE).
> **heady**, *adj.* provocative, intoxicating, stimulating (EXCITEMENT).
> **heal**, *v.* convalesce, mend, cure (HEALTH, CURE).
> **healer**, *n.* medicine man, witch doctor, shaman (MEDICAL SCIENCE).
>
> ---
>
> **HEALTH**—*N.* **health**, vigor, euphoria, eudaemonia, well-being; trim, bloom, pink, verdure, prime.
>   hygiene, sanitation, prophylaxis.
>   health resort, sanatorium, sanitarium, spa, watering place, rest home, convalescent home, hospital.
>   *V.* **be in health**, enjoy good health, bloom, flourish, thrive.
>   **get well**, convalesce, heal, mend, rally, recover, recuperate, revalesce, get better; cure, heal, restore to health, make well.
>   *Adj.* **healthy**, sound, well, robust, hearty, robustious (*jocose*), trim, trig, hale, fit, blooming, bouncing, strapping, vigorous, whole, wholesome, able-bodied, athletic, eudaemonic, euphoric, tonic.
>   convalescent, recovering, on the mend, recuperating, revalescent.
>   **healthful**, nutritious, salutary, salubrious, wholesome, beneficial; hygienic, sanatory, sanitary, prophylactic.
>   [*concerned about one's health*] **hypochondriac**, valetudinary, atrabilious.
>   **unharmed**, intact, untouched, scatheless, scot-free, sound, spared, unblemished, unbruised, undamaged, unhurt, uninjured, unmarred, unscarred, unscathed, unspoiled, unwounded, whole.
>   See also CURE, MEDICAL SCIENCE, RESTORATION, STRENGTH. *Antonyms*—See DISEASE.
>
> ---
>
> **heap**, *n.* lump, pile, mass (ASSEMBLAGE).
> **heap up**, *v.* pile up, stack, load (STORE).
> **hear**, *v.* give a hearing to, overhear (LISTENING); try, sit in judgment (LAWSUIT).
> **hearing**, *n.* audience, interview, conference (LISTENING); earshot, range (SOUND).
> **hearing aid**, *n.* ear trumpet, auriphone, audiphone (LISTENING).
> **hearsay**, *n.* comment, buzz, report (RUMOR).
> **heart**, *n.* core, pith, kernel (CENTER, INTERIORITY); auricle, ventricle (BLOOD).
> **heartache**, *n.* heavy heart, broken heart, heartbreak (SADNESS).
> **heartbreaking**, *adj.* affecting, heart-rending, moving (PITY).
> **hearten**, *v.* inspire, reassure, encourage (COURAGE).
> **heartfelt**, *adj.* cordial, wholehearted (HONESTY).
> **hearth**, *n.* fireplace, fireside, grate (HEAT); home, homestead, hearthstone (HABITATION).
> **heartless**, *adj.* cruelhearted, flinthearted, hardhearted (CRUELTY); coldhearted, cold-blooded, cold (INSENSITIVITY).
> **heart-shaped**, *adj.* cordiform, cordate (CURVE).
> **heartsick**, *adj.* heartsore, heartstricken, heavyhearted (SADNESS).
> **hearty**, *adj.* healthy, well, robust (HEALTH); cordial, sincere, glowing (FEELING).
>
> ---
>
> **HEAT**—*N.* **heat**, warmth, temperature, calefaction, calescence, incalescence, candescence, incandescence.
>   [*instruments*] thermometer, calorimeter, pyrometer, centigrade *or* Celsius thermometer, Fahrenheit thermometer; thermostat, pyrostat, cryometer.

Word Cards

An excellent way of learning and retaining the meanings of new medical and general terms is to create word cards. To do this, you need to buy index cards that are lined on one side and blank on the other. On the blank side of the index card you write the unknown word. If you wish, you can copy the pronunciation of the word from the dictionary so you can remember how to say it at some later time. On the lined side of the index card, write the definition of the word. In addition, you may want to write a sentence with the word in it to help you remember how the word is actually used.

What you have now created with the index card is a flash card with which you can practice remembering the new word. Because the words are written on index cards, you can carry them anywhere and practice memorizing the words when it is convenient for you. Also, these words are words that you, rather than your instructor, have chosen to learn, so the memorizing process should be more meaningful for you. Finally, the cards are versatile, so you can use them in many ways. You may decide to look at the word and try to recall the definition. Or you may want to look at the definition and try to come up with the word. Whatever you decide, the use of the word cards allows you to be as creative as you wish in learning new medical and general vocabulary words.

EXERCISE 3–11

Directions: Using this textbook or any of your others, choose ten general vocabulary and ten medical vocabulary words and create word cards. Use Figure 3–1 as an example for setting up your cards. Use the two strategies suggested for memorizing the definitions, or invent your own strategies.

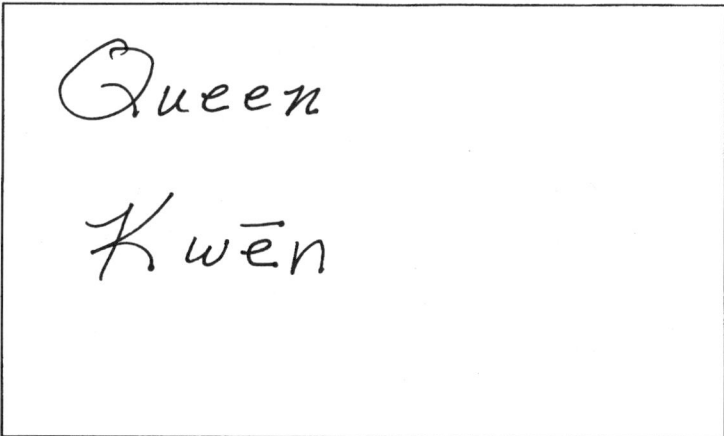

FIGURE 3–1 Example of both sides of a word card.

REVIEWING THE LEARNING STRATEGIES

TO LEARN	**USE THIS STRATEGY**
To develop vocabulary	context clues
	word parts
	dictionaries
	glossaries
	thesauruses
To remember new vocabulary	word cards

Chapter 4

Monitoring and Improving Comprehension

LEARNING OBJECTIVES
VOCABULARY WORDS
VOCABULARY CHECK
WHAT IS MONITORING?
SIX COMPREHENSION IMPROVEMENT STRATEGIES
    Comprehension Improvement Strategy 1:
    Rereading
    Comprehension Improvement Strategy 2:
    Learning Unknown Words
    Comprehension Improvement Strategy 3:
    Making Connections
    Comprehension Improvement Strategy 4:
    Summarizing
    Comprehension Improvement Strategy 5:
    Visualizing
    Comprehension Improvement Strategy 6:
    Researching
USING COMPREHENSION IMPROVEMENT STRATEGIES FOR READING YOUR TEXTBOOK
REVIEWING THE LEARNING STRATEGIES

LEARNING OBJECTIVES

In this chapter you will learn how to
- Become aware of when you do not understand what you are reading
- Use six strategies to improve comprehension

VOCABULARY WORDS

The following vocabulary words are important to your understanding of the ideas in this chapter. These vocabulary words are underscored the first time they are used in the chapter. Read the list of words and definitions. Then check your understanding of these words before you read the chapter.

approximate nearly the same or nearly correct.
associate closely connected.
attending physician a doctor who works in a teaching hospital.
diabetes mellitus a disturbance in the oxidation and utilization of glucose (Miller-Keane, p. 412).
function keys special control keys on the computer keyboard.
invoice a list showing items purchased and how much money is owed.
monitoring asking yourself if you are understanding what you are reading, watching, observing.
pulse rate the pressure on the arteries used for the counting of heartbeats.
reference a book containing information, such as an encyclopedia or a dictionary.
visualize to make a mental picture.

VOCABULARY CHECK

Directions: Choose the vocabulary word that best fits into the sentence.

1. Not knowing the meaning of the word, the student checked the _____ in the back of her textbook.

2. After exercising, he put his fingers on his neck to check his _____.

3. The student needed another _____ in order to get more information for the paper she was writing.

4. She was carefully _____ her reading to be sure she was understanding.

5. Because he has _____, he must be careful not to eat too much cake, cookies, and candy.

6. Along with the items she ordered from the catalogue, she found an _____ in the packaging.

7. Because he knew only the _____ answer, he did not get full credit on the test.

8. When the medical secretary remembered to use the _____ on the computer, his work went faster.

9. The _____ decided on the best care for the patient.
10. As she was studying for the test, she tried to _____ the information on page 25 in her textbook.

WHAT IS MONITORING?

At one time or another you may have realized, after reading many pages in your textbook, that you were not really following or understanding what you had read. Although this can happen to the best readers, if it happens to you too often you may be wasting important studying time and your grades will show this.

A very good strategy for improving your reading is monitoring. When you monitor your reading, you are asking yourself if you are understanding what you are reading. In other words, you are constantly watching and observing to see if you are comprehending what you read. If the reading material is hard, you may have to ask yourself this question at the end of every sentence or paragraph. If the reading material is easier, you may need to ask yourself this question only after every section or page. The important point, however, is that as quickly as possible you become aware of when you are not understanding and then take the needed steps to improve the situation. An explanation of six comprehension-improvement strategies to help you better understand your textbooks follows.

SIX COMPREHENSION-IMPROVEMENT STRATEGIES

Comprehension-Improvement Strategy 1: Rereading

Many good readers have discovered that all it takes to improve their comprehension is to simply reread the passage. Usually with a second reading you are able to understand the ideas better. Sometimes it is helpful to reread the passage aloud. Listening to yourself read helps you to focus on the ideas in the selection.

EXERCISE 4–1

Directions: Read the following passage from Kinn, Woods, and Derge (p. 356, underscore added). Then reread to see if you understand the instructions in the passage better. Try rereading aloud the second time and note whether or not this strategy is helpful for you.

All orders should be placed in the storage area and opened only when you have time to check the contents. Compare the items in the package with your original purchase order and the <u>invoice</u> included with the shipment. Check for correct items, sizes, and styles as well as the number or amount received. Note any back orders and discrepancies. When you are satisfied that the order is correct and complete, make the necessary notations on the inventory and order cards and place the items in their designated storage areas.

1. Did your second reading help you understand the passage better?
   yes_____ no_____
2. Was reading the passage aloud helpful? yes_____ no_____

Comprehension-Improvement Strategy 2: Learning Unknown Words

Being unfamiliar with the vocabulary or terminology in your textbooks may be the reason you are not understanding what you are reading. In some cases, you may be able to figure out the meaning or definition of the unknown word by using the surrounding words in the sentence (see Chapter 3). However, when it comes to learning a health care–related word, it will be necessary to use a dictionary or the glossary at the back of the textbook. When learning the meanings of general vocabulary words, it may be enough just to learn an <u>approximate</u> or nearly correct definition of the word. Then it is okay to use the surrounding words or context to supply a definition. When learning the meanings of technical words, you need to learn an exact definition. Therefore you must use some sort of reference. In either case, it will be necessary to use one of these two strategies to help you learn the meanings of unknown words in order to improve your reading comprehension.

EXERCISE 4–2

Directions: Read the following paragraph from Diehl and Fordney (pp. 27–28) and then write the meanings of any unknown words in the space provided. Show whether you used the context, dictionary, or glossary by writing "C," "D," or "G" next to the definition.

A computer has a keyboard that has <u>*function keys,*</u> which are also called *control* or *command keys*. A *program instruction* can be given by depressing certain keys, and this enters a particular command into a word processing or other type of software program. *Response time,* the time it takes the system to react to a command, varies depending on how sophisticated the equipment is. Besides keyboarding in *data,* it is now possible to handwrite or speak and the data appears automatically on the VDT [video display terminal]. It is also possible to point to a picture on a *touch-sensitive video screen,* and the commands are performed. Computer accessories, such as a *mouse* or a *light pen,* enable the operator to draw images, mark choices, or add and delete text on the VDT. Light pens are used in some facilities to scan the patient's admitting information so that the operator does not have to keyboard in the patient's name and other identifying data.

UNKNOWN WORD	MEANING	STRATEGY
1. _____	_____	_____
2. _____	_____	_____
3. _____	_____	_____
4. _____	_____	_____
5. _____	_____	_____
6. _____	_____	_____
7. _____	_____	_____
8. _____	_____	_____
9. _____	_____	_____
10. _____	_____	_____

Comprehension-Improvement Strategy 3: Making Connections

The best way to understand new information is to connect, or <u>associate</u>, it with facts you already know. When you are monitoring your reading and you become aware that you are not understanding, a good strategy will be to connect the topic of the selection to something you already know. Once this connection is made, you may realize that you know something about the topic already and the reading will be more understandable. The easiest way to use this strategy is to go back to the heading of the selection you do not understand and think about what it reminds you of or what you already know about the topic. See the example headings in bold print below from Kinn, Woods, and Derge and note the connections that were made to each of these headings.

Example 4–1

PULSE RATE (p. 449)

Connection: **My own personal experience having my <u>pulse rate</u> taken by my doctor; taking my own pulse rate after I jog; pulse rate is the counting of heartbeats by feeling the pressure on the artery.**

THE HEART'S NATURAL PACEMAKER (p. 546)

Connection: **The four chambers of the heart: left and right ventricles and the left and right atria, different valves that direct the flow of blood, Uncle Max's pacemaker operation.**

THE LABORATORY (p. 570)

Connection: **My old high school lab, the lab in the movie Frankenstein, microscopes, tubes, testing blood and urine, chemicals, lab coats, and complicated equipment.**

Did you notice that in these examples both facts and personal impressions were used to make the connections? When using the "making connections" strategy, associate whatever knowledge or experience you have with the topic to the heading in order to make what you are reading more understandable.

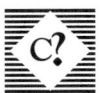

EXERCISE 4–3

Directions: Five bold-printed headings taken from Kinn, Woods, and Derge are shown on p. 58. In the space provided, write you own connections to the headings. Use facts or personal experience to make the connections.

DRESSINGS AND BANDAGES (p. 746)

Connections: _____

_____

_____

ULTRAVIOLET DISINFECTION (p. 412)

Connections: _____

_____

_____

QUALITIES OF A SUPERVISOR (p. 362)

Connections: _____

_____

_____

BILLING METHODS (p. 291)

Connections: _____

_____

_____

MEDICAL ASSISTANT'S ROLE IN THE PEDIATRIC EXAMINATION (p. 508)

Connections: _____

_____

_____

Comprehension-Improvement Strategy 4: Summarizing

When reading your textbooks, you will often see information that is technical and difficult. Sometimes the sentences will be very long and the facts will seem poorly organized and confusing. When this happens, your best strategy is to summarize the passage in your own words. To make a summary, you should briefly write down the main idea and important details from the passage (see Chapters 1 and 2). If the passage is not too long and if there is enough space, you can write the summary in the margin of your textbook. If the misunderstood passage is too long, however, it may be better to write the main ideas and important details in your notebook. When you summarize difficult ideas into your own words, you make the information easier to understand. Once the ideas are easier to understand, they will be easier to learn and you will be a more successful student.

Example 4-2

Directions: Below is an excerpt from a text by Ehrlich and Torres (p. 320). Following that is a summary of this passage. Notice that the writer uses her own words when writing the summary. Also, she summarizes only the main idea and important details.

Infiltration anesthesia involves placement of the anesthetic solution directly into the tissues at the site of the dental procedure. This technique is most frequently used to anesthetize the maxillary teeth.

Infiltration anesthesia is possible in the maxillary teeth because of the more "porous" nature of the alveolus cancellous bone, which allows the solution to reach the apices of the teeth. (The **apices** are the tips of the roots of the teeth. It is here that the nerve enters the tooth.)

Infiltration anesthesia is the putting of the anesthetic solution into the tissues of the tooth that will be worked on. This method of anesthesia is good for the maxillary teeth because they are porous and the solution can easily reach the ends of the root where the nerve enters the tooth.

EXERCISE 4-4

Directions: In the space provided, summarize the following selection from Diehl and Fordney (pp. 15–16). Remember to summarize only the main idea and important details. Use your own words and be brief.

Generally speaking, certain information is not available from the hospital medical record for release to third parties. This includes detailed psychiatric examination information, personal history of the patient or family, and information controlled by state law. If there is a question regarding the content of the medical information to be released, the attending physician should be consulted regarding its accuracy or interpretation. Hospitals prefer to release information by the use of summaries or abstracts or on standard forms recommended by the American Hospital Association or local hospital groups. Duplicating an entire record is expensive; furthermore, control of the record by the hospital would be lost, and the copy might be misused. If the attending physician wishes information from the hospital record, an abstract or copy can be given without the patient's written permission, as long as it is for the physician's own use.

_____

_____

_____

Comprehension-Improvement Strategy 5: Visualizing

Another reason for not understanding what you are reading is that your mind may be wandering to other thoughts when you read your textbook. You may not be concentrating because the room you are studying in is too noisy. Or you may be thinking more about the fight you had with your friend than about what you are reading. If these or similar reasons are not letting you concentrate, then using visualization as a strategy should be helpful.

60 READING STRATEGIES

<u>Some germs under a microscope</u>   <u>Scratching dog</u>
Rickettsiae are microorganisms found in the tissue cells of lice, fleas, ticks and mites and are
<u>being bitten by insects when I work in the garden</u>   <u>Western U.S.A.</u>
transmitted to humans by the bite of these insects. Rickettsial diseases include *Rocky Mountain*
             <u>War-time illness</u>
spotted fever, typhus, Q *fever,* and *trench fever.* These diseases are not common in communities
     <u>Sewers</u>   <u>Sprays</u>   <u>Shots</u>
with good sanitary conditions. They can be prevented by insecticides, vaccines, and
<u>Pills</u>
antibiotics.

FIGURE 4–1   How a reader visualized a selection from Kinn, Woods, and Derge (p. 583).

When you <u>visualize</u>, you make a picture in your mind of what you are reading. As you read more facts from your text, you change the picture in your mind to include the new ideas. In other words, the visualizing strategy is like watching a program on the television set, only you are responsible for making the show happen by deliberately creating a picture in your mind of what you are reading. In Figure 4–1, notice the handwritten notes above the printed lines. These are examples of what one reader visualized as he read the selection.

EXERCISE 4-5

Directions: Read the following excerpt from Kinn, Woods, and Derge, (p. 603). Try to visualize the facts you are reading. Make changes to your mental picture when you read new facts. As in Figure 4–1, write what you visualize above the lines.

Normal urine color is a shade of yellow ranging from pale straw to yellow to amber. Color depends on the concentration of the pigment *urochrome* and the amount of water in the specimen. A dilute specimen should be pale, and a more concentrated specimen should be darker yellow. Variations in color may be caused by diet, medication, and disease.

Comprehension-Improvement Strategy 6: Researching

The most useful way to learn new ideas is to already have some knowledge of the subject. When you have previous knowledge of a subject, you have a base on which to build new facts. Sometimes you may not understand what you are reading because you do not know enough about the topic. If this is the case, your best strategy is to research, or learn more about the subject. One way to do this is to simply read an easier text. Or else you can check an encyclopedia or suitable health care journal in order to build up your base of knowledge. Once you have a greater general understanding about the topic you are reading, understanding your current textbook will be easier.

EXERCISE 4-6

Directions: Knowing what <u>reference</u> to read in order to learn more about your topic will make your research hunt easier. Below are two columns. On the left are different types of references you can use. These references are lettered. In the right-hand column are different topics you may read about in your textbooks. In the spaces in the right-hand column, write the letter of the reference you would use for each topic.

A. Encyclopedia
B. Easier Health Care Textbook
C. Health Care Journal

____ Latest information on AIDS
____ Health Insurance
____ History of Health Care
____ Newest Technique for Assisting with Minor Surgery
____ Job Training
____ General Nutrition

USING COMPREHENSION-IMPROVEMENT STRATEGIES FOR READING YOUR TEXTBOOK

When you are actually reading your textbook and you realize that you are reading without any comprehension, you may need to use one, some, or all of the comprehension-improvement strategies discussed in this chapter. Figure 4-2 is a passage taken from Ehrlich and Torres (pp. 138–139). Above the lines are handwritten notes that describe how one reader uses the different comprehension strategies to help her understand the passage better.

DIABETES MELLITUS *Connections: Aunt Esther's illness, no sweets, amputated foot*

In the diabetic patient, medical complications may occur if the prescribed routine for diabetes is not followed.

SYMPTOMS *Check dictionary*

Diabetic acidosis and insulin shock are two of the most serious complications.

Diabetic Acidosis, also known as hyperglycemic coma, occurs because of an abnormally *Visualize large bowl of sugar* increased level of sugar in the blood. This may occur because the patient has eaten too much sugar-containing food, has not eaten enough insulin, or has an infection.

FIGURE 4-2 Example of how one reader used the various comprehension strategies in a passage from Ehrlich and Torres (pp. 138–139).

Continued on p. 62.

Check encyclopedia

Diabetic acidosis can lead to convulsions, coma, and death. The clinical signs of diabetic acidosis include:

Read aloud {
- Acetone breath (smelling like fruit).
- Warm, dry skin and dry mouth.
- Rapid and weak pulse.
- Air hunger, rapid deep breathing.
- Unresponsiveness to questioning.
- Unconsciousness
}

Summary: diabetes mellitus – 2 major complications
① diabetic acidosis – patient has fruity breath, dry skin and mouth, abnormal pulse & breathing, unresponsive or unconscious
② insulin shock

FIGURE 4–2 Continued

EXERCISE 4–7

Directions: Read the following passage taken from the textbook by Kinn, Woods, and Derge (pp. 326, 328, 330). Using the method shown in Figure 4–2, write above the printed line the names of the comprehension strategies you used to help you understand the following paragraphs better. The comprehension strategies discussed in this chapter are

1. Rereading
2. Learning unknown words
3. Making connections
4. Summarizing
5. Visualizing
6. Researching

Workers' Compensation

Records for the workers' compensation case (sometimes referred to as an "industrial case") should be kept separate from the physician's regular patient histories. If the patient who is seen for an industrial injury has previously been treated as a private patient, a new chart and ledger should be started that will be used only for the treatment rendered under conditions of the Workers' Compensation law.

The insurance carrier may request and is entitled to receive copies of all records pertaining to the industrial injury but not the records of a private patient. Information in the records of a private patient is privileged information and may be released only with the patient's consent.

There could be a lawsuit or a hearing before a referee or Appeals Board for which records are subpoenaed. If separate records are kept, there is no question of privilege involved.

The physician who sees the injured or ill worker first will complete what may be called the Doctor's First Report of Work Injury within the time limit implied by state regulations.... The medical assistant should make a minimum of five copies of this report. The insurance company usually requires at least two copies. One copy goes to the state regulatory body. The employer may get a copy, and one file copy should remain with the physician's record. This report must be personally signed by the physician and should contain the following information:

- The history of the case as obtained from the patient, with notation of any **pre-existing condition** (injuries or diseases).
- The patient's symptoms and physical complaints.
- The complete physical findings, including laboratory and x-ray results.
- A tentative diagnosis.
- An estimate of the type and extent of the disability. In cases in which a permanent disability has resulted, there should be a careful survey, and the extent of disability should be given in detail.
- Treatment indicated, including type, frequency, and duration. It may be necessary to attach a letter giving more detailed information to assist in making an evaluation of the case.
- Whenever possible, the date the patient may be able to return to work, if he or she has been totally disabled.

The insurance company may supply its own billing forms. Payment is usually made on the basis of a fee schedule. Any charges in excess of the fee schedule must be fully explained and documented.

In billing for the service, use the coding system specified in your state. Itemize the statement, including any drugs and dressings used.

In severe or prolonged cases, supplemental reports and billing should be sent to the insurance carrier at least once per month.

At the termination of treatment, a final report and bill are sent to the insurance carrier. Do not bill the patient.

REVIEWING THE LEARNING STRATEGIES

TO LEARN	USE THIS STRATEGY
Monitoring	Ask yourself if you are understanding what you are reading
To improve your reading comprehension	Rereading Learning unknown words Making connections Summarizing Visualizing Researching

Chapter 5

Reading The Textbook

LEARNING OBJECTIVES
VOCABULARY WORDS
VOCABULARY CHECK
SURVEYING THE TEXTBOOK
   Title Page
   Preface
   Table of Contents
   Glossary
   Bibliography
   Appendix
   Index
STRATEGIES FOR READING THE TEXTBOOK
   Strategies to Use Before Reading
      Previewing
      Questioning
   Strategies to Use While Reading
      Asking the 5W Questions
      Assessing Your Health Care Literacy
      Reading Graphic Aids
      Summarizing
   Strategies for Reading Difficult Passages
   Strategies to Use After Reading
REVIEWING READING THE TEXTBOOK

LEARNING OBJECTIVES

In this chapter you will learn how to
- Identify and locate important features in a textbook
- Use strategies to help your concentration and comprehension when you read textbooks

VOCABULARY WORDS

The following vocabulary words are important to your understanding of the ideas in this chapter. These vocabulary words are underscored the first time they are used in the chapter. Read the list of words and definitions. Then check your understanding of these words before you read the chapter.

chaotic pertaining to being in a state of utter confusion.
credentials diplomas or certificates.
discombobulated perplexed or upset.
hypertrophy increase in volume of a tissue or organ produced entirely by enlargement of existing cells.
ingested taken in.
ions charged particles.
plaque food debris on tooth that fosters bacteria.
protein any large organic compound made from one or more polypeptides (Miller-Keane, p. 1228).
secrete to synthesize and release a substance.
statistics numerical data.

VOCABULARY CHECK

Directions: Choose the vocabulary word that best fits into the sentence.

1. The dentist tried to remove the _____ from the patient's tooth.
2. She _____ the vitamins.
3. The glands will _____ a fluid.
4. _____ are charged particles associated with x-rays.
5. The tissue will _____ at a certain age because of hormones.
6. She had to show her _____ before she was allowed to teach.
7. He felt all _____ when he traveled to foreign countries.
8. The student collected all the _____ he could about the number of lettuces grown each year.
9. The zoo was _____ when the animals escaped from their cages.
10. It is important to get enough _____ from your diet.

SURVEYING THE TEXTBOOK

Maybe you have had the experience of walking into a movie theater without knowing anything about the film being shown. Did you sit there for several minutes discombobulated and confused about what you were seeing on the screen? Most of the time we choose to see a movie after we have seen the previews or read reviews in magazines and newspapers. Likewise with reading your textbook. If you just start reading at Chapter 1, you may feel disconnected and bewildered about what you are reading. However, if you survey, or briefly glance through, the entire textbook before you begin your first reading assignment, you will discover that it is similar to seeing movie previews. You will know what you are getting into.

To have the time to adequately survey the text, it will be necessary to buy the book before the semester starts. Many school bookstores have their textbooks on the shelves 2 weeks or so before the semester starts. Buying your textbooks early not only will give you time to become familiar with the books but also will help you avoid the long and chaotic lines of students all buying their books the first day of school.

When you have your textbook, the parts that you will want to survey are

- Title page
- Preface
- Table of Contents
- Glossary
- Bibliography
- Appendix
- Index

Title Page

The title page is found at the very beginning of a book and contains some or all of the following information:

- Title
- Author—name or names and a listing of credentials
- Edition—if there are more than one
- Publisher
- Location or locations of the publisher's main offices

EXERCISE 5–1

Directions: Study the title page on p. 68 and then answer the following questions in the space provided.

1. The complete title of the book is _____.
2. The author's name is _____.
3. The author has _____ degrees.

Third Edition

Clinical Textbook for VETERINARY TECHNICIANS

DENNIS M. McCURNIN, DVM, MS
Diplomate, American College of Veterinary Surgeons
Professor, Department of Veterinary Clinical Sciences
Associate Dean for Clinical and Public Services
Hospital Director, Veterinary Teaching Hospital and Clinics
School of Veterinary Medicine
Louisiana State University
Baton Rouge, Louisiana

W.B. SAUNDERS COMPANY
A Division of Harcourt Brace & Company
PHILADELPHIA   LONDON   TORONTO   MONTREAL   SYDNEY   TOKYO

4. The author works at _____ University.
5. The publisher is _____.
6. The publisher has offices in _____.
7. This is the _____ edition of this text.

Preface

The preface ('prĕf-əs) of a textbook is found after the cover page. The preface is an introduction to the textbook and explains the author's reasons for writing the book and a description of how the book is organized. Sometimes the preface will list the names of people who helped the author write the textbook.

EXERCISE 5-2

Directions: Shown below is a preface from the Flynn textbook *Procedures in Phlebotomy* (p. ix). Read the preface carefully and then answer the following questions.

1. For whom is this book intended? _____
2. What is the general topic for the first section? _____
3. What is the general topic for the second section? _____
4. Where do you find the definitions of boldfaced words? _____
5. What three additional features are included in the textbook? _____

Preface

Procedures in Phlebotomy is intended for students of phlebotomy. These students may be just entering the field, or they may have been practicing the art of blood collection for many years. Whoever wishes to remain abreast of this rapidly changing and expanding field will find this book useful.

Procedures in Phlebotomy is divided into two sections, the first dealing with those topics directly related to blood collection, including an introduction to phlebotomy, with a brief history of the practice and a review of anatomy and physiology. Also in this section is a chapter dedicated to infectious diseases and their prevention, with special attention to Occupational Safety and Health Administration regulations. Most of this section is dedicated to a discussion of the equipment, procedures, and complications of phlebotomy. Finally, for the inquisitive student, there is a special chapter discussing small mammal venipuncture.

The second section covers professional topics such as quality assurance, interpersonal communication, and management issues and topics. This section also contains a chapter dedicated to medico-legal issues with a discussion on Clinical Laboratory Improvement Act of 1988 as it directly applies to phlebotomy.

The reader will find boldfaced terms that are defined in the glossary. Additionally, there are review questions at the end of each chapter to test the reader's comprehension, with answers provided at the back of the book. Of special interest is a 100-item review examination to aid individuals who are preparing for national certification examinations. Finally, a quick reference chart matching the color code of blood collection tubes used for commonly ordered tests is included at the front of the book.

Table of Contents

Surveying the table of contents is useful because it lists the topics you will be studying for the semester. The table of contents is found after the preface. It commonly contains the names of the divisions of the book: units or sections and chapters and the pages on which they start. Sometimes the chapters are divided into more specific topics that are listed as major headings. Page numbers are given for the major headings also. Because the book from which the contents on the opposite page is taken was not divided into sections or units, the contents lists only chapter titles and major headings.

EXERCISE 5-3

Directions: Survey the table of contents from the Beaver textbook *Feline Behavior* on the following pages. Then answer the following questions.

1. The book contains how many chapters? _____
2. What is the title of the fourth chapter? _____
3. On which page does the Hunting Behavior discussion begin? _____
4. In which chapter will you find a discussion of how an adult cat moves? _____
5. The Male Feline Sexual Behavior chapter contains how many major headings? _____

Glossary

The glossary is found at the end of the book and lists words and their definitions that the author believes are important. Occasionally the author will provide a key for pronouncing a word listed in the glossary.

EXERCISE 5-4

Directions: A page from the glossary of the Solomon textbook *Introduction to Human Anatomy and Physiology* (p. 271) is shown on p. 73. Briefly survey the page and answer the following questions.

1. What is the first word defined in the glossary? _____
2. What is the last word defined in the glossary? _____
3. "A contractile <u>protein</u> of the thin filaments within a muscle cell" is the definition of what word? _____
4. The words in a glossary are listed in (numerical, chronological, or alphabetical) order? _____
5. "Ăs ĭd" is the pronunciation of what word? _____

Contents

1
Introduction to Feline Behavior 1
- History of Feline Development 1
- Current Status of the Felid 4
- Introduction to Evaluating Behavior Problems 8

2
Feline Behavior of Sensory and Neural Origin 15
- The Senses 15
- Feline Play Behavior 31
- Feline Learning 37
- Neurologic Origins of Behavior 41
- Sensory and Neural Behavior Problems 43

3
Feline Communicative Behavior 63
- Vocal Communication 63
- Postural Communication 66
- Marking Communication 76
- Communicative Behavior Problems 79

4
Feline Social Behavior 87
- Social Organization 87
- Socialization 95
- Aggression 97
- Social Behavior Problems 102

5
Male Feline Sexual Behavior 121
- Sexual Maturation 121
- Premating Behavior 123
- Mating Behavior 125
- Postmating Behavior 127
- Paternal Behavior 127
- Neural Regulation 128
- Male Sexual Behavior Problems 129

Continued on p. 72.

x / Contents

6
Female Feline Sexual Behavior 141
    Sexual Maturation 141
    Reproductive Cycles 141
    Intraspecies Mating 141
    Pregnancy 147
    Maternal Behavior 153
    Neurologic and Hormonal Controls 157
    Female Sexual Behavior Problems 160

7
Feline Ingestive Behavior 171
    Suckling Ingestive Behavior 171
    Transitional Ingestive Behavior 171
    Hunting Behavior 174
    Food Preferences 180
    Water Consumption 182
    Neural and Hormonal Regulation 184
    Ingestive Behavior Problems 186

8
Eliminative Behavior Development 203
    Adult Urination 205
    Adult Defecation 208
    Eliminative Behavior Problems 208

9
Feline Locomotive Behavior 225
    Fetal Growth and Movements 225
    Infant Growth and Movements 226
    Adult Movements 232
    Resting Behaviors 242
    The Brain and Locomotion 247
    Locomotive Behavior Problems 248

10
Feline Grooming Behavior 255
    Grooming Functions 255
    Grooming Patterns 256
    Neuroendocrine and Grooming Relationships 260
    Grooming Behavior Problems 261

Appendix
    A Phonetics of Feline Vocalization 267
    B Sensory Response Development 268
    C Motor Response Development 269
    D Miscellaneous Response Development 270

Index 271

GLOSSARY

abdomen (**ab**-doe-men) The region of the body between the diaphragm and the pelvis.

abdominal cavity (ab-**dom**-ih-nal) The superior part of the abdominopelvic cavity containing the liver, gallbladder, spleen, stomach, pancreas, and small intestine and part of the large intestine.

abdominopelvic cavity (ab-*dom*-ih-no-**pel**-vic) The lower part of the ventral body cavity below the thoracic cavity.

abduction (ab-**duk**-shun) A movement whereby a body part is drawn away from the main body axis or the axis of a limb.

ABO blood types A system of categorizing blood, based on the presence or absence of specific surface antigens.

abortion (ah-**bor**-shun) Expulsion of an embryo or fetus before it is capable of surviving outside the uterus.

absorption (ab-**sorp**-shun) The passage of material into or through a cell or tissue, as in the movement of digested nutrients from the GI tract into the blood or lymph.

acetylcholine (*as*-ee-til-**koe**-leen) A neurotransmitter released by cholinergic nerves, such as those stimulating skeletal muscle contraction.

Achilles' tendon (ah-**kil**-eez) The tendon of the gastrocnemius and soleus muscle that inserts upon the calcaneus (heel bone).

acid (**as**-id) A proton donor or compound that dissociates in solution to produce hydrogen ions and some type of anion.

acquired immune deficiency syndrome (AIDS) A disease caused by the HIV virus in which a deficiency develops in helper T cells. Symptoms include fever, night sweats, sore throat, coughing, enlarged lymph nodes, body aches, fatigue, and weight loss. No cure is presently known.

acromegaly (*ak*-roe-**meg**-ah-lee) A condition resulting from a hypersecretion of growth hormone in the adult. It is characterized by enlarged bones in the extremities and face along with the enlargement of other tissues.

actin (**ak**-tin) A contractile protein of the thin filaments within a muscle cell.

action potential The electrical activity developed in a muscle or nerve cell during activity; also called a nerve or muscle impulse.

active immunity An acquired immunity resulting from the production of antibodies in response to exposure to antigens.

active transport The movement of substances through cell membranes against concentration gradients. Active transport requires energy expenditure.

acute (a-**kyout**) Having a short and relatively severe course; not chronic.

Adam's apple The thyroid cartilage of the larynx. In males, it is pronounced because of enlargement caused by testosterone.

adduction (ad-**duk**-shun) A movement whereby a body part is drawn toward the main body axis or the axis of a limb.

adenosine triphosphate (ATP) (a-**den**-oh-seen try-**fos**-fate) The energy currency of the cell; a chemical compound used to transfer energy from those biochemical reactions that yield energy to those that require it.

adipose tissue A type of connective tissue characterized by the presence of many fat cells.

adrenal cortex (ah-**dree**-nal **kore**-tekz) The outer part of the adrenal gland. It has three zones, each producing different hormones.

adrenal glands (ah-**dree**-nal) The two glands located superior to the kidneys. They are also known as the suprarenal glands.

adrenal medulla (ah-**dree**-nal meh-**dul**-ah) The inner part of the adrenal gland that secretes catecholamines (epinephrine and norepinephrine) in response to sympathetic stimulation.

adrenocorticotropic hormone (ACTH) (ad-*ree*-no-kore-ti-kow-**trope**-ik) A hormone produced and released by the anterior pituitary that causes the production and release of hormones of the adrenal cortex.

adventitia (*ad*-ven-**tish**-eah) The outermost layer or covering of an organ or structure.

Bibliography

The bibliography can be found at the end of each unit or chapter or at the back of the book. The bibliography lists the titles and authors of all the textbooks the writer used for writing the text. The bibliography can also be called "References."

EXERCISE 5-5

Directions: Survey the references below from the LaFleur-Brooks textbook *Health Unit Coordinating* (p. 469). Then answer the questions that follow.

References

Anthony, Catherine Parker and Alyn, Irene B.: *Structure and Function of the Body*, 5th ed. St. Louis, The C. V. Mosby Co., 1976.
Brunner, Theodore F. and Berkowitz, Luci: *The Elements of Scientific and Specialized Terminology*. Minneapolis, Burgess Publishing Co., 1967.
Chabner, Davi-Ellen: *The Language of Medicine*, 3rd ed. Philadelphia, W. B. Saunders Co., 1984.
Frenay, Sister Mary Agnes Clare and Smith, Helen M.: *Understanding Medical Terminology*, 3rd ed. St. Louis, The Catholic Hospital Association, 1964.
Keane, Claire Brackman: *Essentials of Nursing*, 3rd ed. Philadelphia, W. B. Saunders Co., 1974.
Memmler, Ruth Lundeen and Wood, Dena Lin: *Structure and Function of the Human Body*, 2nd ed. Philadelphia, J. B. Lippincott Co., 1977.
Miller, Benjamin F. and Keane, Claire Brackman: *Encyclopedia and Dictionary of Medicine and Nursing*. Philadelphia, W. B. Saunders Co., 1987.
Mosby's Medical and Nursing Dictionary, 2nd ed. St. Louis, The C. V. Mosby Co., 1986.
Mulvihill, Mary Lou: *Human Disease: A Systemic Approach*, 3rd ed. San Mateo, CA, Appleton & Lange.
Taber's Cyclopedic Medical Dictionary, 13th ed. Philadelphia, F. A. Davis Co., 1977.
The Merck Manual, 12th ed. Rahway, NJ, Merck & Co., Inc., 1972.
The Nurse's Reference Library. Diseases. Horsham, PA, Intermed Communications Inc., 1981.

1. What is the title of the book written by Davi-Ellen Chabner? _____
2. In what year was *Mosby's Medical and Nursing Dictionary* published? _____
3. What edition of Keane's *Essentials of Nursing* was used? _____
4. What is the title of Frenay's textbook? _____
5. The items in a bibliography are listed in (numerical, chronological, or alphabetical) order? _____

Appendix

The appendix that is also found in the back of the textbook contains additional information that the author did not include within the chapter. The appendix is usually ordered by letters; for example, Appendix A, Appendix B, and can contain charts, graphs, or <u>statistics</u>.

EXERCISE 5–6

Directions: Survey Appendix B from the Beaver textbook (p. 268). List the names of the five general sensory responses illustrated in the chart.

1. _____
2. _____
3. _____
4. _____
5. _____

APPENDIX B

Sensory Response Development

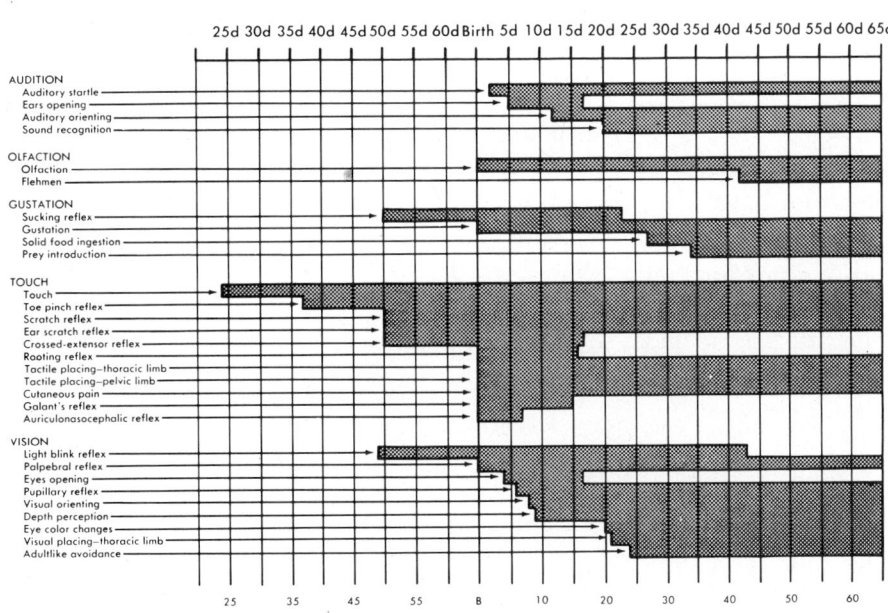

Index

The index is found at the very end of the textbook. It is an alphabetical listing of all the important topics in the text. The index also indicates on what page the topic can be found. For example, "cat, 651–565" means that information about cats can be found on pages 561 **to** 565. Another entry about cats from another textbook can look like this: "cat, 220, 223, 225." This means that information concerning cats can be found on pages 220 **and** 223 **and** 225. Indexes are particularly helpful when you are writing research papers.

EXERCISE 5–7

Directions: Look over the page from the index of the Kinn, Woods, and Derge textbook *The Medical Assistant: Administrative and Clinical* on the opposite page. Then answer the questions that follow.

1. The example index covers items lettered _____.
2. On what page is information about the Kling bandage found? _____
3. Into how many subtopics is "Iodine" divided? _____
4. Can names of people be included in an index? _____
5. List all the pages on which information on "Job Interview" is found. _____

EXERCISE 5–8

Directions: You have now learned how to survey a textbook. Practice surveying by using this textbook or another health care textbook and answer the following questions with "yes" or "no."

1. The title page includes the edition number? _____
2. The preface discusses how many units or chapters the book is divided into? _____
3. The table of contents lists more than 10 chapters? _____
4. The glossary includes the pronunciation of key words? _____
5. The bibliography in the textbook is referred to as "References"? _____
6. An appendix is found at the back of the textbook? _____
7. Some topics in the index are divided into subtopics? _____

Insurance claims *(Continued)*
  requests for assistance with, via telephone, 148
Integument, functions of, 522
Interest, ethics of changing of, Judicial Council opinions on, 44–45
Interferon, in viral disease and cancer therapy, 402
Internal medicine, as specialty practice, 33
  physical examination in, 525–526, *526*
International Classification of Diseases, Ninth Revision, Clinical Modification (ICD-9-CM), 320
  for medical transcription, 203
  in diagnosis-related groups (DRGs), 331
International Nursing Index, 340
International Units (IU), in drug dosage, 777
Interprofessional relations, ethics of, Judicial Council opinions on, 43
Interrogatory, 56
Intestine, surgical bypass of, diet after, 687
Intradermal test, allergy diagnosis with, 518–519
Intraocular pressure, assessment of, 484
  measurement of, 529
Intrauterine device (IUD), 501(t)
  uterine infection from, 495
Inventory, of office furniture and equipment, 355
  of supplies, 357(t)
  personal, biographic data in, 82
    educational data in, 82–83
    employment history in, 82
    extracurricular interests and activities in, 83
    personal goals in, 83
Iodine, deficiency of, 681, 683(t)
  physical examination in, 523
  functions of, 681, 683(t)
  requirements for, 671(t), 684
  sources of, 683(t)
  toxicity from, 683(t)
Iodoform gauze strips, 695, *695*
Ipecac, 772
  in crash tray, 857
  plant sources of, 760
Iris scissors, 696, *698*
Iron, deficiency of, 681, 684(t)
  functions of, 681, 684(t)
  in hemoglobin, 681
  requirements for, 671(t), 681
  sources of, 684(t)
  toxicity from, 684(t)
Irrigation, ear, 536(t)–538(t), 536–537, *538*
  drug administration via, 793
  eye, 532, 532(t)–533(t), *533*
  drug administration via, 793
  wound, patient positioning for, 730
Isocult, for *Streptococcus* screening, 593
Isolation systems, universal precautions vs., in HIV infection prevention, 432–433
Itinerary, travel, 346
Ivan laryngeal metal applicator, 705, *705*

J

Jackknife position, 479, *479*
Jargon, definition of, 4

Jars, sterilization of, 424
Jaundice, 523
  in physical examination, 482
  obstructive, in choledocholithiasis, 525
Jenner, Edward, 19, *19*, 24(t)
  smallpox vaccination discovery by, 19
Job interview, 86–91. See also *Employment.*
  closure in, 91
  conduct of, 88–89, 91
  employment application completion in, 88
  follow-up activities for, *90*, 91
  preliminary steps before, 82
  preparation for, 82–86
    on day of interview, 87–88, *90*
    personal inventory in, 82–83
    resumé in, 83–86
  request for, 86–87, *89*
  unsolicited, 87, *89*
Jock itch, characteristics of, 397(t)
Johns Hopkins University Medical School, early medical education and, 28
Joint Motion: Method of Measuring and Recording, 536
Joints, diseases of, paraffin bath for, 839
  mobility of, active exercise for, 846
    passive exercise for, 846
    range-of-motion exercise for, 846, 848–849
  sprained, heat therapy for, 838
Journal, cash payment, 251
  daily, 247, *247*
  disbursement, 248
  general (daily), 248

K

Kaposi's sarcoma, in AIDS, 430–431
Kelley, Howard A., 28
Kelly hemostat, 696, 701
Ketones, urinary, 608
Ketonuria, 608
Keyboard, computer, definition of, 95
Kidney, diseases of, drug response in, 770
  urine volume changes in, 603
  drug excretion by, 769
  function of, testing of, 511
  in urine formation, 602
Kilocalorie, 669
Kilograms, conversion to pounds of, 462
Klebsiella, as cause of urinary tract infection, 400(t)
Kling bandage, 747
Knee-chest position, 480, *481*
Knee-jerk reflex, 485
Koch, Robert, 24(t), 392, 416
  bacteriologic postulates of, 21
  cholera discovery by, 21
Korotkoff, Nicolai Sergeevich, 460
Korotkoff sounds, during blood pressure measurement, 458, 460–461
  phase I of, 460
  phase II of, 460–461
  phase III of, 461
  phase IV of, 461
  phase V of, 461
Krause nasal snare, 703, *705*
Kwashiorkor, protein deficiency and, 674
Kyphosis, physical examination of, 481, 535

L

Labels, for patient record filing, 222, 222(t)
Labia, herpes simplex of, 496
Labor, stages of, 500
Laboratory, 570–572
  departments of, 570
  equipment maintenance in, 571–572
  hazards in, biologic, 571
    chemical, 570
    physical, 570
  hospital, 570
  legal and ethical responsibilities in, 596
  location of, 570
  microscope in, 572, *572*, 573(t), 574
  nonhospital, 570
  personnel in, 570
  physicians' office, quality assurance in, 596
  procedures performed in, 570
  quality assurance in, 571, 596
  quality control in, 571
  reference, 570
  requisition for testing by, 576, *576*
  rules for, 571
  safety in, 570–571
  test results of, reference values for, 571
  utilization and care of, 354
Laboratory reports, 211
  chronologic order of, 215, *216–217*
Laboratory tests, blood chemistry, 580–582, 581(t)
  for blood glucose levels, 580–581
  for blood urea nitrogen (BUN) levels, 582
  for cholesterol levels, 582
  for serum calcium determination, 581
  for uric acid levels, 581
  chemistry, 581(t)
  electrolyte, 581(t)
  for drug monitoring, 575
  for HIV antibody levels, 575
  for metabolic defects, 575
  lipid, 581(t)
  medical assistant's role in, 570
  obstetric, 581(t)
  panel/profile, 581(t), 582
  proficiency testing program for, 596
  rubella, 575
  screening, 574, 583
  specimen collection for. See *Specimen(s).*
  thyroid, 581(t)
  urine, 574. See also *Urinalysis; Urine.*
  venereal, 497, 574
Laceration, patient information on, 871, 876
  treatment of, 871
Laënnec, René, 24(t)
  development of stethoscope by, 20
Lancet, in capillary puncture, 643
Langenbeck retractor, 707, *707*
Language, medical, mythology and, 16
Laryngeal mirror, 705, *705*
Laser, surgery with, 754–755
  assisting with, 754
  equipment for, 754
  history of, 754
  principles of, 754
  safety precautions in, 754
Laundry, in HIV transmission prevention, 436
Lavatory, utilization and care of, 354

STRATEGIES FOR READING THE TEXTBOOK

Reading textbooks in the health care field requires strategies that are different from reading books for pleasure. You can learn techniques to help you to concentrate on, understand, and remember textbook information. These active reading strategies will help you to stay focused on the reading selection.

Strategies that will help you to read your textbooks with increased understanding are

- Previewing
- Questioning
- Checking health care literacy
- Reading graphic aids
- Summarizing
- Checking comprehension
- Using study guides for review

Strategies to Use Before Reading

Previewing

Before reading an assigned textbook chapter, preview the chapter. Follow these five steps:

1. Read the chapter title and ask yourself what you already know about the topic and what you want to learn about the topic.
2. Read the first paragraph and the last paragraph.
3. Read all boldface headings.
4. Pay attention to key words.
5. Look at all graphic aids such as tables, diagrams, pictures, and graphs.

These five preview steps will create a purpose for your reading. Reading with purpose will help you to concentrate as you read the chapter.

Example 5–1

Directions: Preview the following selection from Chabner's *The Language of Medicine* (p. 556). Examine the answers given for questions 1 to 3. Try to answer questions 4 and 5.

GLANDS

Sebaceous Glands

Sebaceous glands are located in the corium layer of the skin and secrete an oily substance called **sebum.** Sebaceous glands are closely associated with hair follicles, and their ducts open into the hair follicle through which the sebum is released. Figure 5–1 shows the relationship of the sebaceous gland to the hair follicle. The sebaceous glands are influenced by sex hormones, which cause them to hypertrophy at puberty and atrophy in old age.

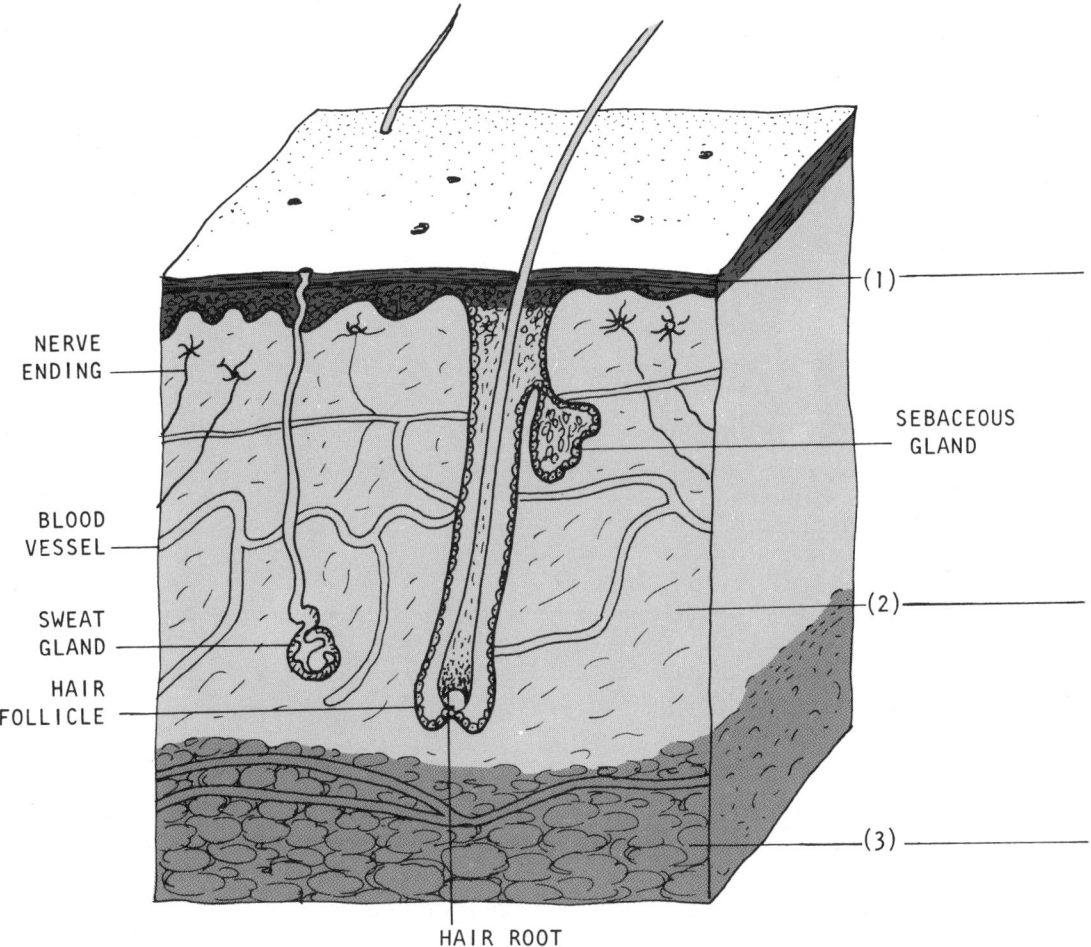

Figure 5–1 The skin. (From Chabner D-E: The Language of Medicine, 4th ed. Philadelphia, W.B. Saunders, 1991, p. 556.)

Sweat Glands

Sweat glands are tiny, coiled glands found on almost all body surfaces (about 2 million in the body). They are most numerous in the palm of the hand (3000 glands per sq in) and on the sole of the foot. Figure 5–1 illustrates how the coiled sweat gland originates deep in the corium and straightens out to extend up through the epidermis. The tiny opening on the surface is called a **pore.**

Sweat, or perspiration, is almost pure water, with dissolved materials such as salt making up less than 1 per cent of the total composition. It is colorless and odorless. The odor produced when sweat accumulates on the skin is due to the action of bacteria on the sweat.

Sweat cools the body as it evaporates into the air. Perspiration is controlled by the sympathetic nervous system, whose nerve fibers are activated by the heart regulatory center in the hypothalamic region of the brain, which stimulates sweating.

A special variety of sweat gland, active only from puberty onward and larger than the ordinary kind, is concentrated in a few areas of the body near the reproductive organs and in the armpits. These glands secrete an odorless sweat, but it contains certain substances that are easily broken down by bacteria on the skin. The breakdown products are responsible for the characteristic human body odor. The milk-producing mammary gland is another type of modified sweat gland; it secretes milk only after the birth of a child.

1. What is the topic of the reading assignment? <u>Glands</u>
2. Write the headings in boldface.

   Glands

   <u>Sebaceous Glands</u>

   <u>Sweat Glands</u>
3. Write the definition of the key word *pore*.

   <u>The tiny opening on the surface</u>
4. Write what you already know about this topic.

   I know about sweat glands
5. Write what you will need to learn about this topic.

   What are other functions of glands?

   How do glands contribute to health?

EXERCISE 5–9

Directions: Preview the following excerpt from a health care textbook (Chabner, pp. 718 and 719). Answer the questions following the selection.

II. RADIOLOGY

A. Characteristics of X-Rays

Several characteristics of x-rays are useful to physicians in the diagnosis and treatment of disease. Some of these characteristics are

1. **Ability to cause exposure of a photographic plate.** If a photographic plate is placed in front of a beam of x-rays, the x-rays, traveling unimpeded through the air, will expose the silver coating of the plate and cause it to blacken.

2. **Ability to penetrate different substances to varying degrees.** X-rays pass through the different types of substances in the human body (air in the lungs, water in blood vessels and lymph, fat around muscles, and metal such as calcium in bones) with varying ease. Air is the least dense substance and exhibits the greatest transmission. Fat is dense, water is next, followed by metal, which is the densest and transmits least. If the x-rays are absorbed (stopped) by the denser body substance (e.g., calcium in bones), they do not reach the photographic plate held behind the patient, and white areas are left in the x-ray film (plate). Figure 5–2 is an example of an x-ray photograph.

   A substance is said to be **radiolucent** if it permits passage of most of the x-rays. Lung tissue (containing air) is an example of a radiolucent substance, and it appears black on an x-ray image. **Radiopaque** substances (bones) are those that absorb most of the x-rays they are exposed to, allowing only a small fraction of the x-rays to reach the x-ray plate. Thus, normally radiopaque, calcium-containing bone appears white on an x-ray image.

3. **Invisibility.** X-rays cannot be detected by sight, sound, or touch. Workers exposed to x-rays must wear a **film badge** to detect and record the amount of radiation to which they have been exposed. The film badge contains a special film that is exposed by x-rays. The amount of blackness on the film is an indication of the amount of x-rays or gamma rays received by the wearer.

4. **Travel in straight lines.** This property allows the formation of precise shadow images on the x-ray plate and also permits x-ray beams to be directed accurately at a tissue site during radiotherapy.

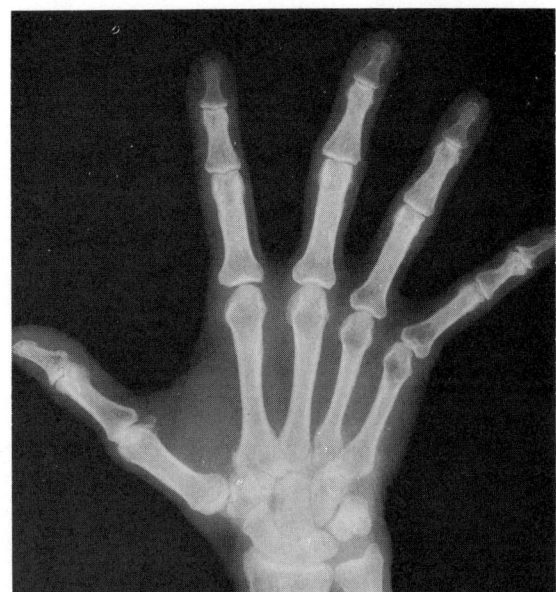

FIGURE 5–2 X-ray photograph (radiograph) of the hand. (From Poznanski AK: The Hand in Radiologic Diagnosis, 2nd ed. Philadelphia, W.B. Saunders, 1984, pp. 1–23.)

   5. **Scattering of radiation.** Scattering occurs when x-rays come in contact with any material. Greater scatter occurs with dense objects and less scatter with those substances that are radiolucent. Scatter can be a serious occupational hazard to those in the vicinity of a source of x-rays, such as an x-ray machine. Also, because scatter can blur images and expose areas of film that otherwise would be in shadow, a grid (containing thin lead strips arranged parallel to the x-ray beams) is placed in front of the film to absorb scattered radiation before it strikes the x-ray film.
   6. **Ionization.** X-rays have the ability to ionize substances through which they pass. Ionization is a chemical process in which the energy of an x-ray beam causes rearrangement and disruption within a substance, so that previously neutral particles are changed to charged particles called **ions**. This strongly ionizing ability of x-rays is a double-edged sword. In x-ray therapy, the ionizing effect of x-rays can help kill cancerous cells and stop tumor growth; however, ionizing x-rays in small doses can affect normal body cells, leading to tissue damage and malignant changes. Thus, persons exposed to high doses of x-ray are at risk of developing leukemia, thyroid tumors, breast cancer, or other malignancies.

   1. What is the topic of the reading assignment? _____
   2. How many characteristics are listed? _____
   3. Write the definition of the key word ions. _____
      _____
   4. Write what you already know about this topic. _____
      _____
   5. Write what you need to learn about this topic. _____
      _____
      _____

Questioning

Try to think about the main ideas that will be covered in the assignment. Ask questions to help you identify these main ideas as you read. Asking questions helps you to read with a purpose. Your goal while reading is to answer your questions. Asking questions will help you to

- Identify the concepts and facts that you still need to learn.
- Think about and evaluate the information you are reading.
- Remember important details.

A good method is to turn boldface headings into questions.

Example 5–2

Directions: Look at the following example of formulating questions from a boldface heading.

Diseases of Red Blood Cells

1. What are the diseases of red blood cells?
2. How are the diseases of red blood cells treated?

Looking for answers to your questions will help you concentrate as you read textbooks.

EXERCISE 5–10

Directions: Read the following heading.

Patient Registration System

Write two questions that you could ask about this heading.

1. _____
2. _____

Strategies to Use While Reading

Asking the 5W Questions

You can use the following 5W questions to help you focus on your textbook assignments. The 5Ws will help you to identify the main ideas and important details as you read. These 5W questions will help you to understand the most important information in the selection. You will not be discouraged by complicated sentence structure and difficult vocabulary if you use the 5W questions to give you the essential information in your reading assignments.

1. Who or what is the assigned reading about? (The answer to this question helps you to identify the topic, or subject, of the reading assignment.)

2. What is the main point being made about the subject? (The answer to this question is the main idea.)

3. When? (The answer to this question helps you to locate the important details.)

4. Where? (The answer to this question helps you to locate the important details.)

5. Why? or How? (The answer to this question helps you to locate the important details.)

At times, not all of the details are given in a selection. Therefore, you may not always find the answers to all of the 5Ws. Use the 5W questions to keep you actively involved as you read.

Read each chapter section by section. Stop at the end of each section to check your comprehension by trying to answer the 5W questions. You might want to write these answers or other notes in the margin of your textbook. Note taking helps you to become an active reader.

Example 5-3

Directions: Read the following excerpt from the Bonewit-West health care textbook *Computer Concepts and Applications for the Medical Office* (p. 101). Review the 5W questions and the answers to these questions.

Time Investment: Because medical management programs perform highly sophisticated tasks, it takes considerable time to learn a program and use it with ease. Most software vendors provide on-site training of staff as well as technical support when problems are encountered. Even with all of this assistance, however, the orientation period can easily last a month or more and the complete conversion process can last as long as 6 months to a year. During this time the medical assistant may experience much frustration when difficulty is encountered in executing a task. However, once the initial training period is completed, most individuals agree the time and patience expended are justified by the outcome.

1. Who or what? *Medical Management Programs*
2. What is the main point being made about the subject? *Takes considerable time to learn the program*
3. When? *1 month to 1 year*
4. Where? *On-site staff training*
5. Why? *Because medical management programs perform highly sophisticated tasks*

EXERCISE 5-11

Directions: Read the following selection from Chabner's textbook (p. 683) and answer the 5W questions.

DNA, located in the nucleus of a cell, controls not only the production of new cells but also the cell's ability to grow by directing the making of new proteins **(protein synthesis)**. When a cell reproduces itself, the DNA material (located within the chromosomes) replicates (copies) itself, so that exactly the same DNA is passed to new cells that are formed. This process is called **mitosis** or **self-replication.**

1. Who or what is the assigned reading about? _____
2. What is the main point being made about the subject? _____
   _____
3. When? _____
4. Where? _____
5. Why or how? _____

Assessing Your Health Care Literacy

Be aware of your literacy level in the health care fields. To be literate in the health care field, you have to have the ability to read the textbooks and write about the information you are learning. You should also be able to apply this information to job related tasks in the health fields.

You may have difficulty with the vocabulary in your textbooks because there are many technical terms to learn. Vocabulary meanings in the health care fields have to be precise. You have to learn technical terms and abbreviations and symbols for these terms to understand the reading material. You cannot simply skip over difficult vocabulary. You should learn new technical words as you come to them when you read your textbooks. When you come across a new technical word in your health care textbooks, apply these strategies:

1. Try to see if the word is defined in context.
2. If you cannot determine the meaning from context clues, use the glossary or index of your textbook.
3. If you cannot find the word meaning within the textbook, use the dictionary of allied health terms or a technical dictionary.
4. When you have found the meanings of the new words, reread the assignment. You will now have a much better understanding of the chapter.

Example 5–4

Read the following excerpt from a health care textbook (Chabner, p. 35). Reread the excerpt after you have learned the meanings of the words in boldface.

Differences in Cells. Cells are different, or specialized, throughout the body to carry out their individual functions. For instance, a **muscle** cell is long and slender and contains fibers that aid it in contracting and relaxing; an **epithelial,** or skin, cell may be square and flat to provide protection; a **nerve** cell may be quite long and have various fibrous extensions that aid in its job of carrying impulses; a **fat** cell contains large empty spaces for fat storage. These are only a few of the many types of cells in the body.

1. *Muscle* cell: long and slender and contains fibers that aid it in contracting and relaxing
2. *Epithelial* cell: skin cell, square and flat to provide protection
3. *Nerve* cell: quite long and has fibrous extensions to help it carry impulses
4. *Fat* cell: contains large empty spaces for fat

Learning the meanings of these terms helps you to understand the main idea of the selection, which is that different cells are specialized to carry out their specific functions.

EXERCISE 5–12

Directions: Read the following excerpt from the Chabner health care textbook (p. 399). Write the meaning of each word in boldface. Reread the excerpt after you have learned the word meanings. Then write the main idea of the selection.

The lungs extend from the collarbone to the **diaphragm** in the thoracic cavity. The diaphragm is a muscular partition that separates the thoracic from the abdominal cavity and aids in the process of breathing. The diaphragm contracts and descends with each **inhalation (inspiration).** The downward movement of the diaphragm enlarges the area in the thoracic cavity and reduces the internal air pressure, so that air flows into the lungs to equalize the pressure. When the lungs are full, the diaphragm relaxes and elevates, making the area in the thoracic cavity smaller, and thus increasing the air pressure in the thorax. Air then is expelled out of the lungs to equalize the pressure; this is called **exhalation (expiration).**

WORD **MEANING**
1. Diaphragm _____
2. Inhalation _____
3. Exhalation _____

MAIN IDEA
4. _____

Reading Graphic Aids

Health care textbooks are filled with graphic aids: pictures, graphs, tables, and diagrams. You should carefully read this material so that you can succeed in your studies.

Graphic materials are designed to be clear so you can use these aids to help you concentrate on and learn new information. The following five strategies allow you to use graphic aids to help you better understand and read your textbooks.

1. Read the title carefully to determine the subject of the graphic aid.
2. Check the vocabulary. Learn the meaning of each word in the headings, labels, and captions so that you will understand the information.
3. Figure out the purpose of the graphic aid. Think about how it relates to the ideas discussed in the chapter. Work back and forth between the picture and

the written text. Determining the relationship between the two will help you to understand the information you need to learn.

4. If the graphic aid has a number or symbol, think about what each item represents.
5. Paraphrase the ideas in the picture into language you understand.

Read graphic aids carefully to help you concentrate on, understand, and remember textbook information.

Example 5–5

Read and study Figure 5–3, a graphic aid from Chabner (p. 398), and the answers that are provided to the questions.

1. What is the subject of the diagram? *Comparison of the diaphragm in inspiration and expiration.*
2. What symbols are being used to illustrate the comparison? *Arrows*
3. Define inspiration. *Breathing in*
4. Define expiration. *Breathing out*
5. When air flows out, is the chest cavity larger or smaller? *Smaller*

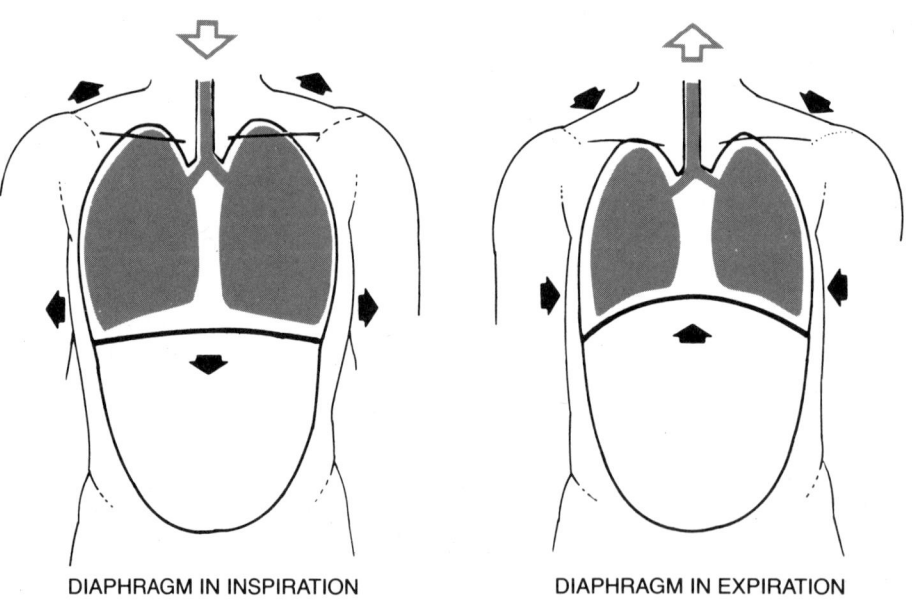

DIAPHRAGM IN INSPIRATION   **DIAPHRAGM IN EXPIRATION**

FIGURE 5–3 Position of the diaphragm during inspiration and expiration. During inspiration air flows in as the chest cavity enlarges. During expiration air flows out as the chest cavity becomes smaller. (From Chabner D-E: The Language of Medicine, 4th ed. Philadelphia, W.B. Saunders, 1991, p. 398.)

EXERCISE 5–13

Directions: Read and study Table 5–1, a graphic aid from the Torres and Ehrlich textbook *Modern Dental Assisting* (p.99). Answer the questions and write your answers in the space provided.

1. What is the title of this table? _____
2. What vitamins are listed in this table? _____
3. Hemorrhages are a deficiency symptom of vitamin _____.
4. What information is summarized in this table? _____
   _____

5. Look for two vocabulary words in Table 5–1 that you need to learn. On page 88 write the words, their definitions, and your source for finding the word meanings.

TABLE 5–1. Fat-Soluble Vitamins

VITAMIN	IMPORTANT FUNCTIONS	BEST SOURCES	DEFICIENCY SYMPTOMS
Vitamin A	Growth Health of the eyes Structure and functioning of the cells of the skin and mucous membranes Promotes health of the oral structures	Fish liver oils Liver Green and yellow vegetables Fruit (yellow) Butter, milk, cream, cheese Egg yolk	Retarded growth Night blindness Increased susceptibility to infections Changes in skin and mucous membranes
Vitamin D	Helps absorb calcium from digestive tract and build calcium and phosphorus into bones and teeth Growth	Vitamin D–irradiated milk Fish liver oil Sunshine on skin	Rickets Poor tooth development
Vitamin E	Protects vitamin A and essential fatty acids from oxidation Aids in the formation of red blood cells, muscles, and other tissues	Wheat germ oil Vegetable oils Green vegetables Milk fat, butter Egg yolk	Undetermined
Vitamin K	Normal clotting of blood Helps maintain normal liver function	Green leafy vegetables Liver Soybean and other vegetable oils Synthesized by intestinal bacteria	Hemorrhages

From Torres HO and Ehrlich A: Modern Dental Assisting, 5th ed. Philadelphia, W.B. Saunders, 1995.

	WORD	DEFINITION	SOURCE
1.	____	_____	_____
2.	____	_____	_____

Summarizing

Check your comprehension by answering the 5W questions. Your answers will give you a summary of each topic. Paraphrase the ideas of the text into language you understand. Make sure that you understand each topic before you go on to the next boldface heading.

Strategies for Reading Difficult Passages

Sometimes, the textbook assignment may seem difficult and you are tempted to give up. Take a short break and then try these strategies to help you interpret complicated reading.

1. Read carefully. Do not skip any information.
2. Work methodically. Much of the information is presented step by step. Follow the order of the selection so that you are not confused.
3. Go over the vocabulary. Make sure that you have learned all the new words.
4. Ask questions. Formulating questions can help you to clarify your thinking.
5. Reread the section, looking for the main idea and the most important details.

Strategies to Use After reading

When you have finished reading the chapter one topic at a time, look at the assignment as a whole.

- Underline the main idea and the important details that you want to remember.
- Write a summary, outline, or map of the main ideas and important details that you can use to review the chapter. This written summary or outline will serve as a study guide.
- Study the important ideas of the chapter. Review underlined text material, summaries, outlines, maps, and notes.
- Answer the review questions at the end of each chapter. Correct your answers.
- Design your own test based on the reading assignments.

Answer the questions on this practice test and correct your answers. Taking practice tests will help you to remember the information so that you will improve your test grades.

EXERCISE 5–14

Directions: Use all the reading strategies you learned in this chapter to concentrate on, understand, and remember textbook information. The questions and directions in this exercise will help you guide your reading of the following selection from a health care textbook (Torres and Ehrlich, p. 114).

PATIENT EDUCATION IN PREVENTIVE DENTISTRY

Patient education is the responsibility of all members of the dental health team as they come into contact with the patient; however, the assistant or hygienist is usually assigned responsibility for providing information, guidance, and motivation.

The major thrusts of patient education in preventive dentistry include

- Presenting a program of personal oral hygiene that the patient will carry out at home on a routine basis
- Counseling to increase the patient's awareness of the role of nutrition in achieving optimum dental and general health
- Creating patient awareness of the need to return regularly for professional prophylaxis, examination, and treatment

In your role as the dental health educator, you must be enthusiastic about helping others learn these skills. You must also be concerned about them as individuals, be sensitive to their needs, and be accepting and tactful in working with them.

A patient education program emphasizes **motivation** and **education.**

Motivation

The dental health team should work to increase the patient's motivational level so he *wants* to learn and apply plaque-control skills. However, ultimately it is the patient who decides what value will be placed on his oral health, and the lower the patient's level of motivation, the less the chance of success for his personal oral hygiene program.

Awareness and Interest

The first step must be to make the patient aware that he has a problem that needs to be solved. Then it is necessary to gain the patient's interest and cooperation in solving the problem.

As an example, the patient may not be aware of how much sugar he is consuming each day. Table 5–2 lists the sugar content of popular foods. (Remember, in addition to the amount of sugar present, the frequency of consuming sugar is also important.)

Education

Once the patient is motivated so that he wants to learn and use these skills, he must learn how to use them correctly. It is here that the dental health educator can best help the patient.

Acceptance

The patient can learn more easily when he feels safe, accepted, and respected. In this setting, encouragement is given freely, and correction is structured in a positive manner. Most important, the patient is never scolded, embarrassed, or teased because of his ignorance or errors.

Action

The least learning occurs when the patient merely sits and listens, as in a lecture. Far more learning occurs when as many of the senses as possible are involved and the patient is actively participating in the process.

TABLE 5–2. Sugar Content of Popular Foods

FOOD	APPROX. MEASURE	TSP. OF SUGAR
Coca Cola	6 oz.	5
Chocolate milk shake	8 oz.	14
Chocolate ice cream soda	Average size	11
Cinnamon bun with raisins	1 average	8
Jelly doughnut	1 average	7
Iced cupcake	1 medium	9
Peach ice cream	1 cup	15
Orange water ice	$\frac{1}{2}$ cup	19
Apple pie	$\frac{1}{6}$ of medium pie	14
Chocolate pudding	$\frac{1}{2}$ cup	9
Raisins	$\frac{5}{8}$ cup	17
Candy bar	Average	8
Fudge, plain	1" square	5
Jelly beans	10	4
Lollipop	1 medium	8

From Torres HO and Ehrlich A: Modern Dental Assisting, 5th ed. Philadelphia, W.B. Saunders, 1995.

Teaching plaque control is an ideal situation for active learner participation. The following are four educational ideas that combine these factors:

- Present the skills to be learned one at a time and as simply as possible. When possible, use visual aids (such as disclosing tablets) to clarify the point.
- Give the patient an opportunity to practice the new skills. For example, provide a toothbrush and guide the patient as he practices the new brushing technique.
- Provide reinforcement and encouragement until the patient has mastered these skills. For example, a disclosing tablet is used again to demonstrate that all of the plaque has been removed.
- Encourage the patient to continue these new actions at home until the desired habit pattern has been formed.

I. Before Reading

   A. Previewing

      1. Read the heading and subheadings to identify the topic. Write the topic in the space provided. _____

      2. Read the first and last paragraphs.

      3. Write the meaning of these key words.

         a. Motivation_____

_____

b. Education _____
_____

4. How many teaspoons of sugar are in 10 jelly beans? _____
5. Think about what you already know about this topic. Write what you still need to know. _____
_____
_____

B. Questioning

6. Based on your preview, formulate questions from the heading of the reading selection. _____
_____
_____

II. While reading

7. Ask the 5W questions. Read the selection with the goal of answering your question. Stop at each boldface heading to check your comprehension.
8. Think about the order of the information. Which did you learn about first, nutritionally sound snacks or snacks to be avoided? _____
9. What is the subject of the table? _____
10. How does this table relate to the written text? _____

A. Summarizing

11. Answer your 5W questions. Remember to check your comprehension as you complete each topic. Paraphrase the author's information in your own words to reinforce your understanding of the information._____
_____
_____
_____
_____

III. After Reading

A. Underline

12. **Underline** the main ideas and important details that you will want to remember.

B. Write
13. **Write** a summary or outline or map the main ideas and important details of the selection.
C. Study
14. **Review** your underlined material and study guides. Design a practice test. Correct your answers.

REVIEWING READING THE TEXTBOOK

TO LEARN	USE THIS STRATEGY
How to identify and locate important information in your textbook	Survey the following features: 1. Title page 2. Preface 3. Table of contents 4. Glossary 5. Bibliography 6. Appendix 7. Index
Previewing	1. Read the title 2. Read the first and last paragraphs 3. Read all boldface headings 4. Pay attention to key words 5. Look at all graphic aids
Questioning	Turn boldface headings into questions
To concentrate while reading	Ask 5W questions
To check health care literacy	Learn technical vocabulary words
To read graphic aids	1. Read the title 2. Check the vocabulary 3. Figure out the purpose of the graphic aid 4. Learn what the numbers or symbols represent 5. Paraphrase the ideas into your own words
To summarize	Answer the 5W questions
How to understand difficult passages	1. Do not skip information 2. Follow the order of the information 3. Learn all new vocabulary words 4. Ask questions 5. Reread the selection
To review the chapter as a whole	Underline, write summary, or map main ideas and important details. Review study guides. Take practice tests.

UNIT II

WRITING STRATEGIES

Many students feel that they need to improve their writing skills. Most students can improve their writing with practice and by learning that writing is a process. Unit II, Writing Strategies, guides students through the steps of the writing process. Chapter 6, Organizing Ideas, will teach you how to use prewriting strategies to develop a plan for writing. Chapter 7, Writing the First Draft, will demonstrate how you put all your ideas on paper by following your writing plan. Chapter 8, Revising the Final Draft, will guide you through the steps of revision, editing, and proofreading. You will also be reminded of some problem areas to avoid in spelling, grammar, capitalization, and punctuation. Following the steps in the writing process will help you to develop an improved final paper.

Chapter 6

Organizing Ideas

LEARNING OBJECTIVES
VOCABULARY WORDS
VOCABULARY CHECK
THE WRITING PROCESS
PREWRITING STRATEGIES
SELECTING A SUBJECT
COLLECTING DETAILS
ORGANIZING YOUR INFORMATION
PLANNING THE MAIN IDEA
DECIDING ON YOUR PURPOSE
ORGANIZING INFORMATION ACCORDING TO PURPOSE
CHOOSING THE FORM
CHOOSING THE AUDIENCE
REVIEWING ORGANIZING IDEAS

LEARNING OBJECTIVES

In this chapter you will learn how to
- Use prewriting strategies
- Develop a plan for writing

VOCABULARY WORDS

The following vocabulary words are important to your understanding of the ideas in this chapter. These vocabulary words are underscored the first time they are used in the chapter. Read the list of words and definitions. Then check your understanding of these words before you read the chapter.

abuse harmful treatment.
audience the people who will read your writing.
brainstorming spontaneously formulating ideas.

E-mail or electronic mail a message sent on a computer.
form the medium for the written message.
narrating telling a story.
prewriting plan for writing.
process the several steps involved in doing something.
purpose why the author is writing.
subject the topic.

VOCABULARY CHECK

Directions: Choose the vocabulary word that best fits into the sentence.

1. Tony learned to use _____ strategies to develop a writing plan.
2. You cannot do everything at once; each step is part of a total _____.
3. Mrs. Jonas decided to use the _____ of a manual when she wrote the directions for the use of the new computer program.
4. Have you established your _____ for writing this outline?
5. As the storyteller was _____ the tale, everyone listened intently.
6. Thelma received your message on _____ before she received the letter.
7. The topic, or _____, of your report is a crucial issue today.
8. The _____ listened to the speaker's report and then criticized the information.
9. Veronica finds _____ helpful as she collects information about her topic.
10. Verbal _____ can be damaging to a child's self esteem.

THE WRITING PROCESS

Many students find it difficult to start a writing assignment. They are overwhelmed by the task of writing because they try to do the planning, drafting, revising, editing, and proofreading in just one step.

Writing is a process of many steps. These steps include the following:

- **Step 1: Prewriting**
  You select a subject, collect details about the subject, and develop your writing plan.
- **Step 2: Writing the First Draft**
  You organize your ideas into sentences and paragraphs.
- **Step 3: Revising**
  You make the changes necessary to improve your writing.
- **Step 4: Editing and Proofreading**
  You examine your writing for any specific errors in spelling, punctuation, gram-

mar, or style. Check your paper carefully and correct any errors before you hand in your final draft.

If you learn the strategies involved in each of these steps in the writing process, you will be more successful in completing your writing assignments.

PREWRITING STRATEGIES

<u>Prewriting</u> strategies help you to develop a plan for writing. This plan will be your guide when you are ready to write your first draft. Your writing plan should include the following:

1. The <u>Subject</u>: The subject answers the question **who?** or **what?** The subject is the topic you will write about.
2. The <u>Purpose</u>: The purpose answers the question **why?** Why are you writing? Are you writing to **explain**, to **describe**, to **persuade**, or to **narrate?**
3. <u>Form</u>: Form answers the question **what?** What are you writing? Form is the medium through which you express your ideas.
4. <u>Audience</u>: The people who read your writing make up the audience. Think about your readers. You should always direct your information to a specific audience for clear, direct writing.

If you begin all your writing assignments by following this plan, you will be getting off to a good start.

Example 6–1

One student's writing plan:

Subject: Child <u>abuse</u>

Purpose: To persuade your readers of the danger of child abuse

Form: Report

Audience: Nursing Assistants

EXERCISE 6–1

Directions: Develop your own writing plan. Fill in the following information:

Subject: _____

Purpose: _____

Form: _____

Audience: _____

SELECTING A SUBJECT

Think about who or what you want to write about. Then list words or ideas that relate to your subject. This step is called <u>brainstorming</u>. It means that you are thinking of everything you know about your chosen subject so that you can collect information about this topic.

COLLECTING DETAILS

An effective strategy for collecting details about your subject is to ask and answer the 5W questions.

Example 6–2

Ask and answer the 5W questions:

1. **Who or what?** Child abuse.
2. **What is the main point being made about the subject?** Child abuse is a major cause of child injury and death.
3. **When?** Currently on the increase.
4. **Where?** The United States.
5. **Why or how?** Abusive parents and failure of health professionals to report previous, less serious injuries.

EXERCISE 6–2

Directions: Collect details about your subject by asking and answering the 5W questions.

Who or what? _____

What is the main point being made about the subject? _____
_____

When? _____
Where? _____
Why or how? _____

ORGANIZING YOUR INFORMATION

Once you have answered the 5W questions, you are ready to organize your information. You can organize the details around your subject by

- **Mapping**
- **Listing**
- **Writing a topic outline**

Example 6-3

Different ways a student could organize details around a subject:

1. **Mapping:** Map your ideas. Begin to map your ideas with your subject in the middle. Add the details that relate to your subject.

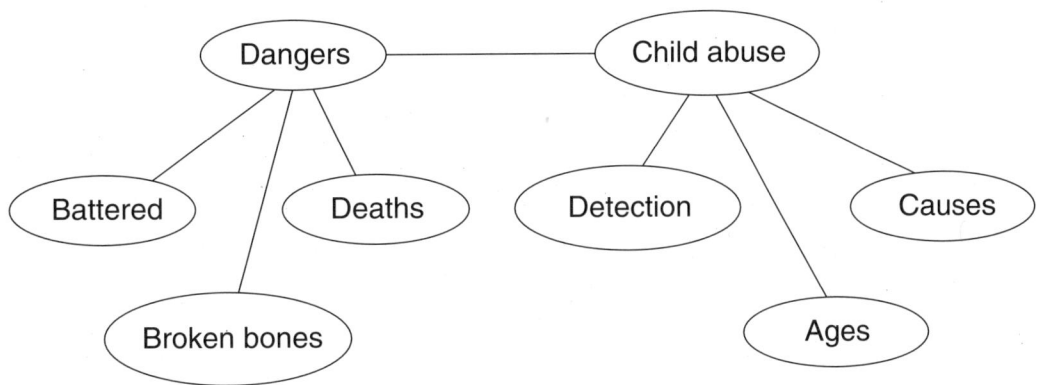

2. **Listing:** Child abuse is a major cause of injury and death to children.
   - Burns
   - Bruises
   - Broken bones
   - Sexual abuse
   - Death
   - Prevention
3. **Writing a topic outline:** Dangers to children caused by child abuse.
   a. Major physical injuries
      (1) Burns
      (2) Bruises
      (3) Broken bones
   b. Lasting emotional trauma
      (1) Sexual abuse
      (2) Emotional abuse
   c. High death rates
   d. How to prevent abuse
      (1) Early detection
      (2) Immediate reporting

EXERCISE 6-3

Directions: Review your collection of details that you gathered by asking and answering the 5W questions. Decide which method of organizing details around your subject will work the best for you. Organize your details by mapping, listing, or writing a topic outline.

PLANNING THE MAIN IDEA

Enlarge your subject into a main idea by answering the first 2 of the 5W questions:

- **Who** or **what** are you writing about? = **Subject**
- **What** do you want to say about the subject? = **Main Idea**

Example 6-4

- **Who** or **what?** = Child abuse
- **What** is being said about child abuse? = Child abuse is a major cause of children's injury and death in the United States.

EXERCISE 6-4

Directions: Fill in the following information so that you can formulate the main idea of your writing:

- **Who** or **what?** _____
- **What** are you saying about the subject? _____

DECIDING ON YOUR PURPOSE

Why are you writing? Your purpose should be related to your main idea. For example, if a writer wants to convey to readers that child abuse is a major cause of children's injury and death, the purpose would be to **persuade** the readers of all the dangers of child abuse. The facts collected would be included to sway the reader toward the writer's point of view. The facts and examples that are given are collected to persuade your readers to agree with your opinion.

Example 6–5

The details collected are to **persuade** the reader that child abuse is dangerous.

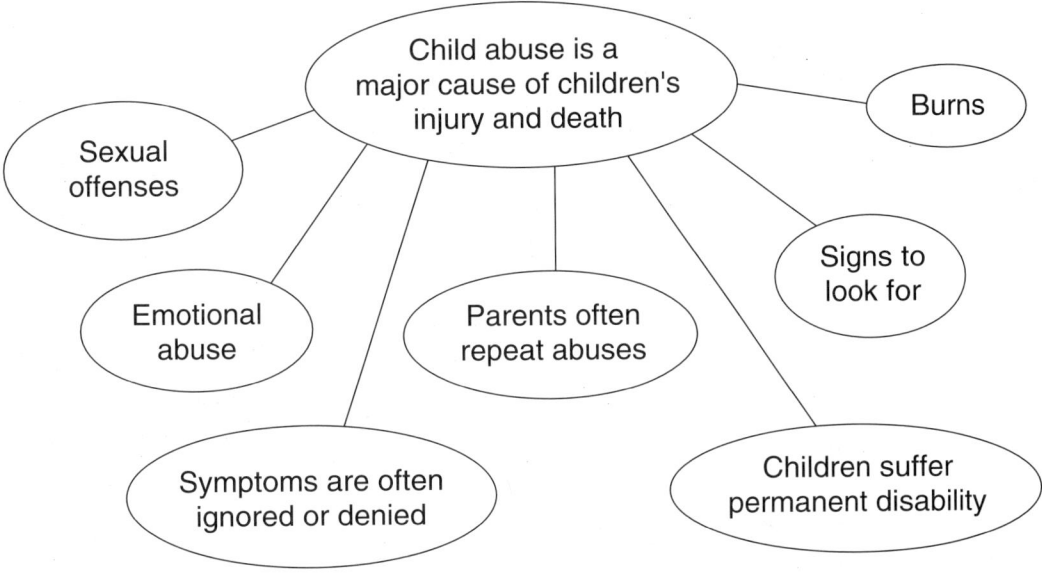

EXERCISE 6–5

Directions: Choose your purpose. Why are you writing? Fill in your map, list, or outline so that the details you collect will reflect your purpose.

ORGANIZING INFORMATION ACCORDING TO PURPOSE

Your organization should be related to your purpose in writing. Choose a plan of organization that will fulfill your purpose. Some types of organization plans are:

- **Describing:** You give many details. You might be describing people, places, or objects.
- **Explaining:** You are explaining "how to" or "giving causes" or "definitions." When you are explaining, the facts you choose give information about the object or process you are writing about.
- **Persuading:** You are persuading when you are trying to convince someone that he or she should agree with your opinion. You might be persuading when you are writing about reasons for following procedures or for changing existing conditions. When you are persuading, you collect details to back up your opinion.
- <u>Narrating</u>: You are narrating when you are giving details about an experience you want to share. You might narrate an encounter with a patient or an employer. When you are narrating, sequence is important.

TABLE 6-1 Some Sample Forms for Writing

Descriptions	Requests
Directions	Case studies
Letters	E-mail
Memos	Lab reports
Pamphlets	Observation reports
Brochures	Patient histories or profiles
Captions for pictures	Summaries
Charts	Add other forms _____
Proposals	_____
Reports	_____

CHOOSING THE FORM

Once you have chosen your main idea, purpose, and organization plan, think about the most effective form to use to communicate your ideas. Look over Table 6–1 and choose the form that would best convey your message.

EXERCISE 6-6

Directions: Choose the form that would communicate your main idea most effectively. _____

Write why you have chosen this form. _____

CHOOSING THE AUDIENCE

Who will read your writing? Will your reader be your instructor, your employer, a coworker, a classmate, or yourself? Your writing will be improved if you direct your message toward a specific audience. Think about your audience when you are organizing your information.

EXERCISE 6-7

Directions: List your audience. Why did you choose this audience? _____

Now it is your turn to be the audience. When you read the following selections, try to uncover the writer's plan. You can then try to model your writing around those plans that you can identify.

Example 6-7

Read the following selection from *EMT Prehospital Care* by Henry and Stapleton (p. 365) and the answers given for the writer's plan.

> Liver disease may be accompanied by jaundiced (yellow) skin or mucous membranes. The earliest jaundice tends to appear at the sclera (the white portion of the eyes) or mucous membranes. Jaundice is caused by a buildup of bilirubin in the blood. Bilirubin is a breakdown product of red blood cells that is processed and excreted by the liver into the small intestines. Extensive liver damage or blockage of the normal excretion (along the pathway of bile ducts) can contribute to jaundice. (Excessive breakdown of red blood cells can also cause jaundice.) Other signs and symptoms of liver failure may include vomiting, lethargy, and anorexia. End stages of liver failure can result in hepatic coma due to a buildup of toxins in the blood, which alters brain function.

Subject: *Signs of liver failure.*
Main Idea: *There are several signs of liver failure.*
Purpose: *Describing.*
Form: *Description and caption under picture.*
Audience: *You.*

EXERCISE 6-8

Directions: Read the following selections and fill in the blanks to identify the writer's plan.

CASE HISTORY

EMTs responded to a call about an "unconscious" patient in an apartment building. On arrival, they discovered an unresponsive 55-year-old man who was found by his neighbor, with a large scalp laceration and a pool of blood surrounding him on the floor. The laceration was not actively bleeding. The man was unresponsive to verbal and painful stimuli, had a blood pressure of 80/60, respirations of 12, a pulse of 80, and a smell of alcohol on his breath. The skin was pale, cool, and dry. A diagnosis of hypovolemic shock was made and PASG were applied, resulting in an improvement in blood pressure to 100/80, with no change in pulse or mental status.

Further assessment and treatment in the hospital confirmed the diagnosis of hypovolemic shock from a scalp laceration and revealed a core body temperature of 31°C. The EMTs noted that the apartment in which the patient was found was of normal temperature. Blood analysis showed that the patient had a significant blood alcohol level. [Henry and Stapleton, p. 494]

Subject: _____

Main Idea: _____
_____

Purpose: _____

Form: _____

Audience: _____

PRINTER PAPER

The type of paper used with a printer is classified as either continuous paper or cut sheets. *Continuous paper* (also called "computer paper") consists of a continuous length of sheets joined with perforations and folded in a zig-zag fashion. Columns of small sprocket holes on its outer edges serve to automatically feed the paper through the printer, thus avoiding the time consuming hand-feeding of individual sheets of paper into the printer. Continuous paper is available in a number of formats: blank sheets, professional letterhead, envelopes, mailing labels, index cards and preprinted forms such as patient statements and insurance claim forms. Continuous preprinted forms are also available in multiple-parts, consisting of an original and one or more copies. This is useful when more than one person needs a copy of the same document (e.g., insurance claims).

After feeding through the printer, continuous paper must be separated at its perforated margins to remove the sprocket holes. Removing the margins of standard continuous paper leaves the edges slightly ragged. A more expensive paper with smaller perforations resulting in much cleaner edges is available and is suitable for professional correspondence.

Cut-sheet paper refers to single sheets of paper as commonly used with a typewriter. This type of paper is also available in a number of formats such as letterhead, bond paper, preprinted forms, envelopes, and so on. [Bonewit-West, pp. 34-35]

Subject: _____

Main Idea: _____

_____

Purpose: _____

Form: _____

Audience: _____

WHEN TO START CPR

CPR performance includes built-in assessment and treatment steps to be used for every apparently unresponsive patient. If breathing is absent or ineffective, rescue breathing should be administered. If the pulse is absent, cardiac compressions should be initiated. As a rescuer you should not concern yourself with the question of "biologic death." If an infant or child has been in cardiac arrest for a prolonged period, you should start CPR and allow hospital personnel to determine whether irreversible brain death has occurred. [Henry and Stapleton, p. 253]

Subject: _____

Main Idea: _____

_____

Purpose: _____

Form: _____

Audience: _____

REVIEWING ORGANIZING IDEAS

TO LEARN	USE THIS STRATEGY
To develop a plan for writing	Use prewriting strategies
To select a subject	Ask yourself who or what you want to write about
To collect details about the subject	Ask the 5W questions
To organize the details	Map, list, or outline your information
To plan the main idea	Ask yourself what you want to say about the subject
To decide on the purpose	Ask yourself why you are writing
To choose an organization plan	Decide whether you want to describe, explain, persuade, or narrate
To select the form	Choose the medium for your writing
To choose the audience	Decide who will read your writing. Direct your writing toward those readers

To construct a writing plan	Outline your
	    Subject
	    Main Idea
	    Purpose
	    Form
	    Audience

Chapter 7

Writing the First Draft

LEARNING OBJECTIVES
VOCABULARY WORDS
VOCABULARY CHECK
INTRODUCTION
GETTING STARTED
GETTING THE MAIN IDEAS ON PAPER
ORGANIZING YOUR THINKING
INCLUDING ALL THE PARTS
FINISHING THE FIRST DRAFT
REVIEWING WRITING THE FIRST DRAFT

LEARNING OBJECTIVES

In this chapter you will learn how to
- Write the first draft

VOCABULARY WORDS

These vocabulary words are important to your understanding the ideas in this chapter. These vocabulary words are underscored the first time they are used in the chapter. Read the list of words and definitions. Then check your understanding of these words before you read the chapter.

confidence self-assurance.
detect to see.
draft a rough version of written work.
emphasis stresses the importance of something.
endangered subject to being destroyed.

expanded expressed in greater detail.
product the end result of the creative effort of writing.
revision rewriting.
sequence the order of events.
slanted biased.

VOCABULARY CHECK

Directions: Choose the vocabulary word that best fits into the sentence.

1. This work is the _____ of many years effort.
2. My first _____ needed to be changed.
3. Diane has the _____ as well as the ability needed to accept the leading role in the play.
4. Margaret's _____ of her first paper was well organized.
5. Barry _____ his ideas so that we could understand his message.
6. Environmentalists want to protect _____ species.
7. That article is _____ towards the writer's point of view.
8. The _____ of the story is easy to follow.
9. It's easy for Raymond to _____ the problem, but does he know how to solve it?
10. The _____ on the cost of health care outweighs other issues.

INTRODUCTION

Writing the first draft is when you, the writer, put all your ideas on paper. Remember, your first draft is not your finished product. Once you learn that writing is a process and that your first draft is not the end product, you will not have to worry about making the first draft perfect. This realization should take away your feelings of anxiety when you have a writing assignment. Remember that the writing process breaks the task of writing into manageable steps.

GETTING STARTED

Sometimes, students find it difficult to get started on the first draft. Begin your first draft while all the ideas are fresh in your mind and you can get all these thoughts on paper. Start your first draft when you have realistically set up enough time to finish. It's best to work on your first draft uninterrupted. Don't attempt to initiate this step of the writing process if you know that in five or ten minutes you'll have to leave for a class or your job. Don't stop your work to answer phone calls or watch television. Find a place to work where you can write freely, away from distractions and interruptions. Realizing that you are not expected to write a perfect first draft should give you the confidence to get started.

Look over your writing plan. You've selected your **subject, purpose, form** and **audience.** Expand this plan by developing your main ideas into sentences and paragraphs. Write freely. Remember, you'll have time to make your changes in the next step in the writing process, revision.

Example 7-1

Look at how one student expanded a writing plan into a first draft.

WRITING PLAN

Subject: Child abuse

Purpose: To persuade reader of the danger of child abuse

Form: Report

Audience: Nursing assistants

Child abuse is a danger to children that results in harmful injury and even death. As nursing assistants, we have to be aware of the symptoms of child abuse. When we examine children who are repeatedly bruised, or accident prone, we should be suspicious. Neglecting to report cases when children are repeatedly being treated for broken bones could lead to greater injury. Child abuse affects children of all ages and crosses all economic groups. If we do not act on our suspicions because we want to protect the parents, the children will be endangered.

EXERCISE 7-1

Directions: As you read this first draft, think about the writing plan. Did the student stick to the writing plan? Yes ___ No ___. If you think changes were made, list the changes:

_____
_____
_____
_____

The student referred back to the collection of details in the map, list, or topic outline developed in the prewriting strategies in Chapter 6. This collection of details helps a writer turn the writing plan into a first draft.

EXERCISE 7-2

Directions: Look at the writing plan you developed in Chapter 6. Check the method you used to collect your details. Did you write:

- A map? _____
- A list? _____
- A topic outline? _____

EXERCISE 7-3

Directions: Use your writing plan and your map, list, or topic outline as your guide to write your first draft. Write freely. Get all your ideas on paper. Remember that you will have time to make changes during the next step in the writing process.

GETTING THE MAIN IDEAS ON PAPER

Did you write all your main ideas on your subject? Did you include all of the details that you collected? Did you choose to eliminate information or did you just forget to include it? Look back to your first step in the writing process. Reread your writing plan and your collection of details. Check your first draft against your prewriting strategies. See if there is anything you need to add to your first draft.

Example 7-2

Examine the student's first draft on the subject of child abuse. This student used the writing plan and map developed in Chapter 6 as a guide to write the first draft.

When the student checked the first draft against the writing plan it was evident that the subject, purpose, and audience followed the plan. However, the tone, or mood, of the draft did not seem appropriate for the chosen form, a report. It seemed that a report should be more detailed.

110 WRITING STRATEGIES

EXERCISE 7-4

Directions: Look again at the map of the student's collection of details from Chapter 6:

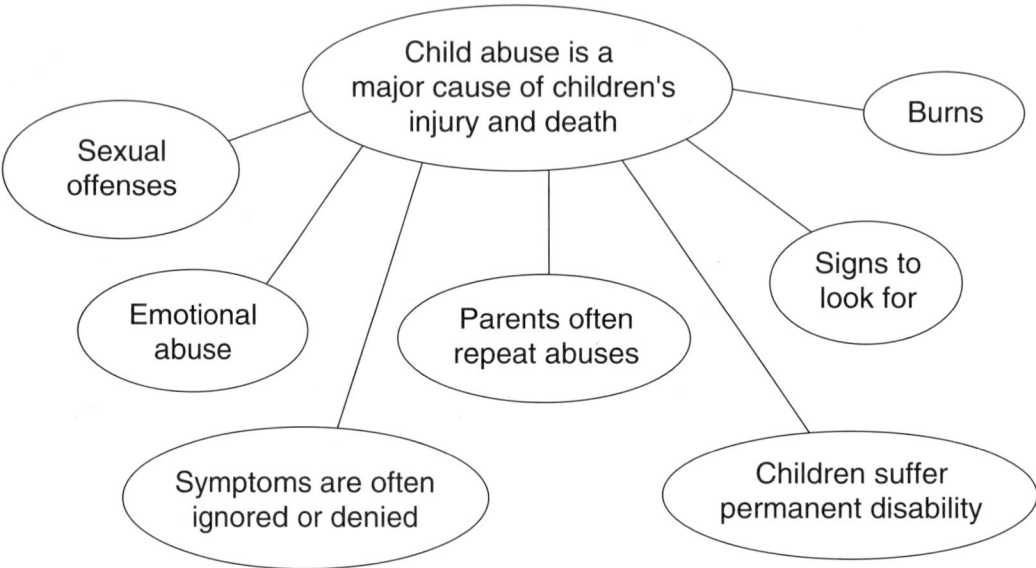

Were all of the details included? Yes ___ No ___. Are more specific details needed for a report? Yes ___ No ___.

The student will have to make these decisions before revising this draft and handing in the final copy.

EXERCISE 7-5

Directions: Check your first draft against your writing plan and collection of details that you used as your guide. Did you follow your plan? Yes ___ No ___. Did you change any of the following?

Subject _____

Purpose _____

Form _____

Audience _____

Did you include all of the information from your collection of details?

Yes ____ No ____.

Did you choose to change any information? Yes ____ No ____.

Did you forget to include any information? Yes ____ No ____.

Using your writing plan as a guide helps you to organize your information when you write your first draft.

ORGANIZING YOUR THINKING

While you are writing a first draft, it is helpful to try to organize your thinking. Think again about your purpose for writing. Do you want to **describe, explain, persuade,** or **narrate.**

Try to write freely while you organize your information according to purpose. When you are **describing,** use adjectives which arouse the senses. Will a reader be able to see, hear, feel, taste or smell when reading your writing? When you choose to **explain** something, you can give reasons and results. Hopefully, your readers will be able to detect a cause-effect relationship. If you compare or contrast things in your explanation, are you telling what something is like by letting the reader know how it is the same as or different from something else? You might choose to explain information by breaking it down into parts or by letting the reader know how something works. When you are writing to **persuade,** your purpose is to convince. Do you **slant** your writing. Slanted writing is writing that is deliberately chosen to sway a reader's opinion. Strong words are used to direct the reader to agree with the writer's opinion. When you are writing to **narrate,** you are telling a story. You might be telling about an experience you had or about an event that influenced you. When you are narrating a story, pay close attention to your sequence of events because logical order is important if a reader is to follow and understand your writing.

Example 7-3

The student who was writing about child abuse chose **persuasion** as a purpose. If you look at the draft, you can find the words that are slanted to convince the reader that child abuse is dangerous. Examine the slanted words which have been italicized in this student's first draft.

Child abuse is a *danger* to children that results in *harmful injury* and even *death*. As nursing assistants, we have to be aware of the symptoms of child abuse. When we examine children who are repeatedly *bruised*, or accident prone, we should be *suspicious*. *Neglecting* to report cases when children are repeatedly being treated for *broken bones* could lead to *greater injury*. Child abuse affects children of all ages and crosses all economic groups. If we do not act on our suspicions because we want to protect the parents, the children will be *endangered*.

EXERCISE 7-6

Directions: Look at your first draft. Check how you organized your information:
- **Describing** _____
- **Explaining** _____
- **Persuading** _____
- **Narrating** _____

EXERCISE 7-7

Directions: Read your first draft again. Circle any words that are examples of slanted writing. Explain why you chose these words to support your purpose in writing.

INCLUDING ALL THE PARTS

When you write your first draft, try to include all the necessary parts. Your writing should include a **beginning, middle,** and **ending.** Each part serves a purpose in your writing. Although you will be checking for these parts in your revision, it is helpful to think of them before you write your ideas.

The **beginning** should get your reader's attention and introduce your subject. The **middle** should support, explain, or describe your subject. The **ending** should summarize your main point and keep your reader thinking about your subject.

Example 7-4

Let's look for a **beginning, middle,** and **ending** in the student's first draft on the subject of child abuse.

Child abuse is a danger to children that results in harmful injury and even death. As nursing assistants, we have to be aware of the symptoms of child abuse. When we examine children who are repeatedly bruised, or accident prone, we should be suspicious. Neglecting to report cases when children are repeatedly being treated for broken bones could lead to greater injury. Child abuse affects children of all ages and crosses all economic groups. If we do not act on our suspicions because we want to protect the parents, the children will be endangered.

The subject and the main idea about the subject ⟶ Child abuse is harmful
is introduced in the first sentence.

Sentences 2, 3 and 4 provide the details which ⟶ Symptoms
support the main idea.
    Bruised
    Accident
    Suspicious
    Broken bones
    Injury
    All ages and economic groups

The last sentence gives <u>emphasis</u> to the importance → Children endangered
of the main idea.

EXERCISE 7–8

Directions: Reread your first draft. Check to see if you have a **beginning, middle,** and **ending.** Underline the beginning and ending. Circle all the details in the middle that support the main idea.

FINISHING THE FIRST DRAFT

Your first draft isn't going to be perfect. Once you have all your main ideas on paper and have thought about the organization of your ideas, you are ready to revise your work. Check for your main ideas and details by looking for the 5Ws in your writing:

- **Who or what?**
- **What is the main point being made about the subject?**
- **When?**
- **Where?**
- **Why or how?**

If you have all the information you need, put your first draft down and take a break before you come back to take the next step in your writing—**revision.**

REVIEWING WRITING THE FIRST DRAFT

TO LEARN	USE THIS STRATEGY
To get started	Follow your writing plan and collection of details
To get your main ideas on paper	Check your writing plan and collection of details
To organize your thinking	Organize your writing according to your purpose: describe, explain, persuade or narrate
To include all the parts	Think about a beginning, middle, and ending as you write
To finish the first draft	Check that you have included all your main ideas by asking and answering the 5W questions

Chapter 8

Rewriting the Final Draft

LEARNING OBJECTIVES
VOCABULARY WORDS
VOCABULARY CHECK
INTRODUCTION
FOLLOWING A PLAN FOR REVISING
USING A REVISING CHECKLIST
USING A COMPUTER TO HELP WITH REVISING
FOLLOWING A PLAN FOR EDITING AND PROOFREADING
USING A CHECKLIST FOR EDITING AND PROOFREADING
LEARNING SOME BASIC SYMBOLS FOR PROOFREADING
PREPARING THE PRESENTATION
AVOIDING TROUBLE SPOTS IN WRITING
   Spelling
      Some Common Spelling Rules
      Commonly Misspelled Words
   Sentence Errors
   Parts of Speech
   Agreement
      Pronouns
      Subjects and Verbs
   Capitalization
   Punctuation
REVIEWING REWRITING THE FINAL DRAFT

LEARNING OBJECTIVES

In this chapter you will learn how to
- Follow a revising plan
- Use a computer to make revising easier
- Follow a plan for editing and proofreading
- Avoid trouble spots in your writing

VOCABULARY WORDS

These vocabulary words are important to your understanding the ideas in this chapter. These vocabulary words are underscored the first time they are used in the chapter. Read the list of words and definitions. Then check your understanding of these words before you read the chapter.

battered bruised.
choppy short sentence.
delete remove.
focused directed.
imperative essential.
mechanics punctuation, sentence style, word choice, capitalization, grammar.
presentation the appearance.
resistant tending to oppose.
tedious boring.
welts a lump on the body caused by a heavy blow.

VOCABULARY CHECK

Directions: Choose the vocabulary word that best fits into the sentence.

1. Marcy _____ her attention on her work.
2. Lewis was asked to _____ the unnecessary information from the proposal.
3. The _____ of Susie's writing had so many errors that it interfered with her message.
4. It is _____ that you finish your assignment before you take the test.
5. Don't be _____ to good advice.
6. Richard's story was so _____ we all stopped listening.
7. The _____ sentences in Maria's paper prevented a smooth reading.
8. The sloppy _____ of your paper will detract from the effort you put into the content.
9. The _____ child was taken to the hospital for treatment.
10. The _____ on the baby's back were not caused by a fall.

INTRODUCTION

After you have developed your writing plan and completed your first draft you are ready for the next step in the writing process. Remember, your first draft is not your final draft. You have to go through the steps of revising, editing, and proofreading before you have a final version of your paper.

Revising is the changes you make to improve your first draft. You will want to look at the main ideas and make some additions or cut some unnecessary details. You might want to change the order of your information. It helps to follow a plan when you are revising. Otherwise, you might not make all the needed improvements to your final draft.

FOLLOWING A PLAN FOR REVISING

You should follow this plan when you are revising your writing:

- Read the first draft several times.
- Think about the changes needed to improve your first draft. For example, ask yourself if you've included all the important ideas. Are any important details missing? Check to see if these ideas are clear, complete, and in the right order.
- Try to improve your writing by evaluating your own work. Look for the parts you want to keep. Look for the parts that need to be changed. You can use a revising checklist to help you evaluate your work and decide what changes need to be made to improve your first draft.

USING A REVISING CHECKLIST

The following checklist should help you to decide what to change as you revise your first draft. Ask yourself:

DID I	**YES**	**NO**
follow my writing plan?	____	____
clearly express my main idea?	____	____
support the main idea with enough details?	____	____
organize the details according to my purpose?	____	____
write a clear beginning, middle, and ending?	____	____
write the ideas in the correct order?	____	____
include unnecessary details?	____	____
repeat ideas?	____	____
fulfill my purpose in writing?	____	____

Answering the questions on the revising checklist will help you to examine the strengths and weaknesses of the first draft. You will now decide how to change your first draft to make it better.

Example 8–1

Let's take another look at the student's first draft on the subject of child abuse:

Child abuse is a danger to children that results in harmful injury and even death. As nursing assistants, we have to be aware of the symptoms of child abuse. When we examine children who are repeatedly bruised, or accident prone, we should be suspicious. Neglecting to report cases when children are repeatedly being treated for broken bones could lead to greater injury. Child abuse affects children of all ages and crosses all economic groups. If we do not act on our suspicions because we want to protect the parents, the children will be endangered.

This is how the student answered the question on the revising checklist:

DID I	YES	NO
follow my writing plan?	Yes, except more specific details are needed to fit the form of a report	
clearly express my main idea?		No, main point should be more directly stated.
support the main idea with enough details?		No, more specific details were needed to make the report complete.
organize the details according to my purpose?	Yes, reasons were given to support conclusion.	
write a clear beginning, middle, and ending?		No, middle needs to be more specific. Ending could be stronger.
write the ideas in the correct order?	Yes	
include unnecessary details?		No
repeat ideas?		No
fulfill my purpose in writing		No, conclusion has to be rewritten to fulfill purpose.

Example 8–2

The following is an example of the first revision:

Child abuse is a danger to children that may result in harmful injury and even death. As nursing assistants, we have to be aware of the symptoms of child abuse. When we examine children who are repeatedly bruised, or accident prone, we should be suspicious. Neglecting to report cases when children are repeatedly being treated for broken bones could lead to greater injury. Two weeks ago, a nine year old child was admitted to the hospital with a broken arm. Upon examination, several older bruises were discovered. This case is now being investigated by social service. This week, an infant was brought in with a head injury. The mother reported that the infant had fallen out of her highchair. However, this same mother brought in a toddler the week before with an arm pulled out of the socket. This toddler also had deep <u>welts</u> across the back and shoulders. The parent claimed not to know how the child got these welts. This case is also being looked into.

Child abuse affects children of all ages and crosses all economic groups.

If you have even the slightest evidence that a child is being abused, report the case to social service. If we do not act on our suspicions because we want to protect the parents, the children will be endangered.

EXERCISE 8–1

Directions: Reread your first draft. Read the revising check list. Answer the questions. Make the needed changes to your first draft.

After you have revised your first draft, look at your revision and make sure that you have made all the needed changes. Is there anything else that you would like to add or <u>delete</u>? Is your subject <u>focused</u>? Does your conclusion sum up the information? Are all the important details included? Take another look at your writing. You may have to make more changes. Sometimes several revisions are needed before a writer is satisfied. Remember not to worry about spelling and <u>mechanics</u> during the revising stage. When you are revising, you are concentrating on the organization of your main ideas and important details.

Example 8–3

Read the student's second revision of the report on child abuse.

Child abuse is a danger to children that may result in harmful injury and even death. As nursing assistants, we have to be aware of the symptoms of child abuse. When we examine children who are repeatedly bruised, or accident prone, we should be suspicious. Neglecting to report cases when children are repeatedly being treated for broken bones could lead to greater injury. Two weeks ago, a nine year old child was admitted to the hospital with a broken arm. Upon examination, several older bruises were discovered. This case is now being investigated by social service. This week, an infant was brought in with a head injury. The mother reported that the infant had fallen out of her highchair. However, this same mother brought in a toddler the week before with an arm pulled out of the socket. This toddler also had deep welts across the back and shoulders. The parent claimed not to know how the child got these welts. Both children had been <u>battered</u>. This case is also being looked into.

Child abuse affects children of all ages and crosses all economic groups. In the last month, two of the seven reported cases of child abuse were from upper middle class homes with both parents.

If you have even the slightest evidence that a child is being abused, report the case to social service. If we do not act on our suspicions because we want to protect the parents, the children will be endangered. Therefore, it is <u>imperative</u> that you report all cases of suspected child abuse to the social service agency.

EXERCISE 8–2

Directions: Read the second revision. Underline any additions you notice. Did the student make any other changes? Yes ____ No ____ Look at the revision checklist again. Did the student make all the needed changes? Yes ___ No ___ Explain your answer.

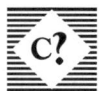

EXERCISE 8–3

Directions: Read your revision. Do you need to make any further changes? If so, revise your paper again. Make all the changes that you think are needed before you go on to the next step in the revision process, editing and proofreading.

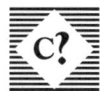

It may take several revisions before you make all the changes that you think are needed to improve your writing. Students are often <u>resistant</u> to revising their papers. Many students make the mistake of trying to avoid the revising step in the writing process. They hand in their first draft as their final draft, and then they are disappointed when their papers receive poor grades.

Students are reluctant to revise papers for many reasons. They mistakenly think that good papers can be written in one step, or they do not want to put in the time needed to make the necessary improvements.

Many students have found that a computer helps them go through the steps of revising. If you don't own a computer, find out if your school and library have computers you can use.

USING A COMPUTER TO HELP WITH REVISING

Many students use the computer from the first step in the writing process—planning—until they hand in their final draft. Other students prefer to do their planning and first drafts on paper and then type their work on the computer to do the revising and editing that is needed before turning in the final draft.

Word processing programs help you use the computer to add ideas and move sentences and even whole pages around. Using a word processor makes revising less <u>tedious</u>. Writing becomes less of a chore and more exciting. Students actually enjoy moving their ideas around. It's fun to see the changes as they appear on the computer screen. Editing is also easier with the computer. Computer programs have spell checks that scan for spelling errors and grammar checks that point out mechanical problems with sentences.

Using a computer will make it much easier for you to make the changes needed to improve your writing.

FOLLOWING A PLAN FOR EDITING AND PROOFREADING

When you have finished revising the ideas in your paper, you are ready for another step in the writing process, editing and proofreading. During editing and proofreading, you make your final changes. You carefully check your writing for errors in spelling and mechanics. You should follow this plan for editing and proofreading your writing: Check

- sentences to determine whether they are smooth or choppy.
- for errors in spelling, punctuation, and grammar.
- your choice of words.
- the presentation of your finished copy.
- your paper one last time to make sure that you have corrected any mistakes.

USING A CHECKLIST FOR EDITING AND PROOFREADING

The following checklist should help you to edit and proofread your writing. Ask yourself:

DID I	**YES**	**NO**
write clear and complete sentences?	___	___
use sentence variety?	___	___
write sentences of different lengths?	___	___
capitalize and punctuate correctly?	___	___
choose vivid, specific words?	___	___
check for repetition of words?	___	___
check for subject-verb agreement	___	___
check for pronoun agreement?	___	___
check for verb tense?	___	___
check spelling errors?	___	___

The questions on this editing and proofreading checklist will help you to make the final corrections needed to improve your writing.

Example 8-4

Let's reread the student's second revision of the report on child abuse:

Child abuse is a danger to children that may result in harmful injury and even death. As nursing assistants, we have to be aware of the symptoms of child abuse. When we examine children who are repeatedly bruised, or accident prone, we should be suspicious. Neglecting to report cases when children are repeatedly being treated for broken bones could lead to greater injury. Two weeks ago, a nine year old child was admitted to the hospital with a broken arm. Upon examination, several older bruises were discovered. This case is now being investigated by social service. This week, an infant was brought in with a head injury. The mother reported that the infant had fallen out of her highchair. However, this same mother brought in a toddler the week before with an arm pulled out of the socket. This toddler also had deep welts across the back and shoulders. The parent claimed not to know how the child got these welts. Both children had been battered. This case is also being looked into.

Child abuse affects children of all ages and crosses all economic groups. In the last month, two of the seven reported cases of child abuse were from upper middle class homes with both parents.

If you have even the slightest evidence that a child is being abused, report the case to social service. If we do not act on our suspicions because we want to protect the parents, the children will be endangered. Therefore, it is <u>imperative</u> that you report all cases of suspected child abuse to the Social service agency.

This is how the student answered the questions on the editing and proofreading checklist.

- Did I write clean and complete sentences? *Yes.*
- Did I use sentence variety? *Sentences 7 and 8 begin the same way.*
- Did I choose vivid, specific words? *Word choice could be improved.*
- Did I use sentences of different lengths? *Yes.*
- Did I avoid repetitions? *No. The words abuse, also, all, repeatedly, and suspected were used too often.*
- Did I capitalize and punctuate correctly? *An exclamation point could be used instead of a period for emphasis. Change Social to lower case.*
- Did I check for subject-verb agreement? *Yes.*
- Did I check for pronoun persons? *No. The report should be kept in second person.*
- Did I check for verb tense? *Yes.*
- Did I check for spelling errors? *Yes.*

Once you have decided on the changes that need to be made, you can use certain tools to help you. You can use spell check and grammar check in your computer word processing program. You can also use a dictionary to check spelling, meaning, and part of speech and a thesaurus to give you choices of words with similar meanings to avoid repetition. Many computer word processing programs include a dictionary and thesaurus.

LEARNING SOME BASIC SYMBOLS FOR PROOFREADING

You can use proofreading symbols to help you mark up your revised paper so that you can make the final changes. Learning these symbols will also help you to understand your instructor's corrections of your writing.

Some common proofreading symbols are

agr agreement.
cap capitalization.
frag sentence fragment.
gram grammar.
nc not clear.
¶ paragraph
p punctuation.

R repetitions.
sp misspelled word.
RO run-on sentence.
TS topic sentence
u usage.
wc word choice.

Example 8–5

Read the student's final draft of the report on child abuse.

Child abuse is a danger to children that may result in harmful injury and even death. As nursing assistants, you have to be aware of the symptoms of child abuse. When you examine children who are frequently bruised, or accident prone, you should be wary. Neglecting to report cases when children are repeatedly being treated for broken bones could lead to greater injury. Two weeks ago, a nine year old child was admitted to the hospital with a broken arm. Upon examination, several older bruises were discovered. Social service is now investigating this case. This week, an infant was brought in with a head injury. The mother reported that the infant had fallen out of her highchair. However, this same mother brought in a toddler the week before with an arm pulled out of the socket. In addition, the toddler had deep welts across the upper back and shoulders. The parent claimed not to know how the child got these welts. Both children had been battered. Social service will explore this matter further.

Child abuse affects children of all ages and crosses every economic group. In the last month, two of the seven reported cases of child abuse were from upper-middle class homes with both parents. If you have even the slightest evidence that a child is being harmed, the case should be reported to social service. If you do not act on your suspicions because you want to protect the parents, the children will be endangered. Therefore, it is imperative that you report all cases of assumed child abuse to the social service agency.

EXERCISE 8–4

Directions: Use the editing and proofreading checklist and the proofreading symbols as guides to correct your revision. Write your final draft.

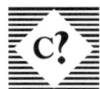

PREPARING THE PRESENTATION

The presentation, or appearance, of your paper is a critical part of the writing process. Whether you write or type your paper, your work should be neat, well spaced, and easy to read. In writing, one cannot separate form from content. A finished paper with a good presentation is an essential part of the writing process.

AVOID TROUBLE SPOTS IN WRITING

When you are proofreading your paper, keep in mind certain areas in which students make errors. If you are aware of these problem areas in writing, you can correct your mistakes before you hand in your final paper.

Spelling

You can avoid making spelling mistakes by learning and applying a few spelling rules.

Some Common Spelling Rules

- **Words ending in "Y":** When you write the plurals of words that end in *y*, change *y* to *i* and add *es*. If the word ends in *ey*, just add *s*.
  baby, babies   turkey, turkeys
- **Consonant Ending:** When you add an ending like *ed* or *ing* to a one-syllable word with a short vowel, the final consonant is usually doubled.
  hop, hopping   tip, tipped
- **"I" Before "E":** *I* before *e* except after *c* or when rhyming with *say* as in *neighbor* and *weigh*.
  belief, conceit, sleigh
- **Silent "E":** If a word ends with a silent *e*, drop the *e* before adding an ending that begins with a vowel. Do not drop the *e* when the ending begins with a consonant.
  hope, hoping, hopeful

Commonly Misspelled Words

You should learn the following words that students often misspell:

Absence	Dilemma	Height
Absent	Disease	Helpful
Accept	Dissatisfied	Hospital
Accident	Dying	
Accommodate		Illegal
Accurate	Embarrassed	Immigrant
Across	Environment	Independent
Advise	Excellence	Intelligence
Already	Exercise	Interfere
Analyze	Exhaust	Itinerary
Apologize	Extremely	
Attendance		Jeopardize
	Feasible	Judgment
Belief	Foreign	
Benefit	Fragile	Knowledge
Benefited	Friend	
Business	Fulfill	Laboratory
		Leisure
Characteristic	Government	
Committee	Grievance	Maintenance
Competition	Guarantee	Medicine
Convenience	Guardian	
Cooperate		Necessary
Criticism	Handicapped	Neighborhood
	Handkerchief	Neither
Decision	Harass	Nuclear
Dependent	Hazardous	
		Occasion
		Occur

Continued on following page.

Omitted
Operate
Opinion

Pamphlet
Persuade
Physical
Physically
Preferred
Prejudice
Professor
Pronunciation
Psychology

Qualitative
Questionnaire

Receipt
Recognize
Recommend

Recurrence
Reference
Remember
Responsibilities

Safety
Schedule
Secretary
Separate
Significant
Suggest
Supervisory
Sympathize

Tedious
Temperature
Temporarily
Tendency
Tomorrow
Tragedy

Transferred
Traveling

Ultimately
Unconscious
Unfortunately
Unnecessary

Vehicle
Violence
Voluntary

Waive
Weigh
Welfare
Witnessed

Yield

Zeros

EXERCISE 8–5

Directions: Choose the correct spelling of the following words:

1.	coppyed	copied	coppied
2.	poked	pokked	pokd
3.	neighbor	nieghbor	nieighbor
4.	guardain	gardian	guardian
5.	handkercheif	hankerchief	handkerchief
6.	easier	easyier	easyer
7.	hopeless	hoppless	hopeles
8.	judgement	judgment	juddgment
9.	temperture	temperature	temparature
10.	dryed	dried	dryied

Words Often Confused

Read over the following commonly misused words. This list should help you find the right words to use in your writing.

accept to receive.
except other than.

allowed permitted.
aloud with a speaking voice.

already previously.
all ready completely ready.

capital the seat of government.
  chief.
  accumulated wealth.
capitol a building that usually houses some part of government.

choose to select.
chose selected.

council a group called together for certain tasks.
counsel advise.
  to give advice.

desert a dry region.
  to leave.
dessert the final course of a meal.

it's the contraction meaning "it is."
its the possessive form of "it."

loose free from restrictions.
lose to misplace.
  to fail to win.

principal a school administrator.
  most important.
principle a rule.

stationary a fixed position.
stationery writing paper.

than compares two things.
then tells when.

their possessive form of they.
there indicates place or direction.
they're a contraction meaning "they are."

to indicates direction.
too also.
  very.
two the number "2."

who's the contraction meaning "who is."
whose the possessive form of "who."

you're the contraction meaning "you are."
your the possessive form of "you."

EXERCISE 8-6

Directions: Choose the correct word in each sentence:

1. _____ (Who's, Whose) picking you up from school today?

2. I have to order new _____ (stationary, stationery) to write my thank-you notes.

3. Mr. Miller is the _____ (principal, principle) of my school.

4. Yesterday the team _____ (choose, chose) Allan to be the captain.

5. Everyone _____ (accept, except) Elizabeth was invited to the party.

6. _____ (Their, There, They're) going to be late for the movie.

7. Are you _____ (allowed, aloud) to take out three books from the library?

8. These suitcases are _____ (to, too, two) heavy for me to carry.

9. Chocolate cake is my favorite _____ (desert, dessert).

10. Try not to _____ (loose, lose).

Sentence Errors

A sentence is made up of a subject and verb and expresses a complete thought. Check for sentence errors. Some common errors are sentence fragments and run-on sentences.

A fragment is a group of words that does not make a complete sentence.
Example: Thinks he can win.
This fragment is missing a subject. You can correct this fragment by adding a subject.
Corrected Sentence: My brother thinks he can win.
A run-on sentence is when two sentences are joined without punctuation or a connecting word.
Example: I thought he would never leave he just kept talking.
Corrected Sentence: I thought he would never leave. He just kept talking.

EXERCISE 8–7

Directions: Label each group of words as *fragment, run-on,* or *correct sentence*.

1. To fly a plane. _____

2. Many infections can be prevented. _____

3. Because the virus wasn't treated correctly. _____

4. This test is too difficult I should have studied harder. _____

5. I am allergic to chocolate it makes me break out in hives. _____

6. Call the supervisor if you have a problem with this patient. _____

7. During the intermission. _____

8. People were inoculated. _____

9. The orderly brought ice-cream to the tonsillectomy patient she enjoyed it. _____

10. Hopeful for a complete recovery. _____

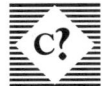

Parts of Speech

Learning the parts of speech will help you to know how to use words correctly in a sentence. Read over the following chart to learn how to use the parts of speech.

PARTS OF SPEECH	USE	EXAMPLES
noun	names	pen, Lewis
pronoun	taking the place of a noun	them, us, herself
adjective	describes a noun or pronoun	red, tallest
verb	action, linking, helping	watched, is, has been writing
adverb	describes a verb, an adjective, or another adverb	slowly, better
preposition	relates a noun or pronoun to another word; begins a phrase	among, around, on
conjunction	joins words	and, but, or
interjection	shows strong feeling	Ouch!

EXERCISE 8–8

Directions: Write the correct part of speech of each italicized word in the following paragraph.

Marcia was having difficulty studying *for* her midterm exams. *Her family* and *work* responsibilities *were interfering* with the hours she needed for study. Studying, working, *and* child care were hard to juggle. Marcia knew she could do *better* in school if she had more time for herself. Sometimes, she felt like crying *"help!"*

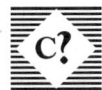

Agreement

Pronouns

Pronouns must agree in person and number with the words they replace.
   Example: John told Sonya and Mary to meet him at work.
   He told them to meet him at work.
   Example: Sylvia instructed the employees on how to operate the computer.
   She instructed them on how to operate it.

Subjects and Verbs

Subjects and verbs should agree in number. If the subject is singular, the verb should be singular. If the subject is plural, the verb should be plural. In the following examples the subject is in italic type and the verb is in boldface type.
   Example: Mindy and Helen **were** absent.
   Example: Either of the doctors **is** qualified to perform the surgery.
   The following words take a singular verb:

Anyone	Everybody	One
Everyone	Each	Someone
Anybody	Either	Neither

EXERCISE 8–9

Directions: Choose the right answer for each of these sentences.

1. Does anyone _____ (live, lives) here?
2. He and I _____ (was, were) at home.
3. One of my friends _____ (is, are) coming to visit.
4. Elijah took _____ (his, him) car to the station.
5. Jackie and Matthew were hoping _____ (they, he) could get a ride to the game.
6. When the medicine expires _____ (it, its) is no longer effective.
7. Everybody _____ (expects, expect) to pass the course.
8. Katherine left _____ (her, hers) book at home.
9. The patient left _____ (his, him) insurance form at home.
10. Antonio _____ (follow, follows) instructions correctly.

Capitalization

Capitalize

- the first word of a sentence
- proper nouns and adjectives

Example: *Celena* traveled to *England* and enjoyed touring the *English* countryside.

Punctuation

Read the following chart to learn how to use punctuation correctly.

.	Period	End of sentence that makes a statement, command, or request
		After abbreviated title or initial
?	Question mark	End of sentence that asks a question
!	Exclamation mark	End of sentence that shows emotion
,	Comma	Items in a series
		In dates, addresses, and numbers
		After introductory expressions
		Around nonessential material
		To set off interruptions
		In direct address
'	Apostrophe	To form the possessive of singular and plural nouns
		In contractions
;	Semicolon	Between two closely related independent clauses unless they are joined by the connecting words (and, but, nor, yet, or, for, so)
:	Colon	After a complete statement when a list or long quotation follows
--	Dash	To show a change of thought or emphasis
" "	Quotation marks	Around the exact words of a speaker
		The name of a short story, poem, essay, or TV program

EXERCISE 8-10

Directions: Put the correct capitalization and punctuation in the following paragraph.

Rosa is taking english lessons so that she will be able to get a better job. She is hoping to improve her skills in reading writing and conversation when she finishes this course she will be able to enter a community college. Will this course give her skills she needs to succeed She will have to meet the following requirements taking notes, understanding lectures and comprehending her textbooks. rosa hopes to become a technician when she moves to philadelphia in two years.

REVIEWING REWRITING THE FINAL DRAFT

TO LEARN	USE THIS STRATEGY
Make necessary changes to your first draft	Follow a plan for revising
Decide what changes are necessary	Use a revising checklist
Make additional changes	Reread your revision
Make revising easier	Use a word-processing program
Make the needed changes in spelling and mechanics	Use an editing and proofreading checklist
Mark your paper so you will remember to make all your changes to prepare your final draft	Use proofreading symbols
Prepare the final presentation	Remember that form cannot be separated from content
Avoid trouble spots in your writing	Review some basic rules and do practice exercises in spelling, sentences, parts of speech, agreement, capitalization, and punctuation

UNIT III

MATHEMATICS STRATEGIES

You may be one of many students who are anxious at the thought of doing mathematics in the health sciences. This unit has been written to ease this anxiety and to teach you the strategies for solving basic math functions. Chapter 9, Learning Computation Skills, will teach you the mathematical foundation of multiplying and dividing whole numbers. Also, you will learn the strategies for solving fraction, decimal, percentage, ratio, and proportion problems. Chapter 10, Understanding Algebra, Geometry, and the Metric System, will go one gentle step further and teach you the basics of algebra, geometry, and performing conversions in the metric system. Unit 3 will conclude with Chapter 11, Solving Word Problems. In this chapter, you will learn how to solve word problems by identifying the various terms that will indicate the operation to perform in word problems. Although Unit 3, Mathematics Strategies, is not intended to be a complete course in math, it is hoped that it will provide a good reintroduction to math. Once you finish all the exercises in this unit, your confidence should be strong and your interest should be sparked for learning more.

Chapter 9

Learning Computation Skills

LEARNING OBJECTIVES
VOCABULARY WORDS
VOCABULARY CHECK
MULTIPLICATION
DIVISION
FRACTIONS
    Reducing to the Lowest Term
    Raising to a Higher Term
    Adding and Subtracting Fractions
    Multiplying Fractions
    Dividing Fractions
DECIMALS
    Adding and Subtracting Decimals
    Multiplying Decimals
    Dividing Decimals
    Changing Decimals to Fractions
    Changing Fractions to Decimals
PERCENTAGES
    Changing Percentages to Fractions
    Changing Fractions to Percentages
    Changing Percentages to Decimals
    Changing Decimals to Percentages
    Doing Problems With Percentages
RATIOS
PROPORTIONS
REVIEWING THE LEARNING STRATEGIES

LEARNING OBJECTIVES

In this chapter you will learn how to
- Memorize multiplication and division facts
- Solve problems using fractions, decimals, percentages, ratios, and proportions

VOCABULARY WORDS

The following vocabulary words are important to your understanding of the ideas in this chapter. These vocabulary words are underscored the first time they are used in the chapter. Read the list of words and definitions. Then check your understanding of these words before you read the chapter.

caret a punctuation mark that shows in what place an item will be inserted.
common belonging to or shared by two or more mathematical entities.
comparison showing similarities of two or more items.
conversion the act of changing or transforming.
denominator the part of a fraction below the line that signifies division.
diagonal passing from the upper left to the lower right or the upper right to the lower left.
numerator the part of a fraction above the line that signifies division.
reverse to go in an opposite direction.
typical having the nature or being part of a type.
values numerical quantities.

VOCABULARY CHECK

Directions: Choose the vocabulary word that best fits into the sentence.

1. The checks in her wallet had different _____.
2. It was bright and sunny; it was a _____ summer day.
3. The children will march in one direction; then they will _____ their march to a different direction.
4. The top part of a fraction is the _____.
5. The stripes did not go up and down or side to side; they went on a _____.
6. The bottom part of a fraction is the _____.
7. He checked a _____ chart to change Fahrenheit into Celsius.
8. All the fish looked alike so they were considered a _____ type.
9. He left out the word "medicine" so he wrote a _____ and inserted the word in the proper place.
10. The _____ of the twins showed that they were identical.

MULTIPLICATION

Multiplication is the fast way of adding similar numbers over and over again. You can recognize a multiplication problem when you see the × sign. To do multiplication problems well, you must memorize the multiplication tables. As an example, the multiplication table for 3 looks like the following:

$$0 \times 3 = 0 \qquad 7 \times 3 = 21$$
$$1 \times 3 = 3 \qquad 8 \times 3 = 24$$
$$2 \times 3 = 6 \qquad 9 \times 3 = 27$$
$$3 \times 3 = 9 \qquad 10 \times 3 = 30$$
$$4 \times 3 = 12 \qquad 11 \times 3 = 33$$
$$5 \times 3 = 15 \qquad 12 \times 3 = 36$$
$$6 \times 3 = 18$$

You can create similar multiplication tables for any number. However, there is a better strategy for learning the multiplication tables—making and learning the multiplication chart (see Table 9–1).

The method for using this chart is as follows:

- You are asked to figure out how many ounces of medicine Ms. Grande takes per week. You know that she takes 3 ounces a day.
- In your mind you see the problem as 7 × 3 = ?, where 7 stands for the number of days in a week and 3 stands for the number of ounces of medicine Ms. Grande takes per day.
- In the top shaded row, put your right finger on the number 7.
- In the shaded column to the left, put your left finger on the number 3.
- Slowly move your right finger down and your left finger to the right until they meet. The number at which both fingers meet is the correct answer.
- "21 oz." is the answer to this problem.

TABLE 9–1. Multiplication Chart

×	1	2	3	4	5	6	7	8	9	10	11	12
1	1	2	3	4	5	6	7	8	9	10	11	12
2	2	4	6	8	10	12	14	16	18	20	22	24
3	3	6	9	12	15	18	21	24	27	30	33	36
4	4	8	12	16	20	24	28	32	36	40	44	48
5	5	10	15	20	25	30	35	40	45	50	55	60
6	6	12	18	24	30	36	42	48	54	60	66	72
7	7	14	21	28	35	42	49	56	63	70	77	84
8	8	16	24	32	40	48	56	64	72	80	88	96
9	9	18	27	36	45	54	63	72	81	90	99	108
10	10	20	30	40	50	60	70	80	90	100	110	120
11	11	22	33	44	55	66	77	88	99	110	121	132
12	12	24	36	48	60	72	84	96	108	120	132	144

Although a multiplication chart is very handy, it does not substitute for learning the tables by heart. Memorizing the multiplication tables until you know them as well as your name will make your personal and student life easier. To help you learn the tables, try making flash cards or find a computer program that will make the learning task enjoyable.

DIVISION

Like multiplication, you use division to solve many common, daily arithmetic problems. You can write division problems two ways:

$$10 \div 2 = 5$$

In this example the number 10 is divided by 2. In other words, you always divide the number after the sign into the number that goes before the sign. The second way to write division problems looks like this:

$$2\overline{)10}^{\,5}$$

In this example, you divide the number that is inside the box by the number that is outside the box. If you have learned your multiplication tables well, you will have an easier time with division. You may have noticed in the first example that if you read the problem from right to left, it reads like a multiplication problem. Consider the following:

- Mr. Sheldon, a medical secretary, was asked to split a $3000 bonus among the three employees working in Dr. Joseph's office.
- Mr. Sheldon knows that 1000 × 3 = 3000.
- He reverses the procedure and divided 3000 by 3.
- Each employee will get $1000.

If you learn the multiplication tables thoroughly, you will be able to do more complicated multiplication and division problems.

EXERCISE 9–1

Directions: Spend some time learning the multiplication chart (Table 9–1). Then fill in the chart at the top of p. 137. You may want to memorize one table at a time and then fill in the chart as you learn that table. Remember that learning the multiplication tables by heart will help you with both multiplication and division problems.

×	1	2	3	4	5	6	7	8	9	10	11	12
1												
2												
3												
4												
5												
6												
7												
8												
9												
10												
11												
12												

FRACTIONS

Fractions represent parts of a whole. You go to school 5 days out of 7 days. When this is written as a fraction, it looks like this:

$$\frac{5}{7}$$

In this example the number 5 on top is called the <u>numerator</u>. The numerator tells you how many parts of the whole. The number 7 on the bottom is called the <u>denominator</u>. The denominator tells you how many parts make up a whole.

This example of a fraction is called a **proper fraction.** A proper fraction is when the numerator is smaller than the denominator and has a value less than 1.

Consider this next fraction:

$$\frac{4}{2}$$

This is an example of an **improper fraction.** When the numerator is larger than the denominator, you have an improper fraction.

Sometimes you may see a whole number written with a fraction next to it. It will look like this:

$$13 \frac{6}{12}$$

This is called a **mixed number.**

Reducing to the Lowest Term

Sometimes when working with fractions it is necessary to reduce them to their lowest terms. This means dividing the numerator and the denominator by the same number until you cannot go any further. Study the following problem:

$$\frac{50}{100}$$

- What number is needed to divide both the 50 and 100 so that the answer comes out evenly?
- Try 25. 50 divided by 25 is 2. 100 divided by 25 is 4. The answer so far looks like this:

$$\frac{2}{4}$$

- Is it still possible to reduce this fraction? Is there still another number that can be divided equally into both the 2 and the 4?
- Try 2: 2 goes into 2 once; 2 goes into 4 twice. The answer now is:

$$\frac{1}{2}$$

The lowest term for

$$\frac{50}{100}$$

is

$$\frac{1}{2}$$

Raising to a Higher Term

- Similarly, any fraction can be changed to a higher term by multiplying both the numerator and the denominator by the same number.

$$\frac{9}{18} = \frac{27}{54}$$

$$9 \times 3 = 27 \text{ and } 18 \times 3 = 54$$

Adding and Subtracting Fractions

To add and subtract with fractions that have the same denominator, you add or subtract only the numerator and copy the common denominator to finish the problem.

$$\frac{5}{11} + \frac{3}{11} = \frac{8}{11}$$

$$\frac{9}{64} - \frac{1}{64} = \frac{8}{64}$$

However, if the denominators are different, you need to find the lowest common denominator. The lowest common denominator is the smallest number that can be divided evenly by the denominators of all the fractions in the problem. For example:

$$\frac{2}{3} \qquad \frac{5}{6} \qquad \frac{3}{9}$$

- Think of the smallest number that can be divided evenly by 3, 6, 9.

    $3 \times 6 = 18$ $6 \times 3 = 18$ $9 \times 2 = 18$.

Or

    $18 \div 3 = 6$ $18 \div 6 = 3$ $18 \div 9 = 2$

18 is the lowest common denominator. The problem now looks like this:

$$\frac{(2)}{18} \qquad \frac{(5)}{18} \qquad \frac{(3)}{18}$$

- To finish the problem you must take one more important step. **Whatever you do to the denominator you must do to the numerator.**
- In the first fraction, you multiplied 3 by 6 to get the lowest common denominator of 18. Now you must do the same to the numerator 2. $2 \times 6 = 12$. The fraction is now

$$\frac{12}{18}$$

- In the second fraction you multiplied the denominator 6 by 3 to get the lowest common denominator of 18. Now you must do the same to the numerator 5. $5 \times 3 = 15$. The fraction is now

$$\frac{15}{18}$$

- In the third fraction you multiplied the denominator 9 by 2 to get the lowest common denominator of 18. Now you must do the same to the numerator 3. $3 \times 2 = 6$. The fraction is now

$$\frac{6}{18}$$

The fractions now look like this:

$$\frac{12}{18} \qquad \frac{15}{18} \qquad \frac{6}{18}$$

- These fractions are now ready to be added or subtracted.

Multiplying Fractions

To multiply fractions you simply multiply the numerators and then the denominators. For example:

$$\frac{4}{7} \times \frac{10}{10} = \frac{40}{70}$$

If you are working with mixed numbers, it is important to change them into improper fractions before multiplying or dividing. Look at the following:

$$2\frac{4}{8}$$

- To change this mixed number into an improper fraction, first multiply the denominator by the whole number.

$$8 \times 2 = 16$$

- Next add the numerator of 4 to the 16.

$$16 + 4 = 20$$

- Finally copy the original denominator so the fraction now looks like this:

$$\frac{20}{8}$$

- The mixed number has now been changed to an improper fraction.

Dividing Fractions

To divide fractions, you do the following two steps:

$$\frac{4}{16} \div \frac{5}{15}$$

First you <u>reverse</u> the second fraction. In other words, the 15 becomes the numerator and the 5 becomes the denominator.

$$\frac{15}{5}$$

Then you change the division sign to a multiplication sign and multiply the numerators and then the denominators to get the answer.

$$\frac{4}{16} \times \frac{15}{5} = \frac{60}{80} = \frac{3}{4}$$

Sometimes, if the numbers are large, you may want to reduce them in a multiplication or division problem. Remember to work on a <u>diagonal</u> across the signs.

$$\frac{10}{20} \times \frac{5}{40} \times \frac{1}{10} =$$

$$\frac{\cancel{10}^{1}}{\cancel{20}_{4}} \times \frac{\cancel{5}^{1}}{40} \times \frac{1}{\cancel{10}_{1}} =$$

$$\frac{1}{4} \times \frac{1}{40} \times \frac{1}{1} = \frac{1}{160}$$

EXERCISE 9–2

Directions: Do the following fraction problems. Pay careful attention to the signs so that you perform the correct function. Remember to find the lowest common denominators if necessary and change any mixed numbers to improper fractions.

1. Reduce $\frac{12}{48}$
2. Determine the missing numerator: $\frac{2}{3} = \frac{?}{36}$
3. Change to an improper fraction: $9\frac{2}{14} =$
4. $\frac{9}{11} - \frac{7}{11} =$
5. $\frac{4}{28} + \frac{9}{28} + \frac{14}{28} =$
6. $\frac{1}{3} \times \frac{1}{2} =$
7. $\frac{1}{3} \div \frac{1}{2} =$
8. $\frac{5}{14} \times \frac{7}{25} =$
9. $4\frac{8}{10} \div \frac{4}{5} =$
10. $2\frac{2}{4} \times 1\frac{5}{20} =$

DECIMALS

Decimal numbers are similar to fractions. They both describe parts of a whole number. However, there are two differences between decimals and fractions. The first difference is that denominators of decimals can be only 10, 100, 1000, etc. The second difference is that a decimal point or period is used to separate the whole number from the fraction. In the following example, note the difference between decimals and fractions of the same number.

$$\frac{2}{10} = 0.2$$

$$\frac{80}{100} = 0.80$$

$$\frac{425}{1000} = 0.425$$

$$\frac{734}{10000} = 7.0034$$

The way you read a decimal is determined by how many numbers are to the right of the decimal point. The first example, 0.2, is read "two tenths." The second example, 0.80, is read "eighty hundredths." The third example, 0.425, is read "four hundred twenty-five thousandths." And the last example, 7.0034 is read "seven **and** thirty-four ten thousandths."

Adding and Subtracting Decimals

When you add or subtract decimals, it is necessary to write the problem so that all the decimal points are lined up in a straight row. Then add or subtract decimal numbers the same way you would add or subtract whole numbers.

$$
\begin{array}{r} 4.258 \\ 9.636 \\ \hline 13.894 \end{array}
\qquad
\begin{array}{r} 90.58 \\ 82.21 \\ 8.37 \\ \hline \end{array}
$$

If you are adding or subtracting decimals, use zeros to fill in the places without a number after you align the decimal points.

$$
\begin{array}{r} 21.55 \\ +\,62.2\mathbf{0} \\ \hline \end{array}
\qquad
\begin{array}{r} 21.55 \\ 62.2\mathbf{0} \\ \hline 83.75 \end{array}
\qquad
\begin{array}{r} 9.4707 \\ -\,4.26\mathbf{00} \\ \hline \end{array}
\qquad
\begin{array}{r} 9.4707 \\ 4.26\mathbf{00} \\ \hline 5.2107 \end{array}
$$

Multiplying Decimals

When you multiply decimal numbers, multiply the same way you would with whole numbers. Then count all the numbers to the right of the decimal point in both rows of numbers in the problem. Put the decimal point that number of places in the answer.

$$
\begin{array}{r} 0.798 \\ \times\,6.4 \\ \hline 5.1072 \end{array}
$$
(3 numbers to right of decimal point)
(1 number to right of decimal point)
(4 numbers to right of decimal point)

Dividing Decimals

Dividing decimal numbers is similar to dividing whole numbers. If the number outside the box is a whole number, place the decimal point in the answer in the same decimal place as the number inside the box.

$$
4\overline{)0.8} = 0.2
$$

If the number outside the box is a decimal, change this decimal number to a whole number by moving the decimal point to the right of the last number. Use a caret (^) to show the new place of the decimal. If the number inside the box is also a decimal number, move the decimal point the same amount of numbers as you did the outside number. Also use a caret to show you have moved the decimal point. If necessary add zeros to get the same number of decimal places.

$$.400_\wedge \overline{\smash{)}80.000_\wedge}^{200.}$$

Notice that the decimal point in the answer is placed exactly over the new position of the decimal point of the number inside the box.

Changing Decimals to Fractions

To change a decimal to a fraction, write the numbers in the decimal as the numerator and write the name of the decimal (tenths, hundredths, thousandths, etc.) as the denominator. Reduce the fraction if necessary.

$$0.50 = \frac{50}{100} = \frac{1}{2}$$

Changing Fractions to Decimals

To change a fraction to a decimal, divide the numerator by the denominator. The dividing line of a fraction means "divided by." To divide the numerator by the denominator, it will be necessary to add a decimal point and one or more zeros to the numerator. Carry the decimal point up to the answer.

$$\frac{1}{2} \qquad\qquad 2\overline{\smash{)}1.0}^{0.5}$$

EXERCISE 9–3

Directions: Solve the following decimal problems.
Add the following decimals:

a. 5.439 + 7.63 + 1.257 =

b. 0.428 + 0.029 + 8.35 =

Subtract the following decimals:

c. 21.719 – 5.83 =

d. 103.8 – 62.45 =

Multiply the following decimals:

e. 943.27 × 0.5 =

f. 1.3294 × 0.566 =

Divide the following decimals:

g. 70 ÷ 0.25 =

h. 160 ÷ 0.40 =

Change the following decimals to fractions. Reduce the fraction if necessary.

i. 0.020   0.8   0.45

Change the following fractions to decimals:

j. $\frac{4}{5}$ $\frac{6}{80}$ $\frac{50}{250}$

PERCENTAGES

Percentage numbers, like fractions and decimals, represent a part of the whole. The percentage represents hundredths and is indicated by the percent sign (%). Thus 47 hundredths can be written as

$$\frac{47}{100}, 0.47, \text{ or } 47\%$$

When doing percentage problems, you should change the percentage number to either a fraction or a decimal number and then solve the problem. Table 9–2 is a <u>conversion</u> chart of some of the more common percentages.

Changing Percentages to Fractions

To change a percentage to a fraction, use the number in the percentage as the numerator and put 100 as the denominator. Reduce the fraction if necessary.

$$35\% = \frac{35}{100} = \frac{7}{20}$$

Changing Fractions to Percentages

The easiest way to change a fraction to a percentage is to change the fraction to a decimal number first.

$$75\overline{)3.00}^{\,0.04} \qquad 0.04 = \frac{4}{100} = 40\%$$

Changing Percentages to Decimals

To change a percentage number to a decimal number, erase the percent sign and move the decimal point two places to the left.

$$51\% = 0.51$$

TABLE 9-2. Converting Percentages to Fractions and Decimals

PERCENT		FRACTION		DECIMAL
25%	=	$\frac{1}{4}$	=	0.25
50%	=	$\frac{1}{2}$	=	0.5
75%	=	$\frac{3}{4}$	=	0.75
12.5%	=	$\frac{1}{8}$	=	0.125
37.5%	=	$\frac{3}{8}$	=	0.375
62.5%	=	$\frac{5}{8}$	=	0.625
87.5%	=	$\frac{7}{8}$	=	0.875
$33\frac{1}{3}$%	=	$\frac{1}{3}$	=	$0.33\frac{1}{3}$
$66\frac{2}{3}$%	=	$\frac{2}{3}$	=	$0.66\frac{2}{3}$
20%	=	$\frac{1}{5}$	=	0.2
40%	=	$\frac{2}{5}$	=	0.4
60%	=	$\frac{3}{5}$	=	0.6
80%	=	$\frac{4}{5}$	=	0.8
10%	=	$\frac{1}{10}$	=	0.1
30%	=	$\frac{3}{10}$	=	0.3
70%	=	$\frac{7}{10}$	=	0.7
90%	=	$\frac{9}{10}$	=	0.9
$16\frac{2}{3}$%	=	$\frac{1}{6}$	=	$0.16\frac{2}{3}$
$83\frac{1}{3}$%	=	$\frac{5}{6}$	=	$0.83\frac{1}{3}$

Changing Decimals to Percentages

To change decimal numbers to percentage numbers, move the decimal point two places to the right and write in the percent sign.

$$0.76 = 76\%$$

Doing Problems With Percentages

To find a percentage of a whole number, change the percentage to a fraction or a decimal and then multiply by the whole number.

What is 25% of 500?

$$25\% = \frac{25}{100}$$

$$\frac{25}{100} \times 500 = 125$$

or

What is 8.5% of 250?

$$8.5\% = 0.085$$

$$0.085 \times 250 = 21.25$$

To find what percentage one number is of another number, turn the numbers in the problem into a fraction and change the fraction to a percentage.

5 is what percentage of 50?

$$\frac{5}{50} = \frac{1}{10}$$

$$\frac{1}{10} = 0.1 = 10\%$$

To find the whole number when a percentage is given, divide the whole number by the percentage. Change the percentage to a fraction.

10% of what number is 100?

$$10\% = \frac{1}{10}$$

$$100 \div \frac{1}{10} = \frac{100}{1} \times \frac{10}{1} = 1000$$

EXERCISE 9-4

Directions: Fill in the following chart. Check your work with the conversion chart in Table 9-2. Then solve problems 11 through 15.

Percent	Fraction	Decimal
1. 50%		
2.		0.125
3.	$\frac{1}{6}$	
4.		0.7
5. 60%		
6.	$\frac{2}{5}$	
7.		$0.66\frac{2}{3}$
8.	$\frac{3}{8}$	
9. 80%		
10.	$\frac{1}{4}$	

11. What is 8% of 75?
12. 18 is what percent of 16?
13. 40% of what number is 48?
14. 27 is what percent of 72?
15. 6.25% of 300 =

RATIOS

A ratio is a <u>comparison</u> of two numbers using division. A ratio can be written in three ways:

1. 16 to 32
2. $\frac{16}{32} = \frac{1}{2}$
3. 16:32

Regardless of how you write the ratio, you would read it as "16 to 32." Read the following and find out how you would solve a ratio problem.

- Of Chloe's 28 teeth, 4 have crowns on them. Determine the ratio of crowned teeth to uncrowned teeth.
- Use the 4 crowned teeth as the numerator and the total number of teeth as the denominator and reduce the fraction. $\frac{4}{28} = \frac{1}{7}$
- $\frac{1}{7}$ of Chloe's teeth are crowned.

EXERCISE 9-5

Directions: Solve the following ratio problems. Choose any of the ways to express your answer. If necessary, reduce fractions to their lowest terms.

1. At the veterinary school there are 10 instructors for 400 students. What is the ratio of instructors to students?
2. Out of 25 typed pages, the medical typist had to redo 5 of them because of errors. What is the ratio of redone pages to correct pages?
3. The laboratory assistant discovered that 6 of the 54 microscopes needed repairs. What is the ratio of working microscopes to broken ones?
4. Of the 228 graduates of the medical assistant program, 19 found jobs immediately after graduation. What is the ratio of working graduates to nonworking graduates?
5. Prudence cleaned 15 of the rat cages out of a total of 50. What is the ratio of clean cages to dirty ones?

PROPORTIONS

A proportion is a statement that two ratios are equal. A proportion can be written in three ways:

1. 1 to 2 = 5 to 10
2. $\frac{1}{2} = \frac{5}{10}$
3. 1:2 = 5:10

All three of these proportions are read as "1 is to 2 as 5 is to 10." Below is what a <u>typical</u> proportion problem would look like. Determine the missing number in the following proportion:

$$\frac{?}{10} = \frac{3}{30}$$

To find the missing number, figure out what number you would multiply 10 by to get 30. The answer is 3. Earlier in this chapter you were told that whatever number you use to multiply in the denominator you must use for that numerator. So what number multiplied by 3 would equal 3? The answer is 1. The proportion equation now looks like this:

$$\frac{?}{10} = \frac{3}{30} \qquad \frac{1}{10} = \frac{3}{30}$$

LEARNING COMPUTATION SKILLS **149**

EXERCISE 9–6

Directions: Write each of the following statements as a proportion.

1. 4 is to 12 as 1 is to 3.
2. 16 is to 40 as 2 is to 5.
3. 35 is to 30 as 7 is to 6.
4. 108 is to 24 as 9 is to 2.
5. 77 is to 99 as 7 is to 9.

EXERCISE 9–7

Directions: Solve the following problems by finding the value of the unknown number (?). Remember that the number that was used to determine the denominator should also be used to determine the numerator.

1. $\frac{4}{8} = \frac{?}{16}$
2. $\frac{5}{1} = \frac{35}{?}$
3. $\frac{45}{?} = \frac{5}{9}$
4. $\frac{?}{7} = \frac{18}{42}$
5. $\frac{7}{12} = \frac{?}{108}$
6. $\frac{40}{?} = \frac{4}{12}$
7. $\frac{18}{35} = \frac{108}{?}$
8. $\frac{51}{25} = \frac{?}{1000}$
9. $\frac{?}{76} = \frac{66}{228}$
10. $\frac{62}{909} = \frac{?}{1818}$

REVIEWING THE LEARNING STRATEGIES

TO LEARN	USE THIS STRATEGY
Multiplication and division	Memorize the multiplication chart
Fractions	Learn to recognize the numerator, denominator, proper and improper fractions, mixed numbers, lowest terms, and the common denominator
Decimals	Learn about place holding, reading decimal numbers, changing fractions to decimal numbers, and changing decimal numbers to fractions
Percentages	Learn about reading percentages and changing percentages to decimals or fractions
Ratios	Learn the definition of *ratio* and to read and write ratios
Proportions	Learn the definition of *proportion* and how to read and write proportions

Chapter 10

Understanding Algebra, Geometry, and the Metric System

LEARNING OBJECTIVES
VOCABULARY WORDS
VOCABULARY CHECK
ALGEBRA
    Adding Signed Numbers
    Subtracting Signed Numbers
    Multiplying Signed Numbers
    Dividing Signed Numbers
    Solving Equations
    Working with Equations
    Using Addition in Equations
    Using Subtraction in Equations
    Using Multiplication in Equations
    Using Division in Equations
    Checking Your Answer

GEOMETRY
    Basic Geometry Terms
    Circles
        Finding the Diameter of a Circle
        Finding the Radius of a Circle
        Determining the Area of a Circle
    Triangles
        Types of Triangles
    Squares
        Finding the Perimeter of a Square
        Finding the Area of a Square
    Rectangles
        Finding the Perimeter of a Rectangle
        Finding the Area of a Rectangle
THE METRIC SYSTEM

UNDERSTANDING ALGEBRA, GEOMETRY, AND THE METRIC SYSTEM

LEARNING OBJECTIVES

In this chapter you will learn how to
- Add, subtract, multiply, and divide signed numbers
- Solve for the unknown in an equation
- Recognize four different triangles
- Find the perimeter, radius, and area of circles, squares, and rectangles
- Determine equivalent measures of the English and metric systems of measurement

VOCABULARY WORDS

The following vocabulary words are important to your understanding of the ideas in this chapter. These vocabulary words are underscored the first time they are used in the chapter. Read the list of words and definitions. Then check your understanding of these words before you read the chapter.

concentrate focus.
concepts ideas.
equation a mathematical expression of equality.
exponent a number written above and to the right of a number that shows how many times the number is to be multiplied by itself, for example, $4^3 = 4 \times 4 \times 4$.
extends stretches forward.
identical the same.
indicate demonstrate.
inverse opposite.
procedure steps taken in a logical manner to accomplish something.
variable a letter or symbol that represents a number of undetermined value, for example, $3x = 6$.

VOCABULARY CHECK

Directions: Choose the vocabulary word that best fits into the sentence.

1. The _____ reminded us how many times the number was multiplied by itself.
2. The arm of the octopus _____ way beyond its body.
3. The dental assistant was able to follow the dental _____ perfectly.
4. The _____ of adding is subtracting.
5. If you _____ while reading your textbook, you will do better on exams.
6. The algebraic _____ was hard to solve.
7. The student was nervous about learning all the different medical theories and _____.

8. The signs will _____ which direction to go.
9. The letter in the algebra problem represented the _____.
10. The nursing assistant students were wearing _____ uniforms.

ALGEBRA

Although many students get nervous at the mention of "algebra," they should realize that it is just a continuation of basic math skills. There are two ways that algebra differs from regular arithmetic: The first difference is that when you are working with algebra problems, letters will sometimes be substituted for numbers. Thus you may see a problem that would look like this:

$$a + b =$$

The second difference is that when doing algebra problems you will be working with negative numbers. A negative number is any number that has a value less than zero. When you do arithmetic problems, you are using only positive numbers, that is, any number that has a value greater than zero or zero. To see the difference between negative and positive numbers, refer to the following:

$$^-10\ ^-9\ ^-8\ ^-7\ ^-6\ ^-5\ ^-4\ ^-3\ ^-2\ ^-1\ 0\ ^+1\ ^+2\ ^+3\ ^+4\ ^+5\ ^+6\ ^+7\ ^+8\ ^+9\ ^+10$$

Number Line of Negative and Positive Numbers

The numbers to the left of zero are the negative numbers. To <u>indicate</u> a negative number, use a negative sign ($^-$). (Do not confuse negative signs with minus signs.) The numbers on the right are the positive numbers. To indicate a positive number, use a positive sign ($^+$). **If a number is unsigned, assume that it is positive.** Did you notice in the Number Line of Negative and Positive Numbers that the zero was unsigned? Zeros are neither positive nor negative. They do not require a sign.

Adding Signed Numbers

When you do algebra problems, you will add, subtract, multiply, and divide. However, since you are working with signed numbers, doing these operations will be different from what you remember doing with arithmetic. Here are the two strategies for adding signed numbers.

1. When adding numbers with signs that are the same, add and put the sign of the numbers in the answer.

$$^+3 + ^+6 = ^+9$$
$$^-3 + ^-6 = ^-9$$

2. When adding numbers with different signs, subtract and put the sign of the largest number in the answer.

$$^-8 - {}^+2 = {}^-6$$
$$^+5 - {}^-1 = {}^+4$$

Occasionally you will be asked to add more than two signed numbers. Here are the strategies for adding more than two numbers with mixed signs:

1. Add the numbers with positive signs.
2. Add the numbers with negative signs.
3. Subtract the two subtotals and use the sign of the largest total in your answer.

$$^-6 + {}^+3 + {}^-4 + {}^+8$$
$$^+3 + {}^+8 = {}^+11$$
$$^-6 + {}^-4 = {}^-10$$
$$^+11 + {}^-10 = {}^+1$$

EXERCISE 10-1

Directions: Solve the following addition problems. Pay close attention to the signs. If they are the same in the problem, add and copy the sign into the answer. If the signs are different in the problem, subtract and copy the sign of the larger number in the answer. When adding many signed numbers, add the positive numbers first and then the negative numbers. Subtract the subtotal and copy the sign of the largest subtotal into your answer.

1. $^+4 + {}^+1 =$
2. $^-5 + {}^-7 =$
3. $^+6 + {}^-3 =$
4. $25 + 10 =$
5. $^-66 + {}^-40 =$
6. $800 + {}^-245 =$
7. $^+3 + {}^+7 + {}^-8 + {}^-1 =$
8. $^-37 + {}^+86 + {}^-91 + {}^+10 =$
9. $^+108 + {}^+22 + {}^+439 + {}^-151 =$
10. $^-751 + {}^-488 + {}^-296 + {}^-300 =$

Subtracting Signed Numbers

Again, when you subtract signed numbers, the <u>procedure</u> is different than when you subtract in arithmetic. There are two steps for subtracting signed numbers.

1. When subtracting signed numbers, change the sign of the number being subtracted to the opposite sign.
2. Then *add* the numbers. The numbers in the following problem are in parentheses so you can clearly see the sign that will tell you what operation to do.

$$(^-9) - (^+5) =$$
$$(^-9) + (^-5) =$$
$$(^-9) + (^-5) = {}^-14$$

and

$$(^+12) - (^+2) =$$
$$(^+12) + (^-2) =$$
$$(^+12) + (^-2) = {}^+10$$

EXERCISE 10-2

Directions: Solve the following problems. Remember to change the sign of the second number to its opposite and then follow the same strategies for adding signed numbers.

1. $(^-4) - (^-1) =$
2. $(8) - (^-7) =$
3. $(^+13) - (^-13) =$
4. $(^-89) - (^-89) =$
5. $(^-751) - (232) =$
6. $(1359) - (780) =$
7. $(41,225) - (6,921) =$
8. $(^-34,109) - (29,999) =$
9. $(^+1,000,000) - (^-1,000,000) =$
10. $(^-2,000,000) - (^-1,000,000) =$

Multiplying Signed Numbers

To multiply signed numbers, you do the same as you would in arithmetic. However, to determine what sign to put in the answer, follow these two strategies:

1. If the signs in the numbers you are multiplying are the same, use the positive sign in the answer.

$$(^+25)(^+4) = {}^+100$$

2. If the signs in the numbers you are multiplying are different, use the negative sign in the answer.

$$(^+10)(^-5) = ^-50$$

You may have noticed in these problems that the × sign was not used to indicate multiplication. Instead, there are three ways to signal a multiplication problem in algebra.

1. The numbers will be in parentheses with no sign between them.

$$(2)(7)$$

2. A letter and a number will be next to each other.

$$3b$$

3. There will be a dot between the numbers. This way is discouraged because it could be misread as a decimal number.

$$2 \cdot 7$$

When you need to multiply more than two numbers, multiply the first two numbers and get a subtotal. Then use this subtotal to multiply with the third number.

$$(4)(2)(^-3)$$
$$(8)(^-3) = ^-24$$

When you are multiplying, what sign do you use for the answer? To determine the sign, *concentrate* on the negative signs. If there is an even number (2, 4, 6, etc.) of negative signs in the original problem, make the answer positive ($^+$). If there is an odd number (1, 3, 5, etc.) of negative signs in the problem, make the answer negative ($^-$). Look again at the problem above. There were how many negative signs in the original problem? One is the answer. One is an odd number, so put a negative sign in the answer.

$$(4)(2)(^-3) =$$
$$(8)(^-3) = ^-24$$

and

$$(^-10)(^-2)(^+2) =$$
$$(20)(2) =$$
$$(20)(2) = {}^+40$$

Count the number of negative signs in the original problem. Two is the answer. Since two is an even number, use a positive sign for the answer.

EXERCISE 10-3

Directions: Solve the following problems. Pay attention to the signs in the problem so you will know what sign to use in the answer.

1. (4)(2) =
2. (⁻7)(3) =
3. (16)(28) =
4. (⁻135)(⁻65) =
5. (⁻202)(10) =
6. (⁻1000)(⁻88) =
7. (⁻2)(3)(⁻4) =
8. (10)(⁻5)(2) =
9. (⁻12)(⁻3)(⁺14)(⁺2) =
10. (40)(50)(60)(⁻70) =

Dividing Signed Numbers

Dividing signed numbers is similar to multiplying signed numbers. You will need to figure out what sign to put in the answer the same way you did for the multiplication problems. If the signs in the problem are different, use the negative sign in the answer. If the signs in the problem are similar, use the positive sign in the answer.

$$^-30 \div {}^+10 = {}^-3$$
$$\frac{^-20}{^-5} = {}^+4$$

Note that the second problem is set up like a fraction. The line means "divided by." So the problem reads "⁻20 divided by ⁻5."

EXERCISE 10-4

Directions: Solve the following problems. Pay attention to the signs so you will know what sign to use in the answer.

1. ⁻2 ÷ ⁻6 =
2. ⁻5 ÷ 25 =
3. 100 ÷ 1000 =
4. 75 ÷ ⁻600 =

5. $^-384 \div {}^-32 =$

6. $\frac{^-8}{^-4} =$

7. $\frac{^-55}{^+11} =$

8. $\frac{90}{20} =$

9. $\frac{150}{^-30} =$

10. $\frac{^-222}{^-111} =$

Solving Equations

As was mentioned earlier in this chapter, one of the main differences between algebra and arithmetic is that algebra uses both numbers and letters in problems. An algebraic expression that uses numbers and letters and shows how two statements are equal is called an <u>equation</u>. An equation can look like the following:

$$a + 2 = 10$$
$$m - 2 = 15$$
$$20 = 5c$$
$$\frac{9}{b} = 3$$

Working With Equations

When working with equations, it is your responsibility to find the value of the letter or, in other words, what number the letter in the equation stands for. The letter in the equation is called the "unknown" or <u>variable</u>.

- An equation is said to have two sides—a right side and a left side. The equal sign (=) separates the right and left sides.
- To solve equations, you must use <u>inverse</u> operations.
- Addition is the opposite, or inverse, of subtraction.
- Subtraction is the opposite, or inverse, of addition.
- Multiplication is the opposite, or inverse, of division.
- Division is the opposite, or inverse, of multiplication.
- To solve an equation, perform inverse operations on **both sides of the equation** until you get an answer that states "the unknown = a certain value or number."

$$? = 50$$

Using Addition in Equations

Consider the following problem:

$$x + 10 = 15$$

In this example, x is the unknown and 10 is being added to it. To find out what x stands for, do the opposite or inverse operation. The opposite operation of addition is subtraction. Subtract 10 from the left side of the equation and do the same on the right side.

$$x + 10 = 15$$
$$\underline{-10 \quad -10}$$
$$0 \quad\quad 5$$
$$x = 5$$

You know you have solved the equation when the variable is on one side of the equal sign and a number is on the other.

Using Subtraction in Equations

Look at the next example.

$$20 = b - 8$$

You notice that in this problem 8 is being subtracted from b. To solve this equation and find the value of b, do the opposite or inverse operation to both sides of the equation. Addition is the inverse of subtraction.

$$20 = b - 8$$
$$b = 20 + 8$$
$$28 = b$$

Keep in mind the strategy for adding signed numbers. Look at the right side of the equation. When adding unlike signs, subtract and keep the sign of the larger number. The 8s, however, cancel out each other. On the left side, the signs are the same. Add the 20 and the 8; the answer is $28 = b$.

Using Multiplication in Equations

Study the following problem:

$$11s = 33$$

Because this is a multiplication problem, you need to do the inverse operation, which is division. Divide both sides of the equation by 11.

$$\frac{11}{11s} = \frac{33}{11}$$
$$1s = 3 \quad s = 3$$

On the left side of this problem, you divide 11 by 11. The answer, of course, is 1. It is not necessary to write 1 in algebra because the variable stands for 1 automatically.

Remember that your aim in solving equations is having the unknown or variable on one side of the equal sign and a number value on the other side.

Using Division in Equations

Think about this final equation problem.

$$\frac{p}{5} = 15$$

To solve this problem, you will have to do the inverse operation for division. You will have to multiply by 5 on both sides of the equal sign. The example should look like this:

$$\frac{p}{5} = 15$$

$$(5)\frac{p}{5} = 15\,(5)$$

$$p = 75$$

Remember that when you do any inverse multiplication or division on <u>identical</u> numbers, the result will always be one; when you use inverse addition and subtraction on identical numbers, the result will always be zero.

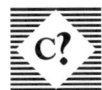

Checking Your Answer

The method for checking your answer when solving an equation is simple. Regardless of the operation you did, substitute the number you arrived at for the unknown in the problem. Consider the last problem.

$$\frac{p}{5} = 15$$

Substitute the 75 you have for your answer for *p*.

$$\frac{75}{5} = 15$$

If the equation is true, you know that you have the right solution.

EXERCISE 10–5

Directions: Solve and check the following equations. Pay attention to what operations you need to do to get the correct answers.

1. $c + 14 = 30$
2. $9 = p + 3$
3. $k - 13 = 3$
4. $25 = m - 5$
5. $36k = 9$

6. $100 = 10v$

7. $\frac{b}{88} = 11$

8. $64 = \frac{k}{7}$

9. $372 = 12n$

10. $\frac{x}{5} = 1$

GEOMETRY

Geometry is the part of mathematics that deals with the measuring of lines, angles, and shapes. As long as you are familiar with certain geometric terms and <u>concepts</u> you should have no trouble doing geometry problems.

Basic Geometry Terms

- A **point** is a precise location in space. Because it cannot be seen, a dot (·) is used to represent a point.

- A **line** is an endless set of points. In geometry, a line with an arrow at each end represents a line.

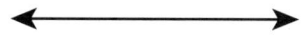

- An **angle** is formed when two straight lines meet at one point. Angles are measured in degrees from 0° to 360°.

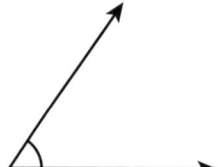

In geometry the common shapes are

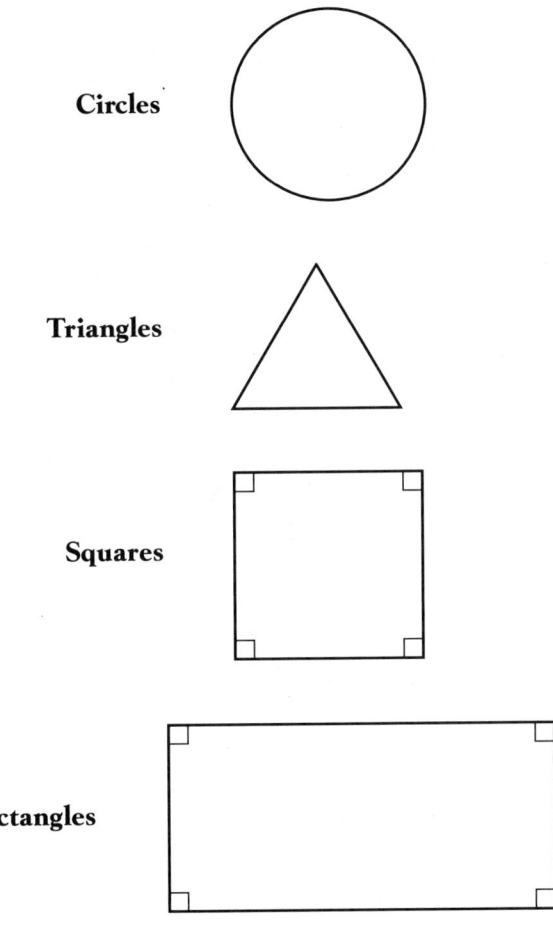

Circles

Triangles

Squares

Rectangles

Circles

A circle is a round shape with points that are an equal distance from the center. The **radius** (r) of the circle is a line that starts at the center and <u>extends</u> to the circle.

The **diameter** (d) is a line that starts at the circle, goes through the radius, and ends at the opposite side of the circle.

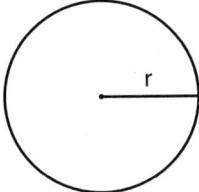 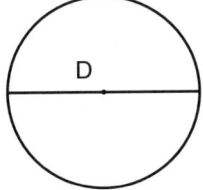

Finding the Diameter of a Circle

The diameter of a circle is twice as long as the radius. Therefore, to find the diameter of a circle, you multiply the radius by 2. Consider the following problem:

What is the diameter of a circle with a 10-inch radius? First, write the formula for finding the diameter. Note that d stands for diameter, r stands for the radius, and (2) means that you multiply the radius by 2.

$$d = r(2)$$

Next substitute a number for its letter. Place 10 in the problem for r.

$$d = 10(2)$$

Complete the problem. Multiply 10 by 2.

$$d = 20$$

The answer is 20 inches.

Finding the Radius of a Circle

To find the radius of a circle when the diameter is given, simply divide the diameter by 2.

$$r = d \div 2$$

Follow the steps for the next problem:
What is the radius of a circle with a diameter of 10 inches?
Since the radius of a circle is half the size of the diameter, divide the diameter by 2.

$$10 \div 2 = 5$$

The answer is 5 inches.

Finding the Circumference of a Circle

The circumference (c) of a circle is the measurement of the distance around the entire circle.

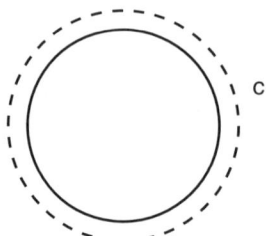

When trying to determine the relationship of the circumference to the diameter of any circle, you must do a ratio (c/d). However, when you use actual numbers to determine the ratio, you will create a nonending decimal. To simplify this fraction, the pi symbol is used (π). The value of pi is approximately 3.14, making the nonending decimal much more manageable.

Determining the Area of a Circle

The area (a) of a circle is all the space within the circle. To determine the area of a circle, you must understand a simple formula:

$$a = (\pi)r^2$$

In this formula, a = area; (π) = pi or 3.14; r^2 = radius multiplied by itself.
Look at the following problem:
If a circle has a radius 10 inches, what is the area?
To solve this problem, you must remove the letters and substitute the numbers given in the problem.

$$a = \pi r^2$$
$$a = 3.14 \, (10 \times 10)$$

Then work the numbers in parenthesis first. The r^2 means that you multiply a number by its own value. In other words, multiply the radius of 10 by 10.

$$10 \times 10 = 100$$

Then multiply the answer by the value of pi.

$$3.14 \, (100) = 314 \text{ inches.}$$

The area of the circle is 314 square inches.

EXERCISE 10–6

Directions: Solve the following problems.

1. What is the radius of a circle with a 20-inch diameter?
2. What is the radius of a circle with a 1-inch diameter?
3. What is the radius of a circle with a $9\frac{1}{2}$ inch diameter?
4. What is the diameter of a circle with a 7-inch radius?
5. What is the diameter of a circle with a 25-inch radius?
6. What is the diameter of a circle with a $\frac{3}{4}$-inch radius?
7. What is the area of a circle with a 5-inch radius?

164 MATHEMATICS STRATEGIES

8. What is the area of a circle with an 11-inch radius?
9. What is the area of a circle with a 25-inch radius?
10. What is the area of a circle with a $\frac{1}{10}$-inch radius?

Triangles

Triangle means "three angles," so all triangles contain three inside angles. These angles are measures in degrees (°). When you add up the number of degrees in a triangle, **it always equals 180 degrees.**

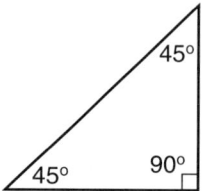

Types of Triangles

An **equilateral** triangle, as its name suggests, has three sides of equal length. Because the three sides are of equal length, the three angles are also equal. In other words, the three angles, which are measured in degrees, consist of the same number of degrees. Since the sum of all angles in a triangle equals 180 degrees, each of the three angles in an equilateral triangle is 180° ÷ 3 = 60°.

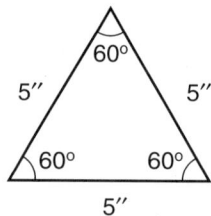

An **isosceles** triangle has two sides of equal length. The angles opposite the equal sides are equal also.

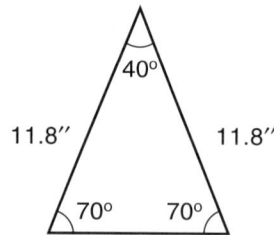

A **right** triangle has an angle that measures 90°. This creates one side that is longer than the other two sides. This side opposite the right angle is called the **hypotenuse.**

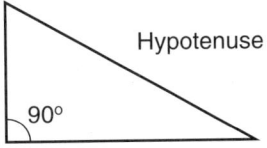

Depending on how it is drawn, an isosceles triangle can also be a right triangle. A **scalene** triangle has no sides that are equal. The angles are unequal also.

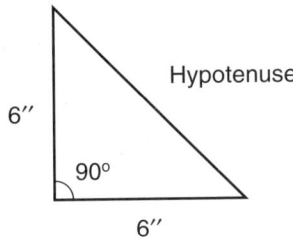
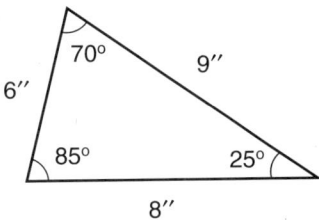

EXERCISE 10–7

Directions: Below is a chart representing three types of triangles—equilateral, isosceles, and scalene. Fill in the chart. Remember that the sum of all angles must equal 180°. The first has been done for you.

TYPE OF TRIANGLE	ANGLE A	ANGLE B	ANGLE C
equilateral	60	60	60
scalene	23	55	
right (isosceles)		45	
	35.5		35.5
	18.2	66	95.8
isosceles	15		
	99.4	3.6	
right			
scalene			
isosceles			

Squares

A square is a shape with four equal sides. The four angles are equal also. The angles of a square are right angles and equal 360°.

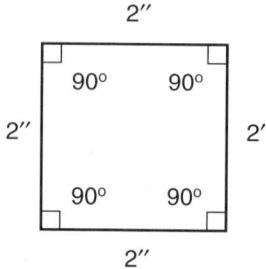

Finding the Perimeter of a Square

The **perimeter** of a square is the entire distance around the edges of the square. You can find the perimeter in two ways. The first way is to measure one side and, since all the sides are equal, add up the lengths of all four sides. The formula for finding the perimeter in this way is:

$$p = s1 + s2 + s3 + s4$$
$$8 = 2 + 2 + 2 + 2$$

In this formula, p stands for perimeter and s for side. The second way of determining the perimeter of a square is to measure one side and then multiply by 4. The formula looks like this:

$$p = 4s$$
$$48 = (4)(12)$$

EXERCISE 10-8

Directions: Find the perimeter for each of the following problems. Use either the addition formula or the multiplication formula.

What is the perimeter of a square that measures:

1. 5 inches?
2. 10.5 inches?
3. $9\frac{1}{4}$ feet?
4. $12\frac{3}{4}$ miles?
5. 100 kilometers?

Finding the Area of a Square

The **area** of a square is how much space is in the inside of the shape. To find the area of a square, measure one side and multiply the number by itself. The formula for finding the area of a square looks like the following where the small 2 is called an <u>exponent</u> and means to "square the number" or multiply it by itself:

$$a = s^2$$
$$a = 3(3) = 9 \text{ square units}$$

(Note that the answer will also be squared.)

EXERCISE 10–9

Directions: Study the above formula for finding the area of a square. Then solve the following problems:
What is the area of a square that measures:

1. 7 inches?
2. 64 feet?
3. $4\frac{1}{2}$ miles?
4. 6,000 kilometers?
5. 2,800 yards?

Rectangles

A rectangle is a shape whose opposite sides are equal in length with all right angles. The shorter sides of a rectangle are the width and the longer sides are the length.

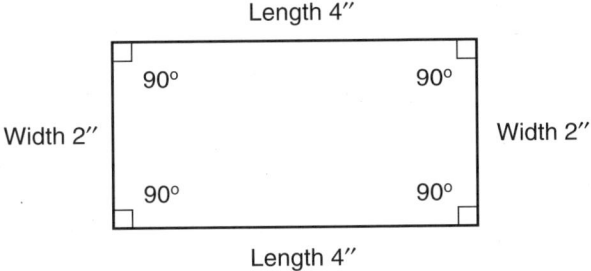

Finding the Perimeter of a Rectangle

To find the perimeter of a rectangle, add up the measurement of all four sides. Remember each side that is opposite will have the same measurement. The formula for finding the perimeter of a rectangle is:

$$p = s1 + s2 + s3 + s4$$
$$p = 2 + 4 + 2 + 4$$
$$p = 12$$

EXERCISE 10-10

Directions: Solve the following perimeter problems:
What is the perimeter of a rectangle with the following measurements?

1. width = 5; length = 8
2. width = 12 inches; length = $1\frac{1}{2}$ feet
3. width = $7\frac{1}{4}$ yards; length = $9\frac{3}{4}$ yards
4. width = 16 kilometers; length = 50 kilometers
5. width = 92 centimeters; length = 186 centimeters

Finding the Area of a Rectangle

To find the area of a rectangle, multiply length by width. The formula for determining the area of a rectangle looks like the following:

$$a = (l)(w)$$
$$a = 4 \times 2$$
$$a = 8$$

EXERCISE 10-11

Directions: Find the area for the following rectangles. Refer to the formula above if necessary.

1. length = 10, width = 4
2. length = 9.5 inches; width = 0.5 inch
3. length = $4\frac{1}{6}$ feet; width = 3 feet
4. length = 21 centimeters; width = 18 centimeters
5. length = 24 miles; width = $\frac{1}{2}$ mile

THE METRIC SYSTEM

The metric system is a system of measurements. Another system of measurements is called the English system. The United States is one of the very few countries that use the English system of measuring. Most of the world, including the health fields, use the metric system of measuring. Therefore, it is very important to be familiar with the metric system. Table 10-1 shows how measurements in the English system and the metric system are equivalent. Since some of the equivalent numbers can be long and

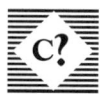

TABLE 10-1. Metric System and English System Conversion Chart

METRIC LENGTHS	ENGLISH LENGTHS
1 meter =	39.37 inches
1 meter =	3.28 feet
1 meter =	1.09 yards
1 centimeter =	0.4 inch
1 millimeter	0.04 inch
1 kilometer	0.62 mile
ENGLISH LENGTHS	**METRIC LENGTHS**
1 inch =	25.4 millimeters
1 inch =	2.54 centimeters
1 inch =	0.0254 meter
1 foot =	0.3 meter
1 yard =	0.91 meter
1 mile =	1.61 kilometers
METRIC LIQUID MEASURES	**ENGLISH LIQUID MEASURES**
1 liter =	1.06 quarts
ENGLISH LIQUID MEASURES	**METRIC LIQUID MEASURES**
1 quart =	0.95 liter
METRIC MEASURE OF WEIGHT	**ENGLISH MEASURE OF WEIGHT**
1 gram =	0.04 ounce
1 kilogram =	2.2 pounds
1 metric ton =	2204.62 pounds
ENGLISH MEASURE OF WEIGHT	**METRIC MEASURE OF WEIGHT**
1 ounce =	28.35 grams
1 pound =	0.45 kilogram
1 short ton (2000 pounds) =	0.91 metric ton
METRIC MEASURE OF AREA	**ENGLISH MEASURE OF AREA**
1 square centimeter =	0.155 square inch
1 square meter =	10.76 square feet
1 square meter =	1.2 square yards
1 square kilometer =	0.39 square mile
ENGLISH MEASURE OF AREA	**METRIC MEASURE OF AREA**
1 square inch =	6.45 square centimeters
1 square foot =	0.09 square meter
1 square yard =	0.84 square meter
1 square mile =	2.59 square kilometers

Copyright © 1995 by W.B. SAUNDERS COMPANY. All rights reserved. Printed in the United States of America.

complicated decimal numbers, they have been rounded off.

To change from the metric system to the English system, multiply the amount of the metric measure by its equivalent in the English system. For example, to change 5 kilometers to miles, multiply 5 kilometers by 0.62 miles.

$$5 \times 0.62 = 3.1 \text{ miles}$$

To change from the English system to the metric system, multiply the amount of the English measure by its equivalent in the metric system. For example, to change 2 inches to centimeters, multiply 2 inches by 2.54 centimeters.

$$2 \times 2.54 = 5.08 \text{ centimeters}$$

EXERCISE 10–12

Directions: Study Table 10–1. Then answer the following questions.

Change the following liters to quarts:

1. 3 liters
2. 18 liters

Change the following square centimeters to square inches:

3. 9 square centimeters
4. 10 square centimeters

Change the following kilometers to miles:

5. 4 kilometers
6. 30 kilometers

Change the following yards to meters:

7. 7 yards
8. 45 yards

Change the following pounds to kilograms:

9. 18 pounds
10. 50 pounds

REVIEWING THE LEARNING STRATEGIES

TO LEARN	USE THIS STRATEGY
Addition of signed numbers with the same sign	Add and use that sign in the answer
Addition of signed numbers with different signs	Subtract and use the sign of the larger number in the answer
Subtraction of signed numbers	Change the sign of the number being subtracted and add
Multiplication of signed numbers	If signs are similar, the product is positive If signs are different, the product is negative
Division of signed numbers	If signs are the same, the quotient is positive If signs are different, the quotient is negative
To solve for the unknown in an equation	Use inverse operations
To find the diameter of a circle	$d = r(2)$
To find the radius of a circle when the diameter is given	$r = d \div 2$
To find the area of a circle	$a = \pi r^2$
About triangles	Review the definitions of equilateral, isosceles, right, and scalene triangles
To find the perimeter of a square	$p = s1 + s2 + s3 + s4,\ p = 4s$
To find the area of a square	$a = s^2$
To find the perimeter of a rectangle	$p = s1 + s2 + s3 + s4$
To find the area of a rectangle	$a = (l)(w)$
To convert from the English system to the metric system or from the metric system to the English system	Review the equivalent chart

Chapter 11

Solving Word Problems

LEARNING OBJECTIVES
VOCABULARY WORDS
VOCABULARY CHECK
CAREFUL READING
FORMULATING QUESTIONS
SIGNAL WORDS
    Signal Words in Addition Problems
    Signal Words in Subtraction Problems
    Signal Words in Multiplication Problems
    Signal Words in Division Problems
PRACTICING WHAT YOU HAVE LEARNED
REVIEWING THE LEARNING STRATEGIES

LEARNING OBJECTIVES

In this chapter you will learn how to
- Carefully read word problems
- Clarify the information in word problems
- Determine the correct operations to use for solving word problems
- Check your answer

VOCABULARY WORDS

The following vocabulary words are important to your understanding of the ideas in this chapter. These vocabulary words are underscored the first time they are used in the chapter. Read the list of words and definitions. Then check your understanding of these words before you read the chapter.

data factual information, usually in number form.
formulate devise.
intimidated made timid or fearful.
logically relating to the ability to use reason.
product the answer in a multiplication problem.
quadrupled made four times greater.
quantity amount or total.
quotient the answer in a division problem.
respectively in the given order.
sum the answer in an addition problem.

VOCABULARY CHECK

Directions: Choose the vocabulary word that best fits into the sentence.

1. He _____ his money by investing wisely.
2. You purchased the right amount; the _____ was perfect.
3. Three is the _____ of 6 divided by 2.
4. He keyed in all the statistical _____ on his computer.
5. The bully _____ the young school child.
6. The _____ of 5 times 5 is 25.
7. The dime and the quarter belonged to Lulu and Mrs. Scheer, _____.
8. Eight is the _____ of 6 plus 2.
9. He worked at the puzzle very _____.
10. They will _____ the complete study schedule.

Example 11–1

Word Problem: The medical secretary typed two reports of 18 pages each. The next day she typed four reports of 21 pages, 11 pages, 16 pages, and 4 pages, <u>respectively</u>. How many times did the medical secretary go to the bubbler?

To many otherwise capable students, all word problems make as much sense as the one above. They are <u>intimidated</u> just by the idea of having to solve even the simplest word problem. The good news is that this does not have to be the case. Once you learn how to read a word problem, <u>formulate</u> your own questions and look for the signal words that will tell you what operation to perform, word problems will no longer seem as confusing as the one above.

CAREFUL READING

The first strategy to use for solving a word problem is to read the problem very carefully. This means that you have to slow down your rate of reading. If there are any words you do not understand, you should look up their meanings in a dictionary if you can. Careful reading of a word problem also means that you may have to read the problem more than once. Remember that there will be no correct solution to the word problem if you do not understand what you are reading and what the words mean.

EXERCISE 11-1

Directions: Below is an example of a word problem. Read the problem carefully. In the space provided, write the strategies you used to make the problem more understandable. Then solve the problem if you can.

Dr. Williams asked his medical secretary to check the electric and gas bills for the office. The reading for last month's electrical meter was 4,295 kilowatt hours, and this month's reading of the electric meter was 5,229 kilowatt hours. How many kilowatt hours were used in Dr. William's office this month? The medical secretary then read the gas meter and remembered that last month's reading was 6,879 hundred cubic feet and that this month's reading was 8,432 hundred cubic feet. How many hundred cubic feet of gas was used this month?

Strategies used to understand this problem: _____

_____

_____

_____

_____

Solutions to this problem: _____

FORMULATING QUESTIONS

Once you feel that you understand the problem, the second strategy for solving word problems is to formulate or create questions to help you begin to solve the problem. The types of questions you can use to aid you in answering the word problems are as follows:

1. What <u>data</u> or numbers are given in the problem?
   Make a list of all the numbers from the word problem on a separate piece of paper. The numbers in a word problem are the heart of the problem. Make sure you are seeing them correctly by rewriting them.
2. What is the question being asked?
   It is important that you recognize the sentence that is asking you to perform a specific mathematical operation. This is a major step in solving the word problem. Table 11-1 lists some of the words used for the question sentence in a word problem.

TABLE 11-1 Some Words Used in the Question Sentence of a Word Problem

QUESTION WORD	EXAMPLE
How	How many are there?
	How much does it cost?
What	What is the total?
Where	Where are the most trees?
When	When will he return?
Which	Which brother is older?
	Which is more expensive?
Who	Who spent the most money?

3. What operation do you use?

   There are words in the problem that will tell you how to solve the word problem. These specific signal words will be discussed later in the chapter.

4. Does my answer make sense?

   This is the question you will use to prove that your answer is correct. In a word problem, you need to check to see whether your answer logically relates to the other numbers in the problem. In other words, you need to determine whether your answer is too large or too small on the basis of the data supplied.

EXERCISE 11-2

Directions: Read the following word problem. Then answer the questions in the space provided.

Serena is reading her physics book. She learns that the speed of sound is 1,088 feet per second. She also learns that the speed of light is 186,324 miles per second. How far does sound travel in 2 hours? How far does light travel in 2 hours?

1. What are the data in the problem? List these numbers.

   _____

   _____

   _____

2. What are the questions being asked?

   _____

   _____

   _____

3. What are the answers to this problem? (Hint: In the problem you were given the length of time in **seconds.** Since you are being asked for the length of time

in **hours,** a greater measure of time, you multiply. Also, there are 3,600 seconds in 1 hour.)

_____
_____

4. Does my answer make sense in relation to the numbers in the problem?

_____

SIGNAL WORDS

As mentioned earlier in this chapter, there are signal words that will tell you what operation to do to solve the word problem. Once you learn to recognize these signal words, you will be able to answer most word problems. The signal words will help you recognize addition, subtraction, multiplication, and division word problems.

Signal Words in Addition Problems

If you see the words in Table 11–2 in a word problem, use addition to get the answer.

EXERCISE 11–3

Directions: Read the following word problems. Answer the questions in the space provided.

A. There are three laboratories in the veterinary school. The first lab has 6 Bunsen burners; the second lab has 5 Bunsen burners and the third lab has 11 Bunsen burners. How many Bunsen burners are in the veterinary school all together?

1. What are the data in this problem?

_____
_____

TABLE 11–2   Addition Signal Words

ADDITION WORD	EXAMPLE
Add	Add the 2 totals together.
Added to	5 was added to 2.
All together	How much was spent all together?
Both	How far did both kids run?
How much	How much did the 3 cats cost?
In all	How many chickens in all were sold?
Increased by	Her waist increased by how many inches?
More than	Peppy has 2 more books than Leslie's 4 books.
Plus	5 rugs plus 4 rugs equal how many rugs?
Sum	The sum of 18 and 19 is what?
Total	What is the total number of fat rats?

2. What question is asked in the problem?

3. What is the question word or words?

4. What are the signal words?

5. What operation do you do to get the answer?

6. What is the answer to the word problem?

7. Does your answer make sense in relation to the numbers in the problem?

B. Three hundred twenty-two persons applied to the dental school in Chicago. Four hundred three persons applied to the dental school in Boston. Six hundred fifty-nine persons applied to the dental school in Atlanta. What is the total number of persons applying to dental schools in Chicago, Boston, and Atlanta?

1. What are the data in this problem?

2. What question is asked in the problem?

3. What is the question word or words?

4. What are the signal words?

5. What operation do you do to get the answer?

6. What is the answer to the word problem?

7. Does your answer make sense in relation to the numbers in the problem?

Signal Words in Subtraction Problems

If you see the words in Table 11–3 in a word problem, use subtraction to get the answer.

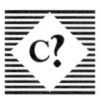

EXERCISE 11–4

Directions: Read the following word problems. Answer the questions in the space provided.

A. Mr. Francis is 5 feet 8 inches tall. Mrs. Francis is smaller than Mr. Francis by 4 inches. How tall is Mrs. Francis?

1. What are the data in this problem?

2. What question is asked in the problem?

3. What is the question word or words?

4. What are the signal words?

5. What operation do you do to get the answer?

TABLE 11-3 Subtraction Signal Words

SUBTRACTION WORDS	EXAMPLE
Decreased by	His allowance was decreased by $2.
Difference	What was the difference in salary?
Fewer	How many fewer dogs are there?
Have left	How many eggs does she have left?
Left over	How much dough was left over?
Less than	He has 6 boats less than his brother.
Remain	17 cups remain out of 20.
Smaller than	Gabrielle is smaller by 6 inches than Josephina.
Subtract	Subtract 10 from 100.
Take away	11 take away 2 equals what?

    6. What is the answer to the word problem?

    7. Does your answer make sense in relation to the numbers in the problem?

B. Benny's studying time has been decreased by 8 hours. Before this, he was able to study 24 hours per week. How many study hours remain for Benny?

    1. What are the data in this problem?

    2. What question is asked in the problem?

    3. What is the question word or words?

    4. What are the signal words?

    5. What operation do you do to get the answer?

180 MATHEMATICS STRATEGIES

6. What is the answer to the word problem?

   _____

7. Does your answer make sense in relation to the numbers in the problem?

   _____

Signal Words in Multiplication Problems

If you see the words in Table 11–4 in a word problem, use multiplication to get the answer.

In addition to these signal words, you may see an occasional word problem that will tell you the <u>quantity</u> of one item and ask you to find the quantity of many items. For example, the problem will give you the price or length of an object and will ask you to find the price or length of 10 objects. Multiply when you see this kind of problem.

EXERCISE 11–5

Directions: Read the following word problems. Answer the questions in the space provided.

A. Jon's rate of reading is 250 words per minute. How many words can he read in an hour?

1. What are the data in this problem?

   _____
   _____

2. What question is asked in the problem?

   _____
   _____
   _____

3. What is the question word or words?

   _____
   _____

4. What are the signal words?

   _____

5. What operation do you do to get the answer?

   _____

TABLE 11-4 Multiplication Signal Words

MULTIPLICATION WORDS	EXAMPLE
Double, triple, etc.	Recently, his salary doubled.
Multiply	Multiply $5 by 4 weeks.
Product (answer in a multiplication problem)	What is the product of 94 multiplied by 6?
Times	What does 9 times 2 equal?

6. What is the answer to the word problem?

7. Does your answer make sense in relation to the numbers in the problem?

B. Carole earned $1000 per week last year. This year she received a raise that quadrupled her salary. How much is she earning now?

1. What are the data in this problem?

2. What question is asked in the problem?

3. What is the question word or words?

4. What are the signal words?

5. What operation do you do to get the answer?

6. What is the answer to the word problem?

7. Does your answer make sense in relation to the numbers in the problem?

Signal Words in Division Problems

If you see the words in Table 11–5 in a word problem, use division to get the answer.

In addition to these signal words, you may see a word problem that tells you the value of many items and asks you to figure out the value of one item. For example, the problem will give you the width or size of many objects and will ask you to figure out the width or size of one object. Use division when you see this kind of problem.

EXERCISE 11–6

Directions: Read the following word problems. Answer the questions in the space provided.

A. Melissa is 9 years 10 months old. Her younger sister Lauren is half of that age. How old is Lauren?

1. What are the data in this problem?

2. What question is asked in the problem?

3. What is the question word or words?

4. What are the signal words?

5. What operation do you do to get the answer?

TABLE 11–5 Division Signal Words

DIVISION WORDS	EXAMPLE
Divide	Divide the cost of the car by 12 months.
Half of	Half of 900 is what?
Separate	Separate the 12 apples into 6 containers.
Quotient (answer in a division problem)	What is the quotient of 81 divided by 9?

6. What is the answer to the word problem?

7. Does your answer make sense in relation to the numbers in the problem?

B. Video tapes were on sale. The cost for 12 videos was $250.00. What was the cost of 1 video?

1. What are the data in this problem?

2. What question is asked in the problem?

3. What is the question word or words?

4. What are the signal words?

5. What operation do you do to get the answer?

6. What is the answer to the word problem?

7. Does your answer make sense in relation to the numbers in the problem?

PRACTICING WHAT YOU HAVE LEARNED

EXERCISE 11–17

Directions: Following are some word problems. Read the problems carefully to make sure you understand what you need to do to correctly answer the questions. On a separate piece of paper, make up your own questions or answer the questions above to clarify the problems further. Look for the question and signal words that will tell you what operations you need to do to answer the questions. Write the answers in the space provided.

1. The LPN was responsible for carrying 5 trays of food on Sunday, 7 trays on Monday, 9 trays on Tuesday, 11 trays on Wednesday, 5 trays again on Thursday, 6 on Friday, and none on Saturday. What is the total number of trays the LPN carried in a week?

    Answer _____

2. How many trays of food did the LPN carry in 13 weeks?

    Answer _____

3. The radiographic technician earns $36,000 per year. What is his monthly salary?

    Answer _____

4. The health care student bought her uniform on sale. The original price was $32.98. The store was willing to reduce the price $2.95. How much does the student have to spend to buy the uniform?

    Answer _____

5. Larry wants to buy a medical dictionary that costs $75.00. He is able to pay half in cash and the rest in equal payments for 6 months. How much are Larry's monthly payments?

    Answer _____

6. Elizabeth is the smartest student in her dental hygienist program. She studies $4\frac{1}{4}$ hours on Monday, $2\frac{1}{2}$ hours on Tuesday, and $8\frac{3}{4}$ hours on both Saturday and Sunday. How many hours does Elizabeth study per week?

    Answer _____

7. There are 245 women in the medical assistant's program and 5 men. What percentage of the class is male?

    Answer _____

8. Tony works in the lab for $8\frac{1}{2}$ hours every day for a week. What is the total number of hours Tony works in the lab?

    Answer _____

9. Mr. Roth made $9\frac{1}{8}$ quarts of the solution. He wants to keep the solution in flasks that hold $1\frac{1}{2}$ quarts each. How many flasks will he need?

   Answer _____

10. The mileage on the ambulance reads 32,980.7 miles. The ambulance is driven 1,003.2 miles more. What is the new mileage?

    Answer _____

11. Lisa runs the 40-yard long hospital corridor in 13.8 seconds. Tom runs the same corridor in 15.9 seconds. How much slower is Tom?

    Answer _____

12. The bus fare to the medical center was raised from $1.00 to $1.25. A student needs to take the bus twice a day, Monday through Friday. How much more will the student spend on bus fare per week?

    Answer _____

13. The cost of 10 cans of soda pop in the hospital cafeteria is $7.70. What is the cost of 1 can of pop?

    Answer _____

14. Blossom typed $\frac{1}{8}$ of the medical report on Monday. She typed $\frac{1}{4}$ of the medical report on Tuesday. How much of the medical report does Blossom need to type to finish it on Wednesday?

    Answer _____

15. Michael uses $2\frac{3}{4}$ ounces of alcohol in a solution. How many ounces of alcohol does he need to make $\frac{1}{4}$ of the solution?

    Answer _____

16. Sara cut gauze that was $1\frac{1}{3}$ yards long into four bandages. How long was each bandage?

    Answer _____

17. The phlebotomy program has 700 students this year. The program's assistant director must order 95 syringes for each of the students. What is the product of 700 times 95?

    Answer _____

18. The head of the dental assistant's program makes $60,000 annually. The financial officer of the program wants to know how much the head of the program makes monthly. What is the quotient of $60,000 divided by 12?

    Answer _____

19. You were assigned 225 pages to read. You finished $\frac{1}{4}$ of them. How many pages remain to be read?

    Answer _____

20. Dr. T. Brown collected $2,265 in patients' fees for one day. He saw 30 patients that day. How much money did each patient pay to the doctor?

    Answer _____

REVIEWING THE LEARNING STRATEGIES

TO LEARN	USE THIS STRATEGY
To read word problems carefully	Slow down reading rate Look up unknown words in the dictionary Reread problem
To clarify word problems	Answer these questions: What are the data given? What is the question being asked?
To determine what mathematical operation to do	Learn signal words for addition, subtraction, multiplication, and division.
To check your answer	Answer this question: Does my answer make sense in relation to the data given in the problem?

UNIT IV

STUDY STRATEGIES

Learning study strategies will help you organize your time and information so that you will become a more efficient learner. You will find that applying these strategies to the subjects you are studying will give you a plan to keep up with your assignments and achieve better grades. Chapter 12, Managing Time, will teach you how to set and prioritize goals, schedule your study time, and eliminate distractions. Chapter 13, Learning Active Listening Skills, will demonstrate how applying active listening strategies will help you to improve your concentration during lectures. Chapter 14, Taking Notes, will give you the strategies you need to focus on the important information in your lectures and textbooks. Chapter 15, Improving Test Scores, will teach you five strategies to help you prepare for and take tests more successfully. Applying the study strategies discussed in this unit will help you to improve your work habits and your test results.

Chapter 12

Managing Time

LEARNING OBJECTIVES
VOCABULARY WORDS
VOCABULARY CHECK
HOW TO MANAGE TIME
SETTING GOALS
PRIORITIZING GOALS
SCHEDULING
    Monthly Calendar
    Weekly Calendar
    Daily Calendar
    To-Do List
ELIMINATING DISTRACTIONS
    External Distractions
    Internal Distractions
MONITORING YOUR ABILITY TO MANAGE TIME
AVOIDING PROCRASTINATION
REVIEWING MANAGING TIME

LEARNING OBJECTIVE

In this chapter you will learn how to
- Organize your time so that you will improve your study habits.

VOCABULARY WORDS

The following vocabulary words are important to your understanding of the ideas in this chapter. These vocabulary words are underscored the first time they are used in the chapter. Read the list of words and definitions. Then check your understanding of these words before you read the chapter.

academic having to do with school or learning.
anxiety emotional pain.
external outside the body.
goals aims, intentions.
internal inside the body.
juggling dealing with several things at one time.
prioritize in order of importance.
procrastination delaying what needs to be done.
recreational having to do with activities designed for relaxation and fun.
tendency leaning toward.

VOCABULARY CHECK

Directions: Choose the vocabulary word that best fits into the sentence.

1. Cynthia was filled with _____ because she was unprepared for her chemistry exam.
2. Tennis is a popular _____ activity.
3. Please _____ your concerns so that we can take care of them in order of importance.
4. _____ home and work responsibilities is often difficult.
5. Tarry has a _____ to manipulate a situation.
6. Maria worked hard to reach all her _____.
7. Jeffrey's habit of _____ prevents him from finishing his assignments on time.
8. _____ events such as work pressures intruded on her personal life.
9. _____ thoughts kept Robert from concentrating on what the speaker was announcing.
10. The school offers a wide range of _____ subjects because it has a varied curriculum.

HOW TO MANAGE TIME

Many students find that they have difficulty getting started on assignments. As the semester goes on, they suddenly realize that they have fallen so far behind that it is difficult to catch up. Learning strategies for managing time will help you to avoid that problem. You will learn how to organize your time by

- Setting goals
- Learning to prioritize

- Scheduling
- Eliminating distractions
- Monitoring your ability to manage time
- Avoiding procrastination

SETTING GOALS

Establish goals for the semester as a whole. What do you want to accomplish by the end of the semester? When setting semester goals, you have to think about all your responsibilities and interests. How many courses are you planning to take during the semester?

Are you working while attending school? Do you work part-time or full-time? Day or evening? What are your home and family responsibilities? Do you have special hobbies, recreational interests, or volunteer activities?

Sometimes you can feel overwhelmed by all that you need to do. A solution is to make a list of your goals like the one that follows. List everything you want to achieve for the semester. Make sure that your goals are balanced. Allow some recreational time. It is not realistic to plan your semester with just study and work.

ONE STUDENT'S SEMESTER GOALS

- Taking full-time schedule at school to become a dental hygienist
- Practice piano 5 hours a week
- Grocery shopping for family
- Volunteer tutoring at public library 1 hour a week
- Part-time job 8 hours a week

EXERCISE 12–1

Directions: Make a list of your semester goals

_____
_____
_____
_____
_____

PRIORITIZING GOALS

Prioritizing goals is placing your goals in order of importance to you. Think about your list of semester goals. Some are more urgent than others. When you are in school, studying for an exam should take priority over going to the movies. Keep in mind that prioritizing will help you to accomplish your most important goals first. Be realistic about what you expect to accomplish in a semester. Decide what goals are most important and focus on achieving those goals.

ONE STUDENT'S PRIORITIZED SEMESTER GOALS

1. Taking full-time schedule at school to become a dental hygienist
2. Grocery shopping for family
3. Working part-time 8 hours a week
4. Practice piano 5 hours a week
5. Volunteer tutoring at public library 1 hour a week

EXERCISE 12–2

Directions Decide what is most important to you and prioritize your list of semester goals.

_____
_____
_____
_____
_____

SCHEDULING

Planning and following a schedule will help you to organize your time. Once you have decided and prioritized your semester goals, you should schedule your time so that you can realistically meet your goals. Using calendars helps you stick to a schedule. Monthly, weekly, and daily calendars will help you plan your time efficiently.

Monthly Calendar

Use monthly calendars to plan long-range assignments. Some helpful information to place on your monthly calendar:

- Test dates
- Vacation dates
- Due dates of reports and projects

EXERCISE 12–3

Directions: Fill in the monthly calendar (Fig. 12–1). List any important test dates or long-range plans on the calendar.

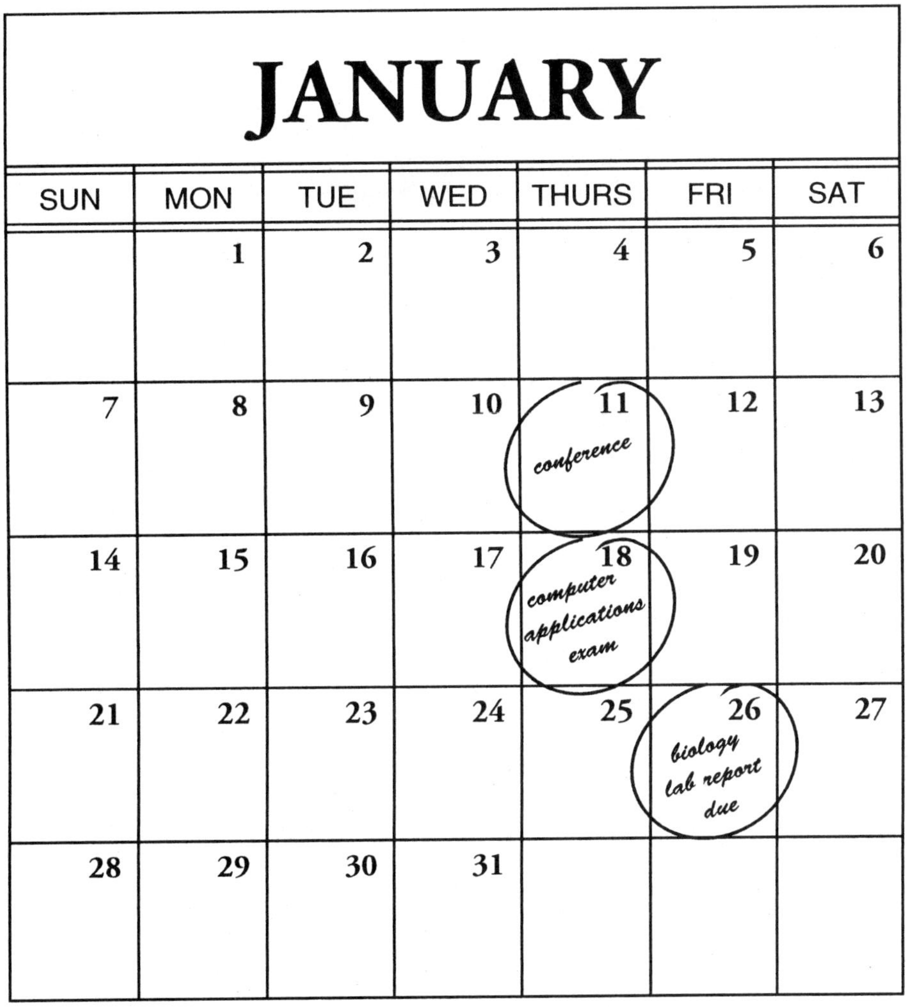

			JANUARY			
SUN	MON	TUE	WED	THURS	FRI	SAT
	1	2	3	4	5	6
7	8	9	10	11 *conference*	12	13
14	15	16	17	18 *computer applications exam*	19	20
21	22	23	24	25	26 *biology lab report due*	27
28	29	30	31			

FIGURE 12–1 A monthly calendar with special assignment dates marked.

Weekly Calendar

Using a weekly calendar will help you to organize your time and to follow a regular schedule. Successful students use weekly calendars to help them work on their assignments at scheduled times. They establish a place to study and a time to study and they follow a regular study plan.

You use a weekly calendar to organize all your activities for the week. You plan your activities at the beginning of each week and follow the schedule as closely as possible. Some of the activities you would put on your weekly schedule are class hours, work hours, mealtimes, sleep time, extracurricular activities, sports practice. Then circle the hours that are free for study. Be realistic. Allow some unscheduled time for relaxing and recreation. Once you have decided *when* you want to study, then you should decide *where* you want to study. Your choice of study place should be quiet, well lit, and free from distractions. Study wherever you will concentrate best, whether it is at home or the library. After you have decided when and where you want to study, you are beginning to get organized. Sticking to the schedule you have planned will help you to manage your time.

EXERCISE 12-4

Directions: Fill in the weekly calendar (Fig. 12–2) at the beginning of the week. As you go through the week, make a check mark next to each task you complete. You will then see at a glance whether you are accomplishing your goals. Remember, you may have to make changes in your calendar as the week progresses, but by planning your week you are learning to manage your time efficiently.

TIME	SUN	MON	TUES	WED	THURS	FRI	SAT
7–8 AM							
8–9							
9–10							
10–11							
11–12							
12–1 PM							
1–2							
2–3							
3–4							
4–5							
5–6							
6–7							
7–8							
8–9							

FIGURE 12–2 A weekly calendar.

Daily Calendar

Use the daily calendar (Fig. 12–3) to help you focus on your priorities. Each night, think about what you want to accomplish the next day. Write a "to-do" list.

To-Do List

A to-do list is your list of everything you want to accomplish the next day. The list includes both <u>academic</u> and nonacademic tasks. Each night, write down everything you need to do on a piece of paper. Be specific as you write your list. Then prioritize your list and transfer this information into the time slots of your daily calendar (Table 12–1).

(✓) When Completed

9:00 – 9:30	
9:30 – 10:00	
10:00 – 10:30	
10:30 – 11:00	
11:00 – 11:30	
11:30 – 12:00	
12:00 – 12:30	
12:30 – 1:00	
1:00 – 1:30	
1:30 – 2:00	
2:00 – 2:30	
2:30 – 3:00	
3:00 – 3:30	
3:30 – 4:00	
4:00 – 4:30	
4:30 – 5:00	
5:00 – 5:30	
5:30 – 6:00	
6:00 – 6:30	
6:30 – 7:00	
7:00 – 7:30	
7:30 – 8:00	
8:00 – 8:30	
8:30 – 9:00	

FIGURE 12–3 A daily calendar.

TABLE 12-1 One Student's To-Do List

TO-DO LIST	PRIORITIZED TO-DO LIST
Do grocery shopping	1. Attend English class
Go to post office	2. Read Chapter 7 in biology text
Read Chapter 7 in biology text	3. Do grocery shopping
Attend English class	4. Practice piano
Practice piano	5. Go to post office

Daily Calendar: Check when completed.

____ 11:00–12:00 English class

____ 2:00–2:30 Do grocery shopping

____ 2:30–3:00 Go to post office

____ 3:30–4:30 Practice piano

____ 5:00–6:30 Read Chapter 7 in biology text

EXERCISE 12-5

Directions: Write a to-do list. Prioritize your list and fill these items into the time slot on your daily calendar. Make a check mark next to each task that you complete.

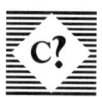

ELIMINATING DISTRACTIONS

Students are often distracted. These distractions, <u>external</u> and <u>internal</u>, waste your time.

External Distractions

External distractions are elements in your surroundings that prevent you from accomplishing your goals. Some external distractions are the telephone, television, computer games, and excessive socializing. Staying on schedule will eliminate the <u>tendency</u> to allow these distractions from taking up too much of your time.

Internal Distractions

Internal distractions are your thoughts and feelings that interfere with your ability to concentrate.

The daily calendar will help you to eliminate internal distractions. You will focus on completing each task rather than wasting your time worrying about things that are out of your control. Sticking to a schedule keeps you organized and focused. Your concentration will improve.

MONITORING YOUR ABILITY TO MANAGE TIME

Managing time will help you to be a successful student. Once you have learned the strategies for managing time, you should stop and ask yourself whether these strategies are working for you. Ask yourself:

- Does my weekly schedule allow enough time for study?
- Am I still wasting too much time?
- Does my daily schedule allow me to take care of my important priorities?
- Am I meeting my semester goals?

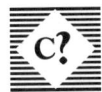

AVOIDING PROCRASTINATION

If you are managing time, you will avoid procrastination, delaying what needs to be done. Do your work now—not later. Procrastination is the greatest source of anxiety for students. You will be more relaxed and your grades will improve if you don't procrastinate. Schedule your difficult assignments first, when your concentration is best. If you can discipline yourself to follow your schedule, you won't get into the habit of procrastination.

Managing your time will help you to be successful in juggling all your responsibilities at home, at work, and in school.

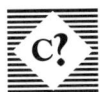

REVIEWING MANAGING TIME

TO LEARN	USE THIS STRATEGY
To set goals	Make a list of your semester goals.
To prioritize goals	Place your goals in order of importance to you.
To schedule	Use monthly, weekly, and daily calendars.
To eliminate distractions	Stay on schedule and concentrate on completing your tasks in order of importance.
To monitor your ability to manage time	Ask yourself whether your schedule is helping you to achieve your goals.
To avoid procrastination	Do work now—not later—stick to your schedule.

Chapter 13

Learning Active Listening Skills

LEARNING OBJECTIVES
VOCABULARY WORDS
VOCABULARY CHECK
UNDERSTANDING THE DIFFERENCE BETWEEN LISTENING AND HEARING
EVALUATING YOUR LISTENING HABITS
LEARNING STRATEGIES FOR ACTIVE LISTENING
MONITORING YOUR LISTENING COMPREHENSION
APPLYING ACTIVE LISTENING STRATEGIES TO SUCCESS IN SCHOOL
REVIEWING ACTIVE LISTENING STRATEGIES

LEARNING OBJECTIVES

In this chapter you will learn how to
- Evaluate your listening habits
- Monitor your listening comprehension
- Learn strategies for active listening
- Apply active listening strategies for success in school

VOCABULARY WORDS

The following vocabulary words are important to your understanding of the ideas in this chapter. These vocabulary words are <u>underscored</u> the first time they are used in the chapter. Read the list of words and definitions. Then check your understanding of these words before you read the chapter.

content the material to be learned in a course.
coworkers fellow employees.

distracted to have attention taken away.
interfere to get in the way of.
highlight emphasize.
journal an account of daily events.
objective lack of feeling toward or against.
passive not active.
rote use of memory without thought.
subject topic or area to be learned.

VOCABULARY CHECK

Directions: Choose the vocabulary word that best fits the sentence.

1. Catherine used a yellow marker to _____ the main ideas in her textbook.

2. My _____ and I have worked together for 5 years.

3. Math is my favorite _____.

4. Steven is easily _____ from his studies.

5. The English instructor assigned the class to write a _____ to keep a record of their daily activities.

6. Jonas didn't really understand the material, he learned it by _____.

7. I find the _____ of my chemistry course more difficult than I expected.

8. I wish you wouldn't _____ in my business.

9. Thelma is not _____ on this subject because she has strong feelings about this topic.

10. Wendy is _____ in class; she doesn't initiate any activity.

UNDERSTANDING THE DIFFERENCE BETWEEN LISTENING AND HEARING

Do you find that you have difficulty concentrating during class lectures? When you are working do you need to have your coworkers repeat instructions to you? Are you easily distracted when someone is speaking to you? If you have answered "yes" to these questions, you are hearing but not listening. When you are hearing, you are aware of sounds, but you are not interpreting these sounds into meaning. Listening involves comprehension. Listening is an active process. Hearing is passive. An active listener concentrates on and understands a speaker's main points. Your success in school and on the job is affected by your ability to be an active listener. You can learn how to focus your attention on a speaker's message.

EVALUATING YOUR LISTENING HABITS

One method of improving your listening skills is to evaluate your habits. Once you are aware of your listening problems, you can try to correct them. Eliminating bad listening habits will help you to learn important information in school and on the job.

Do you have any of the following listening problems?

_____ **Daydreaming.** Does your mind wander during class lectures? Do you find that you miss essential information before you come back to attention? Daydreaming is the most common listening problem. You can learn strategies to focus on a speaker's main ideas and keep your mind on the topic.

_____ **Pretending Attention.** Do you pretend to pay attention in class? Sometimes students are pretending to pay attention, but they are mentally asleep behind open eyes. When you are pretending attention, you are missing all the information. You are occupying a seat in class, but your mind is elsewhere.

_____ **Rote Note Taking.** Do you try to write every word instead of listening for your instructor's main points? When you are finished, you will end up with unfinished sentences and scrambled information. Rote note taking is a listening problem, because you are not focusing on the main ideas and important details.

_____ **Closing off the Subject or Speaker.** Do you turn off subjects or speakers without giving them a chance? Sometimes, you dislike a certain subject, and when you are required to take a course in this content area, you stop listening before the first class begins. Another problem occurs when you decide that you dislike your instructor before the semester begins. You might have heard negative things about this teacher from other students. However, you should be objective. Keep an open mind and give the instructor and the subject a chance. You will be surprised at how much you can learn if you give them your full attention.

_____ **Giving in to Distractions.** Do you get distracted easily? Do you let external noises, conversations, or events disturb you during class lessons? Sometimes, it is difficult to pay attention, but it is your responsibility as a listener to block out these distractions and to concentrate on your instructor's main ideas. Don't allow external distractions to interfere with your learning.

EXERCISE 13-1

Directions: Reread the list of five listening problems. Place a check next to any listening problem that you would like to improve.

LEARNING STRATEGIES FOR ACTIVE LISTENING

Now that you have recognized your listening problems, you can try to solve these problems by learning strategies for active listening.

To improve your listening concentration and comprehension,

- Listen for the main idea.
  Ask yourself: What is the topic of the lecture? What is the most important point being made about this topic?
- Listen for important details.
  Ask yourself: Which facts support the main idea?
- Paraphrase the information.
  Restate the speaker's ideas in your own words. Summarize the speakers message by asking the 5W questions.
  Who or **What** is the lecture about? _____
  What is the main point of the lecture? _____
  When? _____
  Where? _____
  Why or **How**? _____

MONITORING YOUR LISTENING COMPREHENSION

To monitor, or check, your active listening strategies, keep a listening journal for one week. This journal will help you keep track of your listening problems as they take place. You can then check to see if you did anything to correct your listening problem while you were in the situation. Did you remember to apply your active listening strategies? Did these strategies help to improve your concentration? Where you able to better understand your instructor's lecture? This listening journal will help you to check whether you are applying your active listening strategies.

As you can see from one student's listening journal (Fig. 13–1), the student is aware of listening problems and is now monitoring whether these problems were corrected.

EXERCISE 13–2

Directions: Fill in a listening journal (Fig. 13–2) for 1 week of classes. Monitor your listening comprehension. Then, evaluate your listening habits.

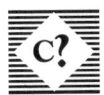

	Class	Type of Listening Problem	Did I Apply Listening Strategies?	Was I Able to Paraphrase and Summarize the Information?
Monday	Biology	Pretending attention	No	No
Tuesday	English	Giving into distractions	Yes	Yes. Main point of lesson was how to revise an essay.
Wednesday	Computer	Closing off to speaker	No	No. I could not follow directions.
Thursday	Math applications	Daydreaming	Yes	No. I already missed important information.
Friday	Part-time job	Closing off to subject	Yes	I understood the directions I had to follow to finish the job.

Figure 13-1 One student's listening journal.

Class	Type of Listening Problem	Did I Apply Listening Strategies?	Was I Able to Paraphrase and Summarize the Information?
Monday			
Tuesday			
Wednesday			
Thursday			
Friday			

Figure 13-2 A listening journal.

APPLYING ACTIVE LISTENING STRATEGIES TO SUCCESS IN SCHOOL

Once you have learned active listening strategies, you can apply these strategies to improve your grades. You can be actively involved in improving your listening skills.

Are you physically and mentally prepared to pay attention in class? If you are tired or hungry, it is difficult to concentrate. Did you do your assignment? Class preparation makes you eager to listen. If you are unprepared, you probably feel uncomfortable and this discomfort interferes with concentration.

Pay attention to your instructor. Look directly at the speaker. Participate in class. Ask questions and listen for the answers. Sit in the front of the room if you have trouble seeing, hearing, or concentrating. Get involved in class discussions. Think about and react to the ideas discussed in class.

Applying active listening strategies will help you to take good notes in class. To take effective notes remember to:

- Listen for main ideas and important details.
- Paraphrase and summarize the information discussed in class.
- Pay extra attention to the instructor's introductory statements and summaries that <u>highlight</u> the most important ideas of the lesson.

Learning active listening strategies will help you to improve your grades. You will learn how to concentrate during class lessons, take better notes, and be actively involved in your success in school.

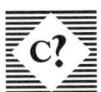

REVIEWING LEARNING STRATEGIES FOR ACTIVE LISTENING

TO LEARN	USE THIS STRATEGY
The difference between listening and hearing	Concentrate on and interpret the speaker's message.
How to evaluate your listening habits	Be aware of five listening problems: • Daydreaming • Pretending attention • Rote note taking • Closing off the subject or speaker • Giving in to distractions
Strategies for active listening	Listen for main ideas and important details. Paraphrase and summarize information.
To monitor your listening comprehension	Keep a listening journal.
To apply active listening strategies to success in school	Be prepared for listening physically and mentally. Take good notes.

Chapter 14

Taking Notes

LEARNING OBJECTIVES
VOCABULARY WORDS
VOCABULARY CHECK
IMPORTANCE OF TAKING GOOD NOTES
USING YOUR NOTES SUCCESSFULLY
TIME MANAGEMENT AND NOTE TAKING
CHOOSING YOUR NOTEBOOK
ORGANIZING YOUR NOTEPAPER
TAKING NOTES FROM YOUR TEXTBOOK
HIGHLIGHTING
MARGIN WRITING
TAKING NOTES FROM YOUR LECTURES
    Instructors' Cues
HOW MANY NOTES TO TAKE
FASTER NOTE TAKING
    Streamlining Your Handwriting
    Abbreviating and Using Symbols
TAPING YOUR LECTURES
STUDYING FROM YOUR NOTES
    Creating Headings
    Other Strategies for Studying Your Notes
REVIEWING THE LEARNING STRATEGIES

LEARNING OBJECTIVES

In this chapter you will learn how to
- Organize your notebook and notepaper
- Take notes from your textbook
- Take notes from your lectures
- Determine how many notes to take
- Take faster notes
- Study from your notes

VOCABULARY WORDS

The following vocabulary words are important to your understanding of the ideas in this chapter. These vocabulary words are underscored the first time they are used in the chapter. Read the list of words and definitions. Then check your understanding of these words before you read the chapter.

cardiac pertaining to the heart (Miller-Keane, p. 250).
chronological arranged in order of time.
complement to complete or make perfect.
condensing making something more compact.
conventional traditional.
indentation the division of a document to create sections.
microcapillary minute vessel connecting arterioles and venules (Miller-Keane, p. 245).
molecules the smallest amount of a substance that possesses its characteristic properties (Miller-Keane, p. 929).
portable able to be carried easily
venipuncture surgical puncture of a vein (Miller-Keane, p. 1597).

VOCABULARY CHECK

Directions: Choose the vocabulary word that best fits into the sentence.

1. A clearly written textbook will _____ a good lecture.
2. To draw blood you need to _____ a vein.
3. The elderly patient died from a _____ arrest.
4. A part of the circulatory system is a _____.
5. When she took brief notes from the lengthy textbook, she was _____ many of the author's ideas.
6. The smaller medical text was more _____ than the larger one.
7. He wrote his entire life history in _____ order.
8. In their chemistry class, the students studied _____ under a very powerful microscope.
9. The _____ of less important ideas was achieved with many margins.
10. The old-fashioned teacher held many _____ ideas about teaching.

IMPORTANCE OF TAKING GOOD NOTES

Your success as a health care student depends almost entirely on how well you take notes from your textbooks and lectures. When it comes to preparing for tests, you must have textbook and lecture notes that adequately record the information you need to learn. Few people have the time to reread the vast amount of material from the textbook to prepare for a midterm or final examination. Few people have the ability to catch and remember every word spoken in a lecture. That is why it is important to have strategies for taking good notes from your books and lectures. You must learn to focus only on the information that is important. You do not want to waste your time recording and remembering facts that may not be necessary to learn. Knowing the strategies for taking good notes will not only save you time but will also enhance your test taking skills.

EXERCISE 14–1

Directions: Below is a checklist for determining how good your present note-taking system is. Check "Yes" or "No."

1. Do I have background knowledge of the textbook or lecture subject?

    Yes_____ No_____

2. Do I see any connection between textbook notes and lecture notes?

    Yes_____ No_____

3. Do I keep current with all my reading assignments?

    Yes_____ No_____

4. Do I attend all lectures?

    Yes_____ No_____

5. Is my notebook well organized?

    Yes_____ No_____

6. Do I have a system for setting up the notebook sheets of paper?

    Yes_____ No_____

7. Do I know how much information to write or highlight?

    Yes_____ No_____

8. Can I tell important facts from unimportant facts?

    Yes_____ No_____

9. Do I take speedy notes?

    Yes_____ No_____

10. Do I have strategies for studying notes?

    Yes_____ No_____

If you answered "no" to most of these questions, you need to learn strategies for taking better notes. This chapter will teach you the strategies for organizing, taking, and studying textbook and lecture notes.

USING YOUR NOTES SUCCESSFULLY

Some students feel it is okay to take notes from their textbooks and lectures and then ignore them until test time. Other students, however, realize that to get good grades you must constantly review your notes. These students realize that textbook notes and lecture notes are interconnected. In order to get the best grades, they use the following strategies:

- Before lectures, take and review textbook notes on the subject of the lecture. This will build your background knowledge of the topic, and the lecture will be that much more understandable.
- After the lecture, review your textbook notes again. This will reinforce your learning the information.
- Before test time, study both the lecture notes and the textbook notes until they are fully learned. This is good test preparation.

TIME MANAGEMENT AND NOTE TAKING

An important aspect to good note taking is time management. This means allowing sufficient time for reading your textbooks and attending all lectures.

- Stay current. Do not fall behind in your textbook reading. You may be responsible for textbook information on exams and once you are behind, you may never be able to catch up. Maintain your scheduling calendars and keep pace with your reading assignments.
- Attend all lectures. Having to borrow someone else's notes is never as good as taking them yourself. If possible, ignore minor physical and emotional upsets and get into the habit of attending all your classes.
- Arrive early for your lectures. This will give you time to organize your notebook for good note taking. Also, you do not want to miss the beginning of the lecture. Many instructors introduce their main points at the very beginning of the class period, so this is something you may not want to skip.

CHOOSING YOUR NOTEBOOK

The first practical step for taking good textbook and lecture notes is buying and setting up your notebook. This will depend on personal preference. The main thing to keep in mind, however, is to organize your notebook so that each subject is kept separated from the other subjects. This may mean buying different 8 x 11 inch spiral notebooks for each subject or spiral notebooks that are divided into three to five sections. The advantage to using spiral notebooks is that they are lightweight and easy to carry. Also, you need to bring only the spiral notebook that is used for a particular daily class. The disadvantage to using a spiral notebook is that you may run out of paper. The manufacturer of these notebooks cannot anticipate how many pages you will actually need. You may find yourself having to buy more than one spiral notebook for each subject. This may prove bothersome and confusing.

An alternative to a spiral notebook is a hard cover loose-leaf binder. If this is your choice, be sure to buy the colorful dividers to keep each of your subjects separate. The advantage to using a loose-leaf binder is that you can control the number of pages for each subject section. If you use more paper in one class than in another, you can always insert more lined paper in that section. The disadvantage to using loose-leaf binders is that, depending on the type, they are not so portable. They may be heavy to carry and may not fit so well into your book bag or backpack. However, you can now purchase for each of your subjects an inexpensive lightweight loose-leaf notebook. Be aware, though, that there is always the possibility that the rings will not close right or will open at the wrong time, and that can mean disarranged or lost notes.

Whatever your preference in notebooks, remember that you must keep notes from each of your subjects separate and distinct from the other subjects. You may also want to consider using different notebooks for lecture notes and textbook notes. Again, the choice is yours.

EXERCISE 14–2

Directions: Think back over your past school years and try to remember whether you used spiral notebooks or loose-leaf binders. In the space below, write some of the advantages or disadvantages you may have found using one type of notebook or another. Use the list as a guide to help you decide which style of notebook is right for you.

_____
_____
_____
_____

ORGANIZING YOUR NOTEPAPER

Whether you are taking textbook or lecture notes, it is important to set up your notepaper in a way that will make your notes understandable when you read them days or weeks later. To organize your lecture notepaper, you must arrive in class a few minutes early to prepare your paper. To organize your textbook notes, plan to begin each study session with setting up your notepapers.

The first strategy to use in organizing your notepaper is numbering and putting the current date on top of each paper. This is important when it comes time to study for exams. By numbering and dating each page, you will know which notes are needed for a specific exam period. You will know which notes to study. Also, if your notes should accidentally get loose, you will have a way of reorganizing them. Keeping your notes in numerical and chronological order is the best way of ensuring that your notes are well organized

Spiral Notebook

Loose-leaf Binder

The next strategy for organizing your notepaper is to draw a line down the page, about an inch and a half from the red left-hand margin (see Fig. 14–1). When taking textbook or lecture notes, leave this space empty. (Note area A in Fig. 14–1.) All your notes should be written in the area marked "B" in Figure 14–1. Later you will write in the area marked "A" if you need to add any information you missed, create headings, or jot down comments and observations you believe are necessary to finish your notes. Organizing your notepaper in this manner will ensure that your notes are complete and useful for test preparation.

EXERCISE 14–3

Directions: At your next lecture or study period, practice organizing your notepaper with the number, date, and second left-hand margin. Then respond to the following statements by checking "Yes" or "No."

1. My notes appear to be better organized now that I number and date them.

    Yes_____ No_____

2. My notes look neater now that I use the second margin for additional notes.

    Yes_____ No_____

3. It is easier to add new information to my notes now that I have the second margin.

    Yes_____ No_____

4. It is more convenient studying for exams now that I organize my notes with numbers, date, and the second left-hand margin.

    Yes_____ No_____

If you answer "Yes" to most of these questions, these strategies for organizing your notepaper are right for you. Continue to use these methods for all your health care classes.

If you answer "No" to most of these questions, keep using these strategies until your next exam. You may be pleasantly surprised to see better test results.

TAKING NOTES FROM YOUR TEXTBOOK

As you probably realize by now, your time as a health care student is very precious. This means that you must use your limited amount of time sensibly. When it comes to reading assignments, you may feel overwhelmed because there is so much to read with so little time to do it in. When it comes to preparing for exams, you do not have the time to reread all the assigned chapters. Therefore you need strategies for taking good notes from your textbook for test preparation. Good textbook notes not only will save

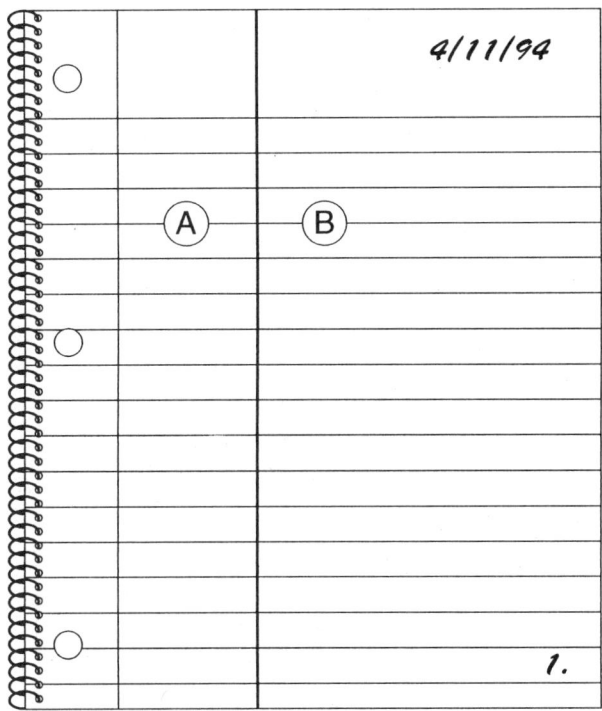

FIGURE 14–1 Notepaper organized with date, number, and hand-drawn second margin.

you time when you are getting ready for tests but will probably result in better test scores. The two strategies for taking textbook notes are

- Highlighting
- Margin writing

HIGHLIGHTING

Highlighting information in your textbook is probably the most popular way of <u>condensing</u> information in your textbook. To highlight important facts, you use a pen, pencil, or special highlighting marker and underline all the sentences you think are meaningful for learning the subject matter. The advantage to using the highlighting strategy is that it saves time. You do not have to rewrite information that is already written. Highlighting is quick and, when done properly, is probably the most efficient way of taking notes from a textbook. The disadvantage to highlighting is that most students tend to overdo it. You have no doubt seen a page in a textbook that is totally highlighted with a yellow marker. What is the point to highlighting every word on the page? The effectiveness of the highlighting strategy is that it is supposed to direct your eyes to only the most important words and ideas on the page. Therefore you must highlight only the most significant facts. To do this, you can use the heading strategy discussed in Chapter 5, Reading The Textbook. To review this strategy,

- Look at the boldfaced headings on each page.
- Turn each boldfaced heading into a question.
- Highlight only those facts that answer the heading question.

Following is an example from *The Medical Assistant: Administrative and Clinical* by Kinn, Woods, and Derge (p. 194) of how a health care student used the heading strategy to guide her highlighting. Notice that she underlined only the facts that answered her heading question.

Example 14–1

CONSULTATION REPORTS

- What are consultation reports?

<u>Physicians who act as consultants</u> are expected to <u>prepare a detailed report of their findings and recommendations and send it to the referring physicians</u>. The *consultation report* is <u>dictated by the consulting physician</u> to be transcribed within the office or by an independent transcriptionist if outside services are used. The consultation <u>report</u> is frequently <u>quite long</u>, and <u>promptness in preparations is important</u>.

EXERCISE 14–4

Directions: Below is an excerpt from Flynn's *Procedures in Phlebotomy* (p. 65). Turn the heading into a question and highlight the facts that answer your question. Remember to stay focused on the question and do not highlight too much. You can use a pen, pencil, or highlighting marker.

BLOOD LANCETS

For difficult patients, including situations that normally call for <u>microcapillary</u> techniques, a blood lancet may be used. This is a small, sterile, disposable instrument used for skin puncture....Lancets are available with a variety of point lengths to help control the depth of puncture, which is especially important in children and infants. A variety of semiautomated devices are commercially available, but the manual lancet is the most commonly used device for microcapillary puncture.

MARGIN WRITING

To <u>complement</u> your highlighting of the important points in your textbook, you may also want to consider writing in the margins of your textbook. Following is a list of suggested items that you may use for margin writing:

- *Headings:* You can divide lengthy passages into more manageable sections by creating your own headings. Write these headings between paragraphs or in the margin where you want to divide the passage.
- *Summaries:* You can summarize or condense lengthy passages into brief summaries by writing in the margins of your book. You will not be able to be wordy because of the limited space. Your margin summaries should cover only the most important information in the passage.

- *Symbols:* Using various symbols can be an easy way of emphasizing important facts from the textbook. Some useful symbols are "T" to show what details your instructor said will appear on tests; "B" to show what information in your textbook corresponds to information your instructor wrote on the board during a lecture; and "R" to designate those sections in the textbook that your teacher may have read aloud and discussed in class. Using symbols like these will help you connect important ideas from your lecture to the material in your textbook.

Following is an example from a textbook by Flynn (pp. 22–24). Notice how one student used headings, summaries, and symbols to emphasize important points in the textbook.

Example 14–2

THE DIGESTIVE SYSTEM

Summary: Enzymes split large food molecules into smaller ones. The liver, pancreas, and small intestine create these enzymes.

For nutrients to be of use, they must be in a form small enough to pass through the membrane that surrounds each cell. It is the digestive system...that receives food and breaks it down into its useful components. As food is moved through the digestive tract by contractions known as *peristalsis* it is mixed with digestive juices that split large <u>molecules</u> into smaller ones. Most of these secretions are *enzymes*, chemicals that catalyze metabolic reactions in the body. Most digestion occurs in the small intestine under the effects of enzymes secreted by the small intestine, along with additional substances contributed by the liver and pancreas. The liver produces bile, which emulsifies fats, and the pancreas contributes a mixture of digestive enzymes. Before delivery to the small intestine, bile is stored in the gallbladder, a small sac under the liver.

food absorbtion

The products of digestion are also absorbed into the circulation in the small intestine. The transfer occurs through the villi, tiny fingerlike projections in the lining of the organ that contain blood capillaries and lacteals of the lymphatic system. The building blocks of proteins and carbohydrates are absorbed directly into the bloodstream; the building blocks of fat enter the lymphatic system. The final step in digestion are the storage of undigested waste and its elimination from the body by the large intestine. *B.*

Continued on following page.

metabolism
The nutrient products of digestion are used by cells to generate energy and manufacture needed substances. All of the chemical reactions that occur within the body are collectively referred to as **metabolism**. Reactions in which complex substances are broken down into smaller components constitute *catabolism*; the building of these small molecules into larger products is termed *anabolism*.

(Margin notes: R. next to "metabolism"; T. next to "catabolism"; T. next to "anabolism".)

EXERCISE 14–5

Directions: In the following passage from Kinn, Woods, and Derge (p. 103), practice emphasizing important details by creating headings, summaries, and symbols. Refer to Example 14–2 if you need help.

APPOINTMENT SCHEDULING

The computer can replace the appointment book, but this is practical only in large practices and clinics. Software for appointment scheduling ranges from relatively simple programs that merely display available and scheduled times to sophisticated systems into which the operator may enter information such as the length and type of appointment required and day and time preferences of the patient; the computer then selects the best appointment time based on inputed information.

The computer can also be used to keep track of future appointments. For example, when a patient calls and inquires about an appointment, the system can search by his or her name to find the time and date. The computer can provide printouts of the daily schedule that include the patients' names and telephone numbers and the reason for their visiting. Multiple copies of these schedules can be made according to the needs of the practice.

A big advantage of computer scheduling is that more than one person can access the system at one time, and the information is available to all operators. In many facilities, employees still maintain an appointment book as a back-up to computer scheduling.

TAKING NOTES FROM YOUR LECTURES

As was mentioned earlier, it is impossible to take down all of the instructor's words during a lecture. You must concentrate on the main ideas and the important details (see Chapters 1 and 2). You should also write down the important information in such a way that days later you will be able to tell at a glance what is the main idea and what is a detail. You can do this by using the indentation strategy. The main ideas should be written next to the second margin and the important details should be indented or written in a few letters to the right. See Figure 14–2.

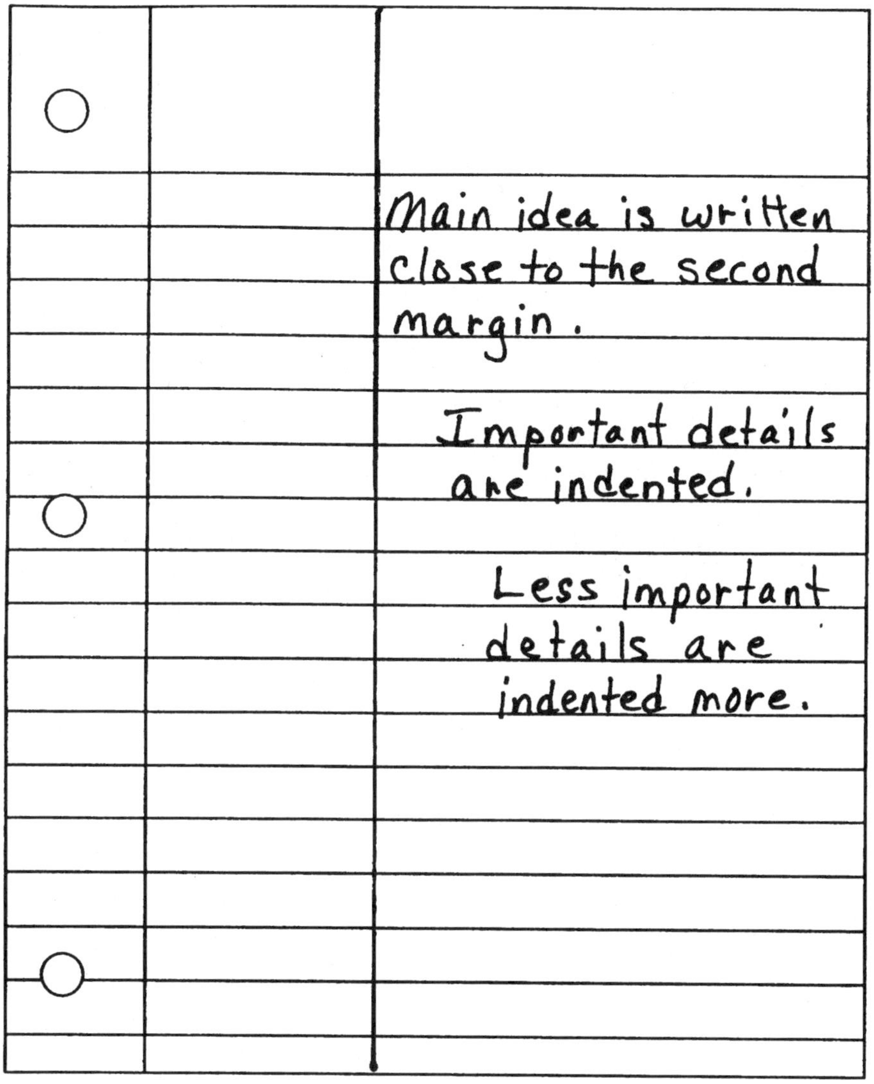

FIGURE 14–2 Indentation strategy.

EXERCISE 14–6

Directions: Following is a selection from LaFleur-Brooks, *Health Unit Coordinating,* p. 349. Using the selection as a lecture, take notes on the sheet of notebook paper on the following page. If it is a main idea, start writing close to the second margin. If it is an important detail, indent. You may want to consider taking notes on less important details and indenting them even more.

Two **medical emergencies**—that is, life threatening situations—that require a cool head, swift action, and good communication by the health unit coordinator are <u>cardiac</u> **arrest** and **respiratory arrest.** (It is common hospital terminology to refer to these as *code arrests*.) In a cardiac arrest the patient's heart contractions are absent or grossly insufficient, and there is no pulse and no blood pressure. In respiratory arrest, the patient may cease to breathe or the respirations become so depressed that the blood cannot receive oxygen and the body cells die. Both conditions require quick action by hospital personnel and the use of emergency equipment. Treatment must be instituted within 3-4 min, since the brain cells deteriorate rapidly from lack of oxygen.

Each hospital nursing unit and department maintains an emergency cart. This is taken to the code arrest patient's room immediately. Fully equipped code arrest carts are also stationed in designated areas of the hospital and are wheeled to the patient's room when a code arrest occurs. These carts contain medications and more equipment than the unit emergency carts. It is important for the health unit coordinator to know the location of the emergency cart and any other emergency equipment so that it can be brought quickly to their nursing unit when needed.

Hospitals have designated hospital personnel who report each code arrest. They are members of the code arrest team. They may be employed in various hospital departments, such as intensive or coronary care, other nursing units, the respiratory care department, pulmonary function department, surgery, and so forth.

Instructors' Cues

Now that you have a system for taking lecture notes, you are left with the decision of determining what information is important to record. Fortunately, your instructor will willingly or unwillingly provide you with cues that should let you know what ideas are significant. By recognizing these cues, you will know what facts to write in your notes and possibly what facts to leave out. Following are the cues most instructors give to indicate meaningful material.

- **Ideas Written on the Board:** Make sure you copy any information the teacher writes on the board. As mentioned earlier, you may want to indicate these facts with a "B" for board in your notes.
- **Verbal Tips:** You may be fortunate to have an instructor who will say, "this will be on the test" or "these are important ideas." Make sure you write these facts accurately and mark these notes with a "T" for test or an "I" for important.
- **Numbering Ideas:** Many teachers may introduce important points by numbering them. They do this by saying "first," "second," "third," etc. If your teacher goes to the trouble of numbering ideas, you should consider them important enough to copy in your notebook.
- **Body Language:** Some instructors will make their voices louder or gesture with their hands to indicate important ideas. Stay alert to these or other body signs that the teacher will use to suggest important ideas.

At the end of the lecture, resist the temptation to stop listening and gather your books. Many times the instructor will summarize the important points at the end of the lecture, so pay attention and stay put until the teacher finishes talking.

HOW MANY NOTES TO TAKE

Many students are puzzled about how many notes they should be writing from their textbooks and lectures. The best strategy in this matter is to know the course requirements and let that help you determine how much to write. If the course deals with broad concepts, you probably will be held responsible for fewer or less detailed notes. If the course presents more factual information, you will need to write greater and more detailed notes.

The best way to determine the requirements of the course is to read the description in the course catalogue, talk with other students who have taken the course, or speak with the instructor directly. Getting this information while the semester is just beginning will help you determine how many notes you should be taking.

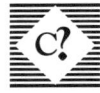

FASTER NOTE TAKING

Many people feel that they would be more successful students if they were able to take lecture notes more quickly. They express frustration at not being able to "catch" all the important points being taught in the classroom. They claim they would do better on tests if their notes were complete. By learning the strategies for faster note taking—streamlining your handwriting and abbreviating and using symbols—these students will improve the rate of their note taking and become better students.

Streamlining Your Handwriting

To take notes more quickly, it is sometimes necessary to make changes in your handwriting. Your note-taking rate will improve if you write in script rather than in printing. When you write in script, one letter connects to the other so that the flow of your writing is faster. However, when you use script, make sure you eliminate any unnecessary strokes or curlicues. Your ability to use a plain streamlined script will greatly enhance your lecture note-taking skills. Following are examples of too fancy a script and a streamlined script.

Streamline your handwriting

Streamline your handwriting

EXERCISE 14–7

Directions: Below is a short excerpt from Solomon, *Introduction to Human Anatomy and Physiology*, p. 47. Using it to substitute for a lecture, rewrite it in your usual handwriting in the space provided. Time yourself. If you see that your handwriting is too elaborate, try rewriting it in a more streamlined fashion. Time yourself again. Notice whether your timing has improved.

The skeleton found in science laboratories consists of dry, dead bones. In the living body, the skeletal system consists of bone, cartilage, and other connective tissues that are alive—their cells must have nutrients and oxygen, they consume energy in their metabolism, they produce waste products, some of their metabolism is regulated by hormones, and they function closely with the muscular system.

Time for first try: _____

Time for second try: _____

Abbreviating and Using Symbols

Another strategy for faster note taking is to use abbreviations or symbols to replace common words. It is much quicker to write "&" for "and" or to spell "patient" "pat." You can use <u>conventional</u> abbreviations and symbols, or you can make up your own. If you make up your own, be sure you remember their meanings. It will do you little good if you use a symbol or abbreviation that you can't understand a few weeks later when you prepare for an exam. Following is a selection from Flynn, p. 92. Note how one student used abbreviations and symbols to create a type of shorthand system for taking notes quickly.

Example 14–3

The glucose tolerance test (GTT) is done on individuals *[ind.]* who are being screened for **diabetes mellitus** or **hypoglycemia**. *[diab. mel. hypogly.]* Although *[altho.]* there is nothing unique about the actual collection process *[coll. proc.]* itself, the number *[#]* of <u>venipunctures</u> *[vent.]* performed in a relatively short period of time makes this test significant *[signif.]*. The purpose *[purp.]* of the test is to determine *[deter.]* the patient's blood glucose level *[pat's. bld. glu. l.]* after the patient *[pat.]* consumes a fixed amount of glucose *[glu.]* (usually 100gm). The test takes from 3 to 5 *[3-5]* hours.

After a patient *[pat.]* has fasted for at least 12 hours, a blood sample *[bld. samp.]* is collected using routine collection procedures *[rout. coll. proced.]*. The blood *[bld.]* may be collected in a plain tube (without any anticoagulant *[anticoag.]*) or in a tube especially designed to preserve glucose levels *[glu. l.]* (e.g., gray-stopped tubes with sodium fluoride and potassium oxalate *[sod. flour. & pot. ox.]*).

EXERCISE 14–8

Directions: The following is a passage from McCurnin, *Clinical Textbook for Veterinary Technicians*, pp. 272–273. Write your own system of abbreviations and symbols in the space between the lines. At the beginning of your next lesson, check to see if you can decode your own system of abbreviations and symbols.

Two methods are available for gloving. *Closed gloving* has the advantage that it minimizes the chances of contaminating the gloves, since the outside of the gloves do not contact the skin. *Open gloving* is at a disadvantage because gloves are relatively easily contaminated by skin contact. Because closed gloving is not always possible (e.g., replacing gloves during surgery), it is necessary for one to be able to glove by the open method.

TAPING YOUR LECTURES

Another strategy for ensuring well-written notes is to tape your lectures with a portable audiocassette recorder. However, before you attempt to do this, get your instructor's permission; some people feel uncomfortable when they know they are being taped. The advantages to taping your lectures are many. First, during your study period you can replay the tape and fill in any missing information. Second, listening to your lectures over and over again is a good strategy for test preparation. Third, you can listen to your lecture tape anytime—as you drive to classes, when you are commuting to school, or at your leisure at home. And, finally, you can have a friend tape a lecture for you if you cannot attend class.

Make sure that your recorder is easy to carry and battery operated. Always remember to carry extra batteries. Buy the long-running blank cassette tapes and sit up front, close to the instructor, so you can get a clear recording. You want your lecture tapes to be as distinct as possible.

STUDYING FROM YOUR NOTES

After a lecture, as soon as you can, review your notes for completeness. This may mean listening to your tape or consulting with a fellow student. Once you feel your notes are as thorough as possible, you should begin to learn these notes in a systematic manner. A wonderful strategy for learning notes is to use the heading method.

Creating Headings

Just as your textbook passages are divided by headings, so should your class notes be divided by headings. Decide where in your notes there is a topic change and, using a different color pen, put in a heading. To create the topic, ask yourself what is this passage mostly about. The answer will be the topic and will work well for a heading. Do this for all the pages in your notebook.

Once you have made headings for all the different topics in your notes, turn these headings into questions. When you are studying for an exam, focus on the information in your notes that will answer the heading question. Below is an example of how a student created headings and questions and highlighted only the important information that answered the heading question.

Example 14–4

- What is this passage mostly about?
- Influenza = Topic = Heading
- What is influenza = Heading question

Influenza virus A produces the most serious form of influenza, with <u>symptoms of fever, chills, headache, myalgia, sore throat, and cough</u>. The <u>onset of symptoms</u> is approximately <u>1 to 4 days after contact</u> with infected respiratory secretions. <u>Infected people shed the virus for 24 hours before the onset of symptoms and for 3 to 4 days during the course of the disease</u>. Death associated with this virus is usually the result of primary influenza pneumonia or a secondary bacterial pneumonia. The influenza viruses that are the cause of epidemics and nosocomial outbreaks change from season to season, and a new vaccine is manufactured each year (Flynn, p. 47).

EXERCISE 14–9

Directions: Following is a passage from Diehl and Fordney, *Medical Typing and Transcribing: Techniques and Procedures*, p. 156. After carefully reading the passage, determine the topic and use it for the heading. Turn the heading into a question and highlight only those facts from the passage that answer the heading question.

When copy is prepared for printing, it is corrected and marked, with correction symbols placed either in the margin or between the lines to indicate the changes to be made. If more than one marginal note is necessary, a slash mark (/) divides the notes. Either or both margins are used.

In proofreading your own copy, you may be more informal, using marginal notes only when there is no room on the single-spaced copy to indicate the change.

While you are a student, your instructor will proofread your work and may mark the copy and use marginal notes in a variety of ways. Therefore, let us examine the proofreading marks as they are used formally and see how we may modify them for our own use. Your instructor may wish to add his or her marking symbols as well.

Other Strategies For Studying Your Notes

You may believe that preparing for an exam means reading and rereading your notes. However, you may have had the experience of sitting at your desk, hour after hour, and "spacing out" when you should have been focusing on your textbook or lecture notes. You probably discovered at test time that all you accomplished was wasting time. Successful students are those who have discovered that more active strategies are necessary for quality test preparation. This means more active note-learning strategies.

An excellent strategy for using your notes to prepare for a test is to create quizzes. At the end of an evening's studying, and before you close the books, make up a quiz covering that day's materials. At the beginning of your next homework session, take the quiz and see how well you have done. Another good studying strategy is to make up a chart of all the information you need to learn. Make a second chart, omitting most of the information except for some guiding facts and try to fill in the chart without looking at the original. Also use your tape recorder and play back the lecture when you are washing dishes or sorting socks. Finally, make flash cards of the important vocabulary words. Print the word on one side of an index card and its definition on the other side. During your study time, look at the word and try to recall the definition. Or, for more variety, look at the definition and try to remember the word. Being creative about taking and studying textbook and lecture notes will go a long way to making you a more successful student.

REVIEWING THE LEARNING STRATEGIES

TO LEARN	USE THIS STRATEGY
Successful use of notes	Time management Careful choice of notebook Notepaper organizing
Note taking from textbook	Highlighting Margin writing
Note taking from lectures	Indenting Interpreting instructor's cues
Length of notes	Learning requirements of course
Faster note taking	Streamlining handwriting Abbreviating and using symbols Taping lectures
Note studying	Creating headings Creating questions Making quizzes Making charts Listening to lecture tapes Making flash cards

Chapter 15

Improving Test Scores

LEARNING OBJECTIVES
VOCABULARY WORDS
VOCABULARY CHECK
HOW TO IMPROVE YOUR TEST SCORES
    Strategy 1: Plan Ahead
    Strategy 2: Keep up with Assignments
    Strategy 3: Study and Learn Material
    Strategy 4: Take the Test Successfully
        Taking Objective Tests
            Learning How to Answer Multiple Choice Questions
            Learning How to Answer Short-Answer Questions
            Learning How to Answer the Matching Question
            Learning How to Answer the True-False Question
            Practice Taking Short-Answer Tests
        Learning Strategies for Taking the Essay Test
            Practice Taking the Essay Test
    Strategy 5: Evaluate Test Results
REVIEWING STRATEGIES FOR IMPROVING TEST SCORES

LEARNING OBJECTIVES

In this chapter you will learn how to
- Improve your test scores
- Use five strategies to help you prepare for and take tests more successfully

VOCABULARY WORDS

The following vocabulary words are important to your understanding of the ideas in this chapter. These vocabulary words are underscored the first time they are used in the chapter. Read the list of words and definitions. Then check your understanding of these words before you read the chapter.

ethicists persons who study morality.
gastrointestinal pertaining to the stomach and intestine.
host an animal or plant that harbors and provides sustenance for another organism.
hypotension lowered blood pressure.
mobilize to put into action.
obligation a commitment to acting in certain ways.
opponents those who disagree.
radiation energy carried by waves or a stream of particles.
transmission passage or transfer of a disease from one person to another.
utility usefulness.

VOCABULARY CHECK

Directions: Choose the vocabulary word that best fits into the sentence.

1. She was suffering from _____, so the doctor gave her medication to raise her blood pressure.

2. The student felt an _____ to study and pass the course.

3. The mechanic was concerned with the _____ of the new tool.

4. Sometimes it is difficult to _____ people to work at improving their environment.

5. A hazard of too much _____ is a severe burn.

6. The scientist was concerned about the _____ of the disease to a new population.

7. The _____ was concerned with the moral issues of the plan.

8. The disease went from a source to a _____.

9. The _____ of the new plan argued for their own point of view.

10. Her stomach pain was caused by a _____ infection.

HOW TO IMPROVE YOUR TEST SCORES

The purpose of tests is evaluation. Tests allow you, the student, and your instructor to find out what you have learned and what you still need to learn.

Of course, students worry about test grades. Doing well on tests is every student's goal. You can learn strategies to improve your grades. However, these strategies have to be applied long before the date of the exam.

Strategy 1: Plan Ahead

Your instructor will assign test dates in advance. Apply your time-management skills. Find out the assignments you need to study for the exam. Make sure that you know which information from your readings, lectures, or labs will be on the test. Then use your monthly, weekly, and daily calendars to schedule enough study time for your exam.

Many students in the health fields are juggling school with busy work and family schedules. Finding time to study can be a problem. Therefore organization is essential. Use your calendars to plan your study time. Stick to your schedule. Don't procrastinate! Avoiding your work today means doing a double assignment the next day.

Cramming, trying to prepare for an exam at the last minute, is not a successful strategy. Cramming increases anxiety. This nervousness often interferes with your test performance.

Do you understand how to plan ahead to schedule enough time to study for tests?
Yes ___   No ___

Strategy 2: Keep Up with Assignments

Assignment should be done on a regular basis. Keep up with all the reading on your class syllabus. Don't fall behind.

Be an active reader. As you read your assignments, **remember** to be an **active reader. Preview** the reading material. **Ask** questions. **Write** summaries and outlines. **Learn** the new **vocabulary** that helps you to understand the ideas in each chapter. Pay attention to **illustrations** and **formulas.**

Do you remember to use your active reading strategies when reading home assignments? Yes ___   No ___

Use Active Listening and Effective Note-taking Strategies. Be prepared for each class session. Don't skip classes. Regular attendance is necessary if you are to understand a sequence of information. In the health fields, details are important. Take accurate notes. Apply active listening strategies. Pay attention to all main ideas and details highlighted in each lecture or lab. Ask questions if you don't understand the material presented. Summarize or outline the material presented in class.

Do you concentrate during class lectures? Yes ___   No ___
Do your class notes help you study for tests? Yes ___   No ___

Strategy 3: Study and Learn Material

Even if you have attended every class and read every assignment, you still have to study before every test.

- Review all class notes, summaries, outlines, and underlined material from your textbooks periodically throughout the course. **Don't cram!**
- Organize information into categories. It will be easier for you to remember organized material.
- Review vocabulary. Definitions are important in helping you learn information in the health fields. In fact, it is helpful to keep a notebook of the words and def-

initions that are highlighted in each chapter. Some students prefer keeping words and definitions on 3 x 5 inch index cards. Learn these definitions before the test.
- Pay attention to illustrations and formulas. Make sure that you understand how these pictures and numbers relate to the ideas in the chapter.
- Use mnemonics, a technique for improving the memory, to help you learn formulas, definitions, or ideas in the text. Mnemonic devices are easily remembered words, sentences, or rhymes that help you to remember more difficult information. Mnemonic devices work by association and help you to remember information that is difficult to organize. Some common mnemonic devices are

Rhymes
i before e except after c
or when sounding like a
as in neighbor and weigh

Acronyms - a word made from the initial letter of the parts of the information to be remembered.
    HOMES - to remember the five Great Lakes
    H - **H**uron
    O - **O**ntario
    M - **M**ichigan
    E - **E**rie
    S - **S**uperior

Try to create mnemonic devices to help you remember information.

Do you find mnemonics a helpful memory tool? Yes ___ No ____

- Don't accept not understanding. Don't give up. Monitor your learning. When you don't understand information, try another approach to learning. Make sure that your study schedule allows you time to ask your instructor or other students to explain difficult ideas to you **before** the test.
- Find out how you learn best. Do you remember information by listening, reading, writing, or discussing the material? Do you find a combination of these methods most effective for learning? Use the learning style that works best for you.
- Design practice tests. Ask your instructor if the test questions will be objective, essay, or both. Answer the questions at the end of each chapter in your textbook.
- Check your answers. Then make up a practice test. Close your book and answer your own test questions. Correct your test. What do you know? What do you still have to learn? Students find that questions on their practice tests often turn up on the actual exam.

List those techniques that you think will help you to study and learn information:

_____
_____
_____
_____

Strategy 4: Take the Test Successfully

Learning how to take a test can improve your test scores. Whether your test is objective or essay, use these strategies:

- Read the test directions carefully before you answer any questions.
- Understand the grading system. Spend extra time on questions that are worth more points.
- Keep track of time.
- Answer the questions that you are sure of first. Then go back to questions that are more difficult for you.
- Answer the questions asked.
- Save time at the end to review your test and make any corrections or additions.
- Write clearly.

Taking Objective Tests

Objective tests are those with multiple-choice, short-answer, matching, or true-false questions. To do well on objective tests, you should learn how to answer four types of questions: multiple-choice, short-answer, matching, and true-false.

LEARNING HOW TO ANSWER MULTIPLE-CHOICE QUESTIONS

When you answer multiple-choice questions, you select one answer from several choices. The following strategies will help you learn how to select the correct answer.

- Statements that contain words like *always*, *every*, *never*, and *all* are usually too broad. They are often incorrect.
- If two choices have the same meaning, they are both incorrect. Therefore, you eliminate both these choices when you select your answer.
- Be aware of directional words such as *but*, *except*, and *however*. They signal opposite meanings.
- To answer multiple-choice questions, you need to know how to:
  - Find the main ideas
  - Find and remember details that support the main idea
  - Draw conclusions
  - Learn vocabulary meanings through context

Example 15–1

Directions: Read the following excerpt from a health care textbook (Bonewit-West, p. 87). Answer the multiple-choice questions based on the selection. Then read the explanation of the answers.

WORD WRAP

Word wrap is a feature which automatically moves a word to the beginning of the next line if it goes past the right margin. Therefore, if the user is in the middle of a word when the right margin is reached, the entire word along with the cursor will automatically drop down to the beginning of the next line. Word wrap increases typing speed because it eliminates having to press a carriage return at the end of each line as is required with a typewriter.

1. Word wrap
   a. is automatic
   b. moves every word to the beginning of each line
   c. just drops the cursor
   d. automatically lifts up to the line above

2. Word wrap moves a word
   a. next to the right margin
   b. to the beginning of each page
   c. to the beginning of the next line
   d. past the left margin

3. Word wrap
   a. increases the number of lines on a computer screen
   b. decreases typing speed
   c. eliminates typing
   d. increases typing speed

The correct answer to number 1 is choice (a). The word *every* in choice (b) makes that answer incorrect. The word *just* in answer (c) eliminates that choice. The answer (d) says *up* and *above* while the text says *down*.

The correct answer to number 2 is choice (c). The answer is *to the next line* not *next to the right margin*. Therefore choice (a) is incorrect. Choice (b) is incorrect because the correct choice is *line* not *page*. The word *left* in choice (d) eliminates that answer choice.

The correct answer to number 3 is (d). Choice (a) is incorrect because the *typing speed* is *increased* not *the number of lines*. The word *decreases* in choice (b) eliminates that choice. The information in choice (c) is incorrect. Typing is not *eliminated*; typing speed is increased.

Answering multiple-choice questions requires careful attention to detail in reading the passage, the questions, and the choices.

EXERCISE 15-1

Directions: Read the following excerpt from a health care text (Bonewit-West, p. 86). Answer the multiple-choice questions based on the selection. Use the strategies you learned for answering multiple-choice questions.

The term *word processing* refers to the process of manipulating words using an electronic device such as a computer. This application is the most common use for microcomputers in both the business and home. Word processing is used in the creation, modification and printing of letters, memos, reports, and other documents. In many respects word processing is similar to typing with a conventional typewriter, however, many functions are available with word processing that are beyond the capability of the typewriter.

The principle advantages of word processing are the rapid and accurate correction of errors and the specialized editing functions not possible with a typewriter (e.g., moving a block of text to another location in the document). Word processing eliminates having to retype the entire document due to errors or having to make carbon copies of a document when an identical form is required.

The hardware required for word processing includes a CPU, monitor, keyboard, and printer. The software requirement is a word processing application program. Examples of commercially available word processing programs include WordPerfect, Microsoft Word and WordStar. Since no two word processing programs are identical, it is important that the user carefully and thoroughly review the program user manual to become completely familiar with its capabilities. In general, all word processing programs perform four basic functions: a) entering text, b) editing text, c) filing text and d) formatting text.

1. Word processing is the process of
    a. manipulating words using an electronic device
    b. buying a computer for home use
    c. using a typewriter for business only
    d. processing information for home study

2. Word processing is
    a. another term for typing
    b. similar to typing
    c. a substitute for typing
    d. easier to learn than typing

3. A difference between typing and word processing is
    a. a typewriter is more suitable for home and office use
    b. a typewriter is used in homes and the word processor is used for business
    c. a word processor has functions beyond the capabilities of the typewriter
    d. a typewriter is easier to use

4. Word processing eliminates
    a. making carbon copies of the document
    b. making copies of the document
    c. typing the document
    d. printing the document

5. Rapid and accurate correction of errors is
    a. an advantage of the typewriter
    b. an advantage of making copies
    c. a disadvantage of word processing
    d. an advantage of word processing

6. Specialized editing functions
    a. are not possible with word processing
    b. are possible with word processing
    c. are always done with a typewriter
    d. are done more easily by retyping

7. Retyping due to errors is
   a. required when word processing
   b. a function of word processing
   c. eliminated by word processing
   d. eliminated by using the typewriter

8. The monitor is an example of
   a. software
   b. word processing programs
   c. text
   d. hardware

9. Two word processing programs
   a. can be identical
   b. are always the same
   c. cannot be the same
   d. cannot be used twice

10. The number of functions performed by all word processing programs is
    a. 1   b. 2   c. 3   d. 4

LEARNING HOW TO ANSWER THE SHORT-ANSWER QUESTIONS

Short-answer questions ask you to fill in the blank. When you decide on an answer, check to see that your answer fits into the sentence in both meaning and grammar.

Example 15–2

Directions: Read the following excerpt from a health care textbook (Purtilo, p. 6). Then answer the short-answer questions based on the excerpt. Read the explanation of the answers.

Ethics is a systematic reflection on and analysis of morality. Thus, ethics is a fundamental part of the life of everyone in society, and takes a specific form when someone assumes the role of "health professional," philosopher, or any other professional role. Philosophers and theologians who study ethics (ethicists) try to understand morality in a systematic way. Many also try to apply it to everyday problems among individuals, in institutions, and in society. To some extent, we all become ethicists when we learn how to use the tools of ethical analysis.

There are two major areas of ethical analysis, metaethics and normative ethics.

1. People who study ethics are called _____.

2. The two major areas of ethical analysis are _____ and _____.

3. Ethics is part of the life of _____.

The answer to question 1 is *ethicists*. If you answered *philosopher* or *theologian*, you would have given an answer that was partly correct.

The answer to question 2 is *metaethics* and *normative ethics*. This answer can be found in the last line of the passage.

The answer to question 3 is *everyone*. If you answered *philosopher* or *theologian*, you again would have been only partly correct.

EXERCISE 15-2

Directions: Read the following excerpt from a health care text (Purtilo, p. 11). Answer the short-answer questions based on the selection. Use the strategies you learned for answering short-answer questions.

TELEOLOGICAL ETHICS

Teleological theories are concerned with consequences. The most important teleological theory for our consideration of health care ethics is utilitarianism. This word takes its root from the idea of utility or usefulness.

In utilitarianism, an act is right if it is useful to bring about the best consequences overall. This approach was developed first by two English philosophers, Jeremy Bentham (1748–1832) and John Stuart Mill (1806–1873). As you can see, roughly they are contemporaries of Kant. In fact, they were vigorous opponents of Kant's position.

Consider Mr. Harvey again. How will the health professionals discern what is the right thing to do on his behalf? From a utilitarian point of view, first they must consider what the good consequence will accomplish. What is the end to which they are striving? One might say something like, "The goal is to restore Mr. Harvey to maximum health within the limits of his impairment," or "the goal is to treat him in such a way that everyone else will be able to have the same treatment as he received," or even "the goal is to be able to live with my own conscience." If all three ends are attainable by one course of action, it should be taken. If not, the most important consequences take priority. One important task of this approach is to distinguish alternative paths of action and then predict as best as possible the consequences of each path. As you can begin to see, this approach, too, has some inherent challenges. How can we predict all the consequences of an act? Moreover, doesn't this approach ignore the fact that at least sometimes humans do think in terms of their duties, rights and responsibilities to one another?

1. Teleological theories are concerned with _____.

2. The most important teleological theory for consideration in health care ethics is _____.

3. Name two philosophers who developed a utilitarian approach: _____ and _____.

4. A _____ point of view considers the end, or goal.

5. The word utility means _____.

6. In utilitarianism, an act is right if it brings about the best _____ overall.

7. List the three goals of health professionals considering Mr. Harvey's case from a utilitarian point of view.

   a. _____

   b. _____

   c. _____

8. Name two philosophers who disagreed with Kant's position: _____ and _____.

9. If all goals cannot be reached by one action, which consequences take priority? _____

10. Teleological ethics ignores the fact that sometimes humans do think in terms of their _____, _____ and _____ to one another.

LEARNING HOW TO ANSWER THE MATCHING QUESTIONS

When answering matching questions, link answers from one column to explanations in another column. Keep track of the answers you have already used. In this way you monitor your progress. Matching questions are often used to link words with definitions or to connect cause-effect relationships.

Example 15-3

Directions: Read the following excerpt from a health care textbook (Purtilo, p. 18). Then answer the *matching* questions based on the excerpt. Read the explanation of the answers. Match the *causes* in column A with the *effects* in column B. There is one extra answer.

HOW DUTIES ARISE

What is an "obligation," anyway? Although most philosophers maintain that it is more than merely a feeling in our everyday lives, we experience it as a commitment to acting in certain ways within our numerous relationships. For example, when I have wronged someone I may feel compelled to make some kind of reparation or restitution, at least in the form of an apology. When I have made a promise I feel compelled to try to keep it. The relationships within which these commitments are perceived may also include my commitment to a group (i.e., to my professional organization, or family), or even to an institution (i.e., to a hospital or other facility in which I am employed). What are some of *your* commitments?

A	**B**
___ 1. A commitment to acting in certain ways	a. Apology
___ 2. Feeling that you wronged someone	b. Obligation
___ 3. Make a promise	c. Commitment to a group
	d. Try to keep it

To answer these questions correctly you would have to understand the relationship between the cause (why) and the result (what) in each column.

The answers are

<u>b</u> 1.

<u>a</u> 2.

<u>d</u> 3.

A commitment to acting in a certain way leads to a feeling of obligation. The feeling that you wronged someone leads to an apology. If you make a promise, the result is that you try to keep it. A commitment to a group is the extra answer. It is not the result of the causes given.

EXERCISE 15-3

Directions: Read the following excerpt from *Computer Concepts and Applications for the Medical Office* by Bonewit-West. Answer the matching questions based on the selection. Use the strategies you learned for answering the matching questions. Match the explanations in column B to the terms in column A. There will be one extra answer.

Based upon size and capability, computers can be classified into three main categories: mainframe computers, minicomputers and microcomputers.

A *mainframe computer* consists of a large central computer system to which numerous terminals are attached. The advantage of a mainframe system is that it can process an enormous amount of data at a very high rate of speed and serve the needs of up to 500 users at a time. Disadvantages include high cost and the necessity that it be housed in a specially-constructed, air conditioned room. Mainframe computers are used primarily by large corporations, hospitals, universities and other facilities with large processing requirements. Exceptionally large medical clinics may use a mainframe, but cost and space requirements make its use in the private-practice medical office impractical.

A *minicomputer* is a midsize system typically used by engineering firms, large medical clinics, and academic institutions. The minicomputer has the same components as a mainframe, but has less memory and fewer capabilities. It is able to support between 10 and 100 users at a time.

A *microcomputer*, also called a personal computer, is a small, general purpose computer that relies on a tiny microprocessor chip to perform its processing functions. Although they do not have the capability or memory of the larger computers, microcomputers are smaller and less expensive than mainframe or minicomputers. Microcomputers are used in the medical office to perform front office procedures, and continuing advances in technology are allowing them to perform an expanding array of more difficult and sophisticated tasks. [pp. 6–7]

A	**B**
___ 1. Minicomputer	a. Can serve needs of up to 500 users at a time
___ 2. Categories of computers	b. Have large processing requirements
___ 3. Mainframe computer	c. Allowing microcomputer to perform more difficult tasks
___ 4. Tiny microprocessor chip	d. Midsize system
___ 5. Advantage of mainframe system	e. Performs processing functions of minicomputers
___ 6. Hospitals	f. Large central computer system
___ 7. How computers are classified	g. Personal computer
___ 8. Advances in technology system	h. Size and capability
___ 9. Disadvantages of mainframe	i. Mainframe computers, minicomputers, and microcomputers
___ 10. Microcomputer	j. Performs processing functions of microcomputers
	k. High cost and space requirements

LEARNING HOW TO ANSWER TRUE-FALSE QUESTIONS

When answering the true-false questions,

- Pay attention to the part of the question that makes it either true or false.
- Pay close attention to detail before you choose your answer.
- Remember that the whole statement has to be correct for the answer choice to be true.
- If part of the statement is incorrect, the answer is false.

Example 15–4

Directions: Read the following excerpt from *EMT Prehospital Care* by Henry and Stapleton; then answer the true-false questions based on the excerpt. Read the explanation of the answers.

Communications. The use of radio codes and proper utilization of the radio itself will be part of your training. Communications over the radio should be short and clear, since long conversations tie up the airwaves and may obstruct other critical messages. The radio is a useful tool to <u>mobilize</u> essential resources, notify hospital personnel of the imminent arrival of an acutely ill patient, and document unusual circumstances that may have medicolegal implications at a later time. For example, a patient who leaves the scene against your advice and without a proper signature on a release form can be documented by radioing the information to the dispatcher. Many systems record all conversations to provide another form of documentation.

Obviously, communication is not limited to radio conversations. You must learn to be an effective communicator in person with patients, family members, and hospital personnel. In this function you will be required to use medical terminology, which is the language of health care systems. [p. 13]

1. _____ Communications over the radio should be long and clear.
2. _____ Communication is limited to radio conversation.
3. _____ Medical terminology is the language of health care systems.
4. _____ You are not required to learn medical terminology.
5. _____ The use of radio codes will be part of your training.

The answer to question 1 is "false" because part of the answer is incorrect. Conversations over the radio should be short, not long. The answer to question 2 is "false." The first sentence of paragraph 2 states that communication is not limited to radio conversations. Be aware of the word **not** when reading. It changes the meaning of the sentence. The answer to questions 3 is true. The information is found in the last sentence in the passage. The answer to question 4 is false. In this case the word **not** in the statement changes the information in the last sentence of the passage, and makes the answer "false." The answer to question 5 is "true." The information can be found in the first sentence.

EXERCISE 15-4

Directions: Read the following excerpt from a health care text (Henry and Stapleton, p. 19). Answer the true-false questions based on the selection. Use the strategies you learned for answering true-false questions.

ABANDONMENT

As an EMT who is part of an EMS system, you assume the responsibility of providing care to an ill or injured patient from the time you arrive on the scene until you transfer the patient to the care of hospital personnel. A special form of litigation that EMTs and other health professionals are subject to is "abandonment." Abandonment occurs when an EMT or other health professional discontinues a patient-provider relationship without giving the patient time or opportunity to obtain substitute treatment. This would include circumstances in which an EMT leaves the patient on the scene in need of emergency care and transportation to a hospital, or in which care is prematurely discontinued.

For a case of abandonment to hold up in court the complainant must first establish that he was owed a duty and that the duty was breached.

Charges of abandonment are also possible in cases in which a patient who refused care was incompetent, such as a child or an adult with an altered mental state. If the EMT suspects that a patient who is refusing care is not capable of making a reasonable judgment, every attempt should be made to transport that patient to the hospital. If the patient adamantly refuses, the EMT should secure the aid of family or police officers. In some instances, it may be appropriate and necessary to take the patient against his or her will. If administrative or legal advice is available in such circumstances, you should avail yourself of this help.

_____ 1. Abandonment is a form of litigation.

_____ 2. Only EMTs are subject to abandonment litigation.

_____ 3. Charges of abandonment is possible in cases in which a person who refuses care is incompetent.

_____ 4. It is never appropriate to take the patient against his will.

_____ 5. As an EMT you are responsible for patient care from the time you arrive on the scene until one week after you transfer the patient to hospital care.

_____ 6. An example of an incompetent patient would be a child or adult with an altered mental state.

_____ 7. Care that is prematurely discontinued is not a case of abandonment.

_____ 8. If an EMT leaves the patient on the scene in need of emergency care, the EMT can be charged with abandonment.

_____ 9. If the patient cannot make a reasonable judgment, every attempt should be made to transport the patient to the hospital

_____ 10. If an incompetent patient refuses care, the EMT should not contact the family.

EXERCISE 15-5

Directions: Read the following excerpt from a health care textbook (Henry and Stapleton, p. 579). Study the material and then answer the objective test questions based on the material.

THE SPREAD OF COMMUNICABLE DISEASES

Infections agents spread from a source to a <u>host</u>. A *source* of infection may be a person, an insect, an object, or another substance that carries or is contaminated by an infectious agent. A *reservoir* is a source in which infectious agents can live and multiply, such as a sewer. For example, the cholera epidemic in London in the 1850s was traced to water supplied from a very polluted portion of the River Thames. During the Middle Ages, the bubonic plague, which killed one of every four people in the world, was carried by rats as well as spread from human to human. An outbreak of typhoid fever was once caused by a cook (Typhoid Mary) who unknowingly carried the disease-causing *Salmonella typhi*.

After a susceptible person or host is infected by a microorganism, the organisms can multiply until symptoms of the disease appear. The time between *contact* with an infectious agent and the onset of signs and symptoms is called the *incubation period*. During the incubation period the host may or may not be infectious to others, depending on the particular infection. The time period during which a person can transmit an infectious disease to others is called the *communicable period*. The communicable period may be before, during, and even after the symptoms of a particular disease occur. A *carrier* is a person who shows no signs of the disease yet harbors an infectious organism; this asymptomatic carrier may be a source of the infection to others (as in the case of Typhoid Mary).

Exposure is a term used to signify one's coming in contact with, but not necessarily being infected by, a disease-causing agent. The type of exposure necessary to transmit disease varies for each infectious agent. Some, such as measles, are highly contagious and can be transmitted simply by being in a room with someone with the disease. Others, such as hepatitis B or HIV, the AIDS virus, are not spread through "casual" contact. Some organisms have a greater infective potential than others.

For example, hepatitis B virus has been found to be more likely than the HIV (AIDS virus) to cause infection if a health workers suffers a stick from a contaminated needle.

In general, the greater the number of microorganisms transmitted to the host, the more significant the exposure. For example, a person receiving a transfusion of contaminated blood has a greater exposure than one suffering a needlestick from the same source.

Not everyone who is exposed to a source of infection becomes sick. Health care workers are exposed to patients with infectious conditions as part of their work. Infectious diseases that are spread by health care workers or within a health care setting are given a special name—*nosocomial infections*. Understanding what factors and conditions of an exposure can lead to actual infection is part of infection control. These factors include mode of transmission, type and duration of contact, host susceptibility, and whether or not appropriate precautions were used.

Part I. After reading this selection, fill in the blanks.

1. Infectious agents spread from a source to a _____.

2. A _____ is a source in which infectious agents can live and multiply.

3. An outbreak of _____ was once caused by a cook.

4. The time between contact with an infectious agent and the onset of signs and symptoms is called the _____.

5. _____ is a term used to signify one's coming in contact with, but not necessarily being infected by, a disease-causing agent.

Part II. Match the letters in column B with the numbers in column A.

A	B
___ 1. HIV	a. highly contagious disease
___ 2. communicable period	b. infectious diseases that are spread by health care workers
___ 3. measles	c. cook who carried disease causing Salmonella Typhus
___ 4. nosocomial infections	d. time period in which one can transmit an infectious disease
___ 5. Typhoid Mary	e. AIDS virus

Part III. Answer the multiple-choice questions based on the passage you have read.

1. A source of infection may be
   a. a person
   b. an insect
   c. an object
   d. all of the above

2. The cholera epidemic in London took place around
   a. 1850
   b. 1580
   c. 1508
   d. 1805

3. The bubonic plague took place in
   a. 1850
   b. the Middle Ages
   c. during the 1700's
   d. the jet age

4. The bubonic plague killed
   a. 4 people in the world
   b. 4,000,000 people
   c. one of every 40 people in the world
   d. one of every 4 people in the world

5. The time between contact with an infectious agent and the onset of signs and symptoms is called
   a. the communicable period
   b. casual contact
   c. the incubation period
   d. lack of exposure

Part IV. Read the following statements. In the space provided write "T" if the statement is true or "F" if the statement is false.

1. The bubonic plague came from a polluted portion of the River Thames. ____

2. During the incubation period, the host is never infectious to others. ____

3. The communicable period may be before, during, and even after the symptoms of a particular disease occur. ____

4. Everyone who is exposed to a source of infection becomes sick. ____

5. The type of exposure necessary to transmit disease is the same for each infectious agent. ____

EXERCISE 15-6

Directions: Read the following excerpt from a health care textbook (Henry and Stapleton, p. 515). Create you own objective test based on the selection. Create five short-answers, five matching, five multiple-choice, and five true-false questions.

ACUTE RADIATION SYNDROME—FACTORS AFFECTING SEVERITY OF EXPOSURE

The severity of a <u>radiation</u> exposure is affected by the strength of the radioactive source, the type of radiation, the duration of exposure, the area of the body exposed, the distance from the radioactive source, the amount of shielding between the source and the victim, and the age and condition of the patient.

ACUTE RADIATION SYNDROME

When high doses of radiation are absorbed over a short period of time, e.g., minutes to hours, signs and symptoms known as "acute radiation syndrome" may be encountered. This syndrome results from damage to the bone marrow, gastrointestinal tract, central nervous system, and cardiovascular system as the dosage increases. For example, at an exposure of 50 rem, patients may have no visible effects, but a small percentage of persons who have been exposed may show a depression of white blood cells and platelets on blood testing. Physical signs and symptoms may first appear at a dose of 100 rem, with nausea and vomiting occurring in a small percentage of exposed persons. At 200 rem most patients show signs of nausea and vomiting, with more profound depression of the bone marrow. At 400 rem about 50% of the exposed individuals die within weeks. An exposure of 600 rem can result in a near 100% death rate if there is no medical intervention.

At doses of 1000 rem, <u>gastrointestinal</u> complications begin to appear as nausea, vomiting, and diarrhea of immediate onset. At doses of 3000 rem there are additional irreversible cardiovascular effects, resulting in irreversible <u>hypotension</u> and a central nervous system syndrome with rapid onset of drowsiness, uncoordination, and convulsions.

Genetic effects may occur at smaller doses. A 5- to 25-rem exposure is the minimal dose detectable by chromosome analysis. The sperm count is reduced in males at doses of 25 rad. Procreation should be avoided for a period of time following exposure. Pregnant women and women who may be pregnant should avoid any exposure to the site of a radiation accident.

Known long-term effects from radiation include cataracts, cancer, alterations in growth and development if the exposure occurs during fetal development, and possibly a shortened life span.

For comparison, note that exposure to natural radioactive sources results in an average of 125 mrem per year. Doses from x-rays vary with the examination, from 66 mrem from a chest x-ray to 10,000 mrem from a lumbar spine examination (four views).

The stronger the radioactive source, the greater is the dose received over a given unit of time for a patient at a fixed distance from the exposure.

TYPES OF RADIATION

As noted previously, gamma radiation and neutrons are the most penetrating forms of radiation. Like x-rays, they pass through all body tissues. Alpha and beta particles do not penetrate through intact skin, and damage is limited with careful decontamination.

Internal contamination with alpha and beta particles requires early medical attention to consider the use of agents to hasten the elimination of the isotope and to block toxic effects on the organs.

DURATION OF EXPOSURE

The duration of exposure is important. Rescuers can gauge the amount of time they have to enter an exposure area if they have knowledge of the exposure rate. For example, if the exposure rate is 100 R/hr, 15 minutes in the area may result in absorption of 25 R. Rescue workers can reduce individual exposure by sharing the time spent in the danger zone. The shorter the time spent in a radiation field, the less radiation the body absorbs.

AREA OF THE BODY EXPOSED

Penetrating radiation affects the cells through which it passes. Limitation of the exposure to an extremity, for example, may limit damage to this area and not result in the radiation syndrome.

Different parts of the body can tolerate different amounts of radiation. The maximal permissible occupational standards for the hands are several times the allowable limit for the gonads or the whole body. The shielding of parts of the body during medical or dental x-rays is an example of limiting body exposure.

DISTANCE FROM THE SOURCE

The greater the distance from the source of radiation, the less the radiation dose that is absorbed. If the source of radiation emanates from a single point, radioactivity falls inversely with the square of the distance. Thus, if one doubles the distance away from the source, the intensity falls off by a factor of four. If radiation sources are scattered, however, this inverse square rule does not apply. However, one always decreases radiation exposure significantly by increasing the distance from the material.

Learning Strategies for Taking the Essay Test

In an essay test, students are expected to state the main ideas and to support those general statements with details. Also, students should be able to draw conclusions from ideas presented. Clear, simple, organized writing, as well as content, often counts toward your grade.

Before writing your answer

- Read the entire test carefully.
- Pay close attention to the directions.
- Look at the point value of each question. You should spend more time on a question worth 30 points than on one worth 10 points.
- Read the questions carefully.

- Understand the question. Are you asked to list, explain, classify, contrast, or sequence information?
- Allow time for reading questions, thinking about, and organizing your answers.
- Arrange your thoughts. Write an outline.

While writing your answer

- State the main idea in a clear topic sentence.
- Support main ideas with relevant details.

After writing your answer

- Read all your answers.
- Check to see that you have answered the questions that were asked.
- Make sure that you have answered all parts of each question.
- Make necessary changes in content, mechanics, and organization.
- Use an editing checklist to help you revise your essay.

Following is an example of an editing checklist:

	YES	NO
CONTENT		
Are the ideas developed?	___	___
Is the presentation logical?	___	___
Are the examples appropriate?	___	___
MECHANICS		
Did you check your choice of words?	___	___
Did you improve the sentence structure?	___	___
Did you make sure your use of punctuation is correct?	___	___
ORGANIZATION		
Does your essay contain		
an introduction?	___	___
a body with supporting evidence?	___	___
a conclusion?	___	___

Example 15-5

Directions: Read the following excerpt from *Ethical Dimensions in the Health Professions* by Purtilo. Review the sample essay question and answer based on the selection.

Sometimes I have heard it said that as part of his or her professional responsibility of self-improvement a health professional has a responsibility to be an exemplar in maintaining a healthy lifestyle. A dietitian who is obese because of dietary habits, a physically unfit physical therapist, a respiratory therapist who smokes cigarettes, a social worker or psychologist who does not attend to social or emotional problems, or a nurse who consistently gets too little sleep soundly is criticized on the basis of being a health professional who should "know better." The health professional *does* know better, knowledge-wise, about the deleterious effects of obesity, unfitness, mental stress, driving oneself, and other abuses or neglects of the body and mind. But what do you think? Should health professionals be more responsible for maintaining a health lifestyle than anyone else? If they have difficulty in these ways do they have a *special* responsibility to do something constructive about it? [p. 77]

Do you think that health professionals should be more responsible for maintaining a healthy lifestyle than other people? Why? Why not?

Sample Answer

NOTE: In the following paragraph the first sentence introduces the topic of the paragraph; the next three sentences provide the supporting details; and the final sentence supplies the conclusions.

Health professionals should be more responsible for maintaining a healthy lifestyle than are people employed in other fields. A person trying to lose weight would not be inspired by an overweight nutritionist. How can a physician who smokes effectively advise a cardiac patient to stop smoking? Social workers who have drinking or drug problems would not be able to deter teenagers from falling into dangerous habits. Health professionals have a responsibility to set a standard and act as positive role models for the people in their care.

EXERCISE 15-7

Directions: Read the following excerpt from the Purtilo health care textbook. Answer the following essay question based on the selection.

PLACEBOS: A SPECIAL CASE OF INFORMATION DISCLOSURE

The issue of placebo use has received some attention from psychiatrists and ethicists, but most literature on placebos has been directed toward physicians. Little research has been done concerning the role of health professionals and the use of placebo medications and procedures and yet nurses and pharmacists, in particular, play a direct and essential part in this particular form of deception in health care practice. Although the health professional is rarely the person who makes the decision to use placebos, he or she may be in a position to dispense or administer the deceptive drug or perform such a procedure. In order to think through clearly the ethical problems that may arise in such a situation, it is important to understand the physician's position in prescribing, and some of the history and psychology of the placebo response.

Placebo comes from the Latin word meaning "I shall please." It can be defined as any therapeutic procedure (or component of one) that is given in spite of the fact that it has no known pharmacologic effect on the condition. A pure placebo is a preparation of an inert substance that is not known to have any pharmacological effect. An impure placebo is an active drug that is being given for its psychological effect in a disorder for which it is not known to be effective, such as antibiotic treatment for a common cold or other viral infection. Administering this kind of placebo carries the risk of real side effects, as well as the interpersonal and professional risks we will discuss in regard to pure placebos.

Physicians rarely give pure placebos, such as sugar pills or saline injections, but when they do, serious ethical issues need to be considered. One important aspect of the practice of giving placebos is what is called the "placebo effect." Virtually all treatments (and some diagnostic studies, as well) have positive effects for some patients over and above the specific effects of their pharmacological mechanisms. Beecher published a classic study in 1955 showing that placebos are effective in treating pain in 35% of patients, regardless of the source of pain or clinical condition of the patient. Modern neuropharmacology research has discovered that the brain produces its own chemicals, which can act as analgesics and relaxants. These chemicals, called endorphins, seem to work better for some people than for others, which may explain scientifically why some people are placebo reactors and others are not. A common error made by health professionals has been the assumption that a symptom (for example, pain) that is successfully treated by a placebo is therefore not real, or "only psychological." The discovery of endorphins gives us a scientific way of understanding some of the very powerful physiological effects of placebos.

The placebo effect may be partly responsible for the success of ancient remedies given by shamans or medicine men. Some of the remedies contained pharmacologically active agents but others did not, and much of the healer's work consisted of rituals and symbols. The fact that they were often successful is a tribute to the power of what we refer to today as the physician-patient relationship, or the "therapeutic partnership."

Modern examples of the placebo effect are the effects of suggestion in decreasing stomach acid in ulcer patients, alleviating bronchospasm in asthma, and lowering blood pressure. The phenomenon of the placebo effect is widespread and powerful enough so that no research trials of new medications or even surgical procedures are considered truly rigorous unless the element of suggestion has been effectively eliminated, as in randomized double blind clinical trials. [pp. 120–121]

Question: Weigh the positive effects against the possible negative effects of administering placebos to patients. Then decide whether you think it is unethical to use placebo medications in patient care.

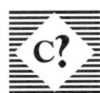

Strategy 5: Evaluate Test Results

Once your test paper is returned, don't just look at your score and throw away the paper. Look at what you know. Look at what you still need to learn. Go back to your notes and text to correct all errors. If you still need help, schedule a conference with your study partner, study group, and/or your instructor. Save all test papers. Use these tests to review for your final exam.

REVIEWING STRATEGIES FOR IMPROVING TEST SCORES

TO LEARN	USE THIS STRATEGY
To plan ahead	Apply time management skills.
To keep up with assignments	Be an active reader.
	Use active listening and effective note taking strategies.
To study and learn material	Review class notes and text, summaries and outlines, and underlined material.
	Organize information into categories.
	Review vocabulary.
	Pay attention to illustrations and formulas.
	Use mnemonics to improve your memory.
	Monitor your learning.
	Discover your best study method.
	Design practice tests.
To take the test successfully	Learn strategies for taking objective tests.
	Learn strategies for taking essay tests.
To evaluate test results	Look at what you know.
	Look at what you still need to learn.

UNIT V

READING SELECTIONS

In Unit V, Reading Selections, you will apply all the strategies you learned in Units I through IV. Each reading selection is an excerpt from a text in the allied health fields. The exercises based on the readings are designed to give you practice in the reading, writing, mathematics, and study strategies that you learned in the other units. Unit V can be used throughout the semester or as a final unit once Chapters 1 to 15 are completed. When you have completed Unit V, you will be prepared to successfully read and study from your textbooks in the allied health fields.

Reading Selection 1

PREVIEW QUESTION
- What are the reasons you chose to enter the allied health care field? What do you expect from your new career?

VOCABULARY

Directions: Locate five words that are new to you in this reading. Write the meaning of each of these words in the space provided.

_____
_____
_____
_____
_____
_____
_____
_____
_____
_____

A career as a medical assistant is challenging and offers variety, job satisfaction, opportunity for service, fair financial reward, and possibility for advancement. It is open to both men and women.

ADVANTAGES

The trained medical assistant is equipped with a flexible, adaptable career. The skills acquired by the medical assistant can be carried all through life, and employment is readily available anywhere in the world that medicine is practiced. Although medical assisting holds many opportunities for young people, it is one career that usually does not have a **mandatory** retirement age. Many medical assistants are still employed far beyond the usual retirement age because physicians realize the value of experienced, mature employees.

From Kinn ME, Woods MA, Derge EF: The Medical Assistant: Administrative and Clinical, 7th ed. Philadelphia, W.B. Saunders, 1993, pp. 6–8.

CAREER OPPORTUNITIES

The delivery of health care has changed dramatically in the last two decades. Increasing health care costs have created a trend away from hospital-based treatment toward the delivery of care in physicians' offices and in outpatient centers. Although doctors have employed assistants in their practices for many years, computerization and technologic advances have created more opportunities for qualified medical assistants and increased their responsibilities; as a result, the need for those trained in this profession has grown.

As the requirements that medical assistants must fulfill have become more clearly defined, the quality of their training has improved and become more accessible. Medical assisting is recognized as an important allied health profession. Employment opportunities in allied health are abundant, extremely varied, and increasing every day because of the growing concern about the availability of health protection for every individual in the United States. More medical assistants are employed by practicing physicians than any other type of allied health care personnel.

As a medical assistant, your work can be **administrative, clinical,** or **technical.** You can be a receptionist in a hospital or physician's office, a transcriptionist, insurance specialist, financial secretary, billing and collection specialist, a clinical assistant involved in patient care, or an emergency technician, to name just a few. You may choose to work for a physician in **solo private practice,** for a medical partnership or **group practice,** a **health maintenance organization (HMO),** a hospital, or a **freestanding emergency center.** The physician(s) may be either in general practice or engaged in a specialty such as surgery, internal medicine, dermatology, obstetrics, pediatrics, psychiatry, or radiology.

There are career opportunities in public health facilities, hospitals, laboratories, medical schools, research institutions and universities as well as in voluntary health agencies and medical firms of all kinds. There are also opportunities for work with such federal agencies as the Department of Veterans Affairs, the United States Health Service, and Armed Forces clinics or hospitals.

Although appropriate training equips you for work in a variety of settings, this text is designed primarily for the person who seeks employment in a medical office or who is already employed as a medical assistant.

Ideally, you should have both administrative and clinical training, even though you may have a personal preference for one or the other. The physician's staff should be able to handle all responsibilities of the office except those requiring the services of a physician or other licensed personnel. Where there are several assistants, each should be able and willing to substitute in an emergency for any of the others. Few physicians in private practice attempt to get along without at least one assistant. The great majority have at least two, and many have five or more.

EARNINGS

What kind of earnings can the medical assistant expect? As in any other career field, there are **regional** differences. There is usually some difference between earnings in **rural** and in **urban** areas. However, as a medical assistant, you can generally expect a satisfactory return on your investment in training, experience, and skill. Physicians have come to realize that a good medical assistant is worth a good salary. Many have learned through bitter experience that "bargain" help is often the most expensive.

The job turnover among medical assistants is surprisingly low. This fact may indicate that medical assistants derive a high degree of satisfaction from their work. Many instances have been reported of medical assistants who were hired when a physician started practice and remained until the physician's retirement.

NECESSARY SKILLS

Every profession or trade has its special vocabulary or **jargon;** the language of medicine must be understood by every allied health professional. The medical assistant must have a basic knowledge of law and ethics as they relate to the medical profession. Additionally, to qualify for administrative duties, the medical assistant must have good handwriting, be a proficient typist, and have good language, communication, and mathematics skills. Knowledge of shorthand is helpful, but in most medical facilities, electronic dictation and word processing are the current trend. Some training in records management is desirable for both the administrative and clinical assistants as are skills in human relations and personal communications. All medical assistants should be trained in cardiopulmonary resuscitation (CPR) and emergency first aid. The clinical medical assistant must be skilled in certain patient care arts and must have the necessary training to perform common medical tests. The laws governing which medical tests a clinical assistant may perform, however, vary from state to state.

DUTIES OF THE MEDICAL ASSISTANT

The duties of the medical assistant vary from one facility to the next, since the schedule must be geared to the type of practice and the working habits of the individual physician. In the office with only one employee, the medical assistant's time is divided between administrative and clinical duties. In the multiple-employee office, the positions tend to be more specialized.

Administrative Duties

A medical assistant's duties are similar to those of any administrative assistant to a top executive, but they have specific medical aspects. They include:

- answering telephones
- scheduling appointments
- interviewing and instructing new patients
- screening nonpatient visitors and salespersons
- explaining the doctor's fees to patients
- opening and sorting mail
- answering routine correspondence
- pulling patient charts for scheduled appointments
- filing reports and correspondence
- making arrangements for patient admission to a hospital and instructing the patient regarding admission
- making financial arrangements with patients
- completing insurance claim forms
- maintaining financial records and files
- preparing and mailing statements
- preparing checks for the doctor's signature
- maintaining a file of paid and unpaid invoices
- preparing and maintaining employees' payroll records (or submitting payroll information to an outside accountant)

Sometimes you may act as an informal editorial assistant to the doctor by helping in the preparation of manuscripts or speeches or by clipping articles from professional journals and assisting with the maintenance of the doctor's personal medical library.

Clinical Duties

Clinical duties are also varied. In general, the medical assistant:

- helps patients prepare for examinations and other office procedures
- takes the medical history
- assists the doctor when requested to do so
- cleans and sterilizes instruments and equipment
- instructs patients regarding preparation for x-ray and laboratory examinations
- keeps the supply cabinets well stocked

You may also collect specimens from patients and either send them to a laboratory or perform certain diagnostic texts for which you have been trained. You may also perform electrocardiography and, depending on state laws, assist in radiography. You may take and record a patient's temperature, pulse rate, respiratory characteristics, blood pressure, height, and weight. You may also prepare treatment or surgical trays and assist with patient treatments or surgery. You may occasionally be called upon to administer emergency first aid.

PAST, PRESENT, AND FUTURE

The first medical assistant was probably a neighbor of a physician who was called to help when an extra pair of hands was needed. As the practice of medicine became more complicated, some physicians hired registered nurses to assist in their office practices. When recordkeeping, data reporting, and an increasing number of business details began to be burdensome, the physician realized a need for an assistant with business training. Slowly, training programs that focused on both administrative and clinical skills began to appear in community and junior colleges. Medical assistant organizations on county and state levels were established. A national organization for medical assistants was formed in 1957, and a few years later, national certification for medical assistants became possible. In recent years, legislation regarding the scope of practice of medical assistants has been enacted in some states. Whether to enter the field of medical assisting is a big decision. Medical assisting is more than just a job—it is a career requiring dedication, integrity, and a commitment to continuing education.

IS MEDICAL ASSISTING FOR YOU?

- Do you have a friendly and pleasant disposition?
- Are you considerate, respectful, and kind?
- Can you view a situation through the eyes of others?

The services performed by a medical assistant are extremely personal. For this reason, the manner in which these services are performed can actually affect the health and welfare of a patient.

- Are you attentive to details?
- Are you accurate and dependable?
- Can you remain calm and accept responsibility during an emergency?

You may be called upon to assume charge of the office when the doctor is out. The doctor must depend on the medical assistant's good judgment when he or she is left alone.

Discretion and concern for the patient are very important. Many patients have chosen other physicians because of a seeming lack of concern on the part of medical assistants. The patient who feels comfortable with the medical assistant will probably feel comfortable with the doctor.

WRITING

Directions: Answer the following question based on the reading selection. Remember to use the following writing strategies:

- Organize ideas
- Write the first draft
- Revise, edit, and proofread to write the final draft

What personal qualities must an individual have to become a successful medical assistant?

COMPREHENSION QUESTIONS

Directions: Answer the multiple-choice questions based on the selection. Use the strategies you learned for answering multiple-choice questions.

1. At 65 years old, or retirement age, a medical assistant
    a. must retire
    b. needs to take a complete medical examination
    c. can continue working
    d. must renew state certification

2. A position as a medical assistant is
    a. available only in the United States and Canada
    b. not available in Africa and Asia
    c. only available in the city where you trained
    d. available anywhere that medicine is practiced

3. A medical assistant's work can be
    a. administrative, clinical, or technical
    b. administrative, clinical, or educational
    c. clinical, technical, or philosophical
    d. clinical, educational, or philosophical

4. The salaries for medical assistants are
    a. the same throughout the country
    b. the same throughout the world
    c. different in rural and urban areas
    d. different depending on your training

5. A medical assistant does not need to know how to
    a. use a computer
    b. prescribe drugs
    c. communicate
    d. write clearly

6. The duties of a medical assistant will
   a. vary from office to office
   b. be uniform from office to office
   c. be independent of the doctor's habits
   d. always be clerical

7. The first medical assistants were probably
   a. physicians' wives
   b. highly trained nurses
   c. other physicians
   d. helpful neighbors

8. After a national organization for medical assistants began
   a. national certification became possible
   b. the clerical aspect of the profession was established
   c. the clinical aspect of the profession was established
   d. international certification became possible

9. To avoid having patients feel that nobody cares, the medical assistant should possess
   a. a mind for details
   b. discretion
   c. intelligence
   d. fairness

10. There is a low turnover among medical assistants because
    a. there are few job openings
    b. medical assistants are afraid of losing their retirement benefits
    c. medical assistants are fearful of getting poor references
    d. medical assistants feel satisfied in their jobs

WORD PROBLEM

Directions: Use the strategies you learned for solving word problems to answer this question:

A medical assistant living in New York City makes $35,000 annually. How much does he make per month? A medical assistant in a farming town in Mississippi makes $9,000 less. How much does she make annually? How much does she make monthly?

Reading Selection 2

> **PREVIEW QUESTION**
> - What questions can you create from the boldface headings?

VOCABULARY

Directions: Locate five words that are new to you in this reading. Write the meaning of each of these words in the space provided.

_____
_____
_____
_____
_____
_____
_____
_____
_____
_____

COMPUTER SOFTWARE

Computers have a *disk operating system* (DOS), which controls the loading and storage of files from and to a computer's memory and to a magnetic disk. There is no standard operating system in the personal computer environment. Some systems are CP/M (control program/microprocessor), MS/DOS (MicroSoft/Disk Operating System), PC-DOS (the IBM PC operating system), and the UNIX system developed by Bell Laboratories. If you are working on a word processor (stand-alone or text editing) or are using a microcomputer, sophisticated word processing software is available as well as English, medical, and pharmaceutical dictionaries. Some word processing packages have macro capabilities, or you can purchase software with a modified keyboard to allow macro or "chording," the simultaneous depression

---

From Diehl MO, Fordney MT: Medical Typing and Transcribing: Techniques and Procedures, 3rd ed. Philadelphia, W.B. Saunders, 1991, pp. 30–32.

of multiple keys. This feature is for frequently used words and phrases. For example, keying in "PE" would appear as "physical examination" on the computer screen. Integrated software packages have *windows* that let you see various functions simultaneously. There are also computer programs that can be activated by voice instead of keyboarding command keys. *Utility programs* are general-purpose software programs that perform activities which are not specific to an application, i.e., spell checkers, line count, macro makers, install *fonts* (the size and style of type), *initialize* a disk (to prepare the magnetic surface of a blank diskette so it can accept data), and so forth. Sometimes a word processing software program will have these utility features incorporated in it. If data is to be stored, a blank disk is initialized and the data is given a file name so it can be *retrieved* from the *file*.

COMPUTER RIBBONS

Cartridge ribbons for printers may look identical, but they can vary considerably in their construction, ink, fabric specifications, print quality, and print durability. The price of the ribbon is not always a good measure of product quality. Generic-brand ribbons are less expensive but may be acceptable, or of poor quality and could cause printer damage. Brand-named ribbons are usually of high quality but also the most expensive. Some features to look for in a good quality ribbon are

1. crisp characters that will not smudge or smear.
2. print quality that is consistent for the life of the ribbon.
3. durable cartridge and ribbon materials.
4. correct and durable packaging to avoid drying out of the ribbon.
5. written guarantee by the dealer to replace or credit defective ribbons.

COMPUTER DISKS

Because you will have important information stored on computer floppy disks, it is wise to take care of them. The information is magnetically recorded. Therefore, any magnetic or electromagnetic field can scramble or destroy data recorded onto a disk. Your telephone, printer, or video terminal contain magnetic fields, so do not place a disk on top of this equipment. Each disk should be properly stored in a protective envelope. If two disks are stored in one envelope, information on one disk can be "imprinted" or transferred onto another. All the disks should be put into a box. The container should be kept away from extreme heat (100°F or above) and out of direct sunlight, since valuable information could be destroyed or the disk could melt. Never attach rubberbands or paper clips to disks because these could bend or damage them.

When labeling a disk, use felt-tip pens when writing on the label if it is affixed to a disk. It is better to fill out the label before adhering it to the disk. Do not stack labels on a disk because this can cause an imbalance in the weight of its surface.

Above all, keep the disks clean and out of the way of possible spills or stains. Therefore, never eat or smoke around the computer area. If a disk must be cleaned, use only tap water.

COMPUTER MODEM

The word *modem* is an acronym for MOdulator DEModulator unit and is a device that converts data into signals for telephone transmission and then (at the receiving end) back again into data. Some transcription services offer this type of telecommunication by hooking their word processing or computer equipment into the telephone lines. Then they can transmit correspondence or reports to an office, clinic, or hospital facility many miles away. Documents transmitted in this way can be revised and edited by the receiving office before they are printed out into a hard copy.

TRANSCRIPTION EQUIPMENT

Dictation and transcription equipment has advanced considerably since the development of electronic and high-*fidelity* recordings. Shorthand has become almost passé because of improved dictating equipment, and the medical transcriptionist can now do other tasks while the physician is dictating reports. There are a variety of models that the physician may use in the office, home, or hospital or while attending conferences. They are as follows:

1. *Digital dictation.* The dictated voice is digitized (converted to a string of O's and I's representing the audio waveform) and stored as data on a computer disk with identifying data (patient and dictator identification and worktype). The data is instantly and selectively accessible before, during, or after transcription. When accessed (from a dictation/transcription station or telephone), the binary digits are converted back to analog waveform to sound just as the original dictation. This type of system features better sound quality, thereby enhancing the dictator's ability to insert or delete for *error-free* dictation. Digital dictation is making analog tape dictation obsolete in the same way that word processors are replacing typewriters.

2. *Voice recognition.* This is transcriptionless dictation and is composed of a computer system equipped with sound sensors. The physician trains the system to understand his or her speech patterns, and the system translates the tones of the human voice into computer commands and text on the screen. The report must be proofread and edited for grammar and punctuation before it is printed and ready for signature.

3. *Telecommunications.* The physician dictates by telephoning from home to the office or the hospital. He or she dials a special number that seizes the transcribing equipment. Physicians may find that they are able to think more quickly and clearly while talking into a telephone-like device rather than into traditional microphone equipment. Phone-in adaptors can be set up to work with a variety of transcribing equipment.

4. *Tank-type machines.* The transcribing unit is located in a remote area with direct input from one or more dictating stations in a building that utilizes telephone-type services. This equipment is popular in the hospital word processing department and uses an *endless loop* system. The transcriptionist does not have to be concerned with the physical transfer of recorded medium from the machine, and only the foot pedal and manual controls on the transcribing units are used. This eliminates the problem of lost reports.

5. *Cassette-changer central recorder.* This holds 15 to 25 cassettes, which can be programmed to change automatically, either by the number of dictators having access to the recorders or by the percentage of tape used. It can also be set up so that each person dictating can be on a separate cassette. Dictators can access the equipment from any telephone, at work or at home.

6. *Desk-top machines.* This is used by the physician and medical transcriptionist in the office. The most common units available include the following:
    a. A *dictation unit,* for dictating purposes only.
    b. A *transcription unit,* designed for the transcriptionist who will transcribe the dictation.
    c. A *combination unit,* which can be used for both dictation and transcription.

7. *Portable dictating machine.* The physician may hand-carry this to a meeting or use it in a car to dictate whenever he or she wishes. It can be wall plug or battery operated. Portable cassette recorders are popular because they can be used at conventions and conferences. Minicassettes or picocasssettes can be played back at the office if the physician has purchased a transcribing unit that features the minicassette adaptor of minicassette or picocassette transcriber.

WRITING

Directions: Answer the following question based on the reading selection. Remember to use the following writing strategies:

- Organize ideas
- Write the first draft
- Revise, edit, and proofread to write the final draft

What role do you see computers playing in the health care professions?

COMPREHENSION QUESTIONS

Directions: Answer the true and false questions based on the selection. Use the strategies you learned for answering true and false questions.

1. DOS stands for digital operating system. T____ F____
2. A macro is used for frequently used words and phrases. T____ F____
3. Fonts refer to the different keys on the keyboard. T____ F____
4. Windows let you see various functions at one time. T____ F____
5. You can assume that an expensive computer ribbon will always be good. T____ F____
6. Information on one computer disk can be transferred to another if they share the same envelope. T____ F____
7. A computer modem relies on a telephone. T____ F____
8. Shorthand is still a much needed skill in the health care professions. T____ F____
9. It is not possible for a computer to recognize human voices yet. T____ F____
10. Portable dictating machines are popular because they can be used at conferences and conventions. T____ F____

WORD PROBLEM

Directions: Use the strategies you learned for solving word problems to answer this question:

Howell General Hospital has 18 cassette-changer central recorders. Each of these recorders holds 15 cassettes. How many cassettes can be used in total? Nine allied health workers have been trained to use these central recorders. How many cassettes can each worker use at one time?

Reading Selection 3

> **PREVIEW QUESTION**
> - What are the three layers of skin, and what are their functions?

VOCABULARY

Directions: Locate five words that are new to you in this reading. Write the meaning of each of these words in the space provided.

_____
_____
_____
_____
_____
_____
_____
_____
_____
_____

THE SKIN

The skin is the body's tough, outer protective covering. Together with its glands, hair, and nails, the skin makes up the **integumentary system** (in-teg"u-**men**'-tar-y). This is the body system with which you are most familiar because it is at least partly exposed to view. Perhaps for this reason we give the skin a lot of attention. We scrub it, cream it, and coat it with makeup; we cut, shave, and curl its hair; and we manicure its nails.

The skin is also important in communication. You may shake hands, stroke, kiss, squeeze, or slap it. Involuntary changes in the skin reflect emotional states. For example, you may blush with embarrassment, blanch with fear or rage, redden with exertion, or sweat excessively when anxious. In addition, the appearance, coloration, temperature, and feel of the skin are important indicators of general health and of many disease states.

From Solomon EP: Introduction to Human Anatomy and Physiology. Philadelphia, W.B. Saunders, 1992, pp 41–43.

The Skin Functions as a Protective Barrier

The skin is the outer boundary of the body—the part in direct contact with the external environment. The 20 or so square feet of skin that cover the body must resist continuous wear and tear, drying, and exposure to cold, heat, and toxic substances. The skin is frequently cut, bruised, or scraped and must be able to heal such wounds. The skin is important in maintaining the balanced internal environment. The skin:

1. Protects the body against injury and against disease organisms. The skin is the body's first line of defense against harmful bacteria and other agents of disease.
2. Receives information about the outside world. Located within the skin are sensory receptors that detect touch, pressure, heat, cold, and pain.
3. Prevents drying out. The cells of the body are bathed in an internal sea, a carefully regulated, dilute salt solution essential to life. We humans move about in the relatively dry environment of air. The skin prevents loss of fluid so that the cells do not dry out.
4. Helps maintain body temperature. Capillary (tiny blood vessels) networks and sweat glands in the skin are an important part of the body's temperature regulating system.
5. Has sweat glands that excrete excess water and some wastes from the body.
6. Contains a compound that is converted to vitamin D when the skin is exposed to the ultraviolet rays of the sun.

The Skin Consists of the Epidermis and Dermis

Skin consists of two main layers: an outer **epidermis** (ep"-ih-**der**'-mus) and an inner **dermis** (**der**'-mus). Beneath the skin is an underlying **subcutaneous layer** (sub-koo-**tay**'-nee-us) (Fig. V-1).

The Epidermis Continuously Replaces Itself

Over most parts of the body the epidermis is only about as thick as a page of this book, yet it consists of several sublayers. The epidermis consists of stratified epithelial tissue. The outer cells of the epidermis continuously wear off. They are immediately replaced by new cells. New epidermal cells are constantly produced in the deepest sublayer of the epidermis. These cells mature as they are pushed toward the outer surface by newer cells beneath. As they move through the outer sublayer of epidermis, the cells die. **Keratin** (ker'a-tin), a tough waterproofing protein, fills most of each cell. The cells at the surface of the skin resemble dead scales. They are closely packed together and serve as a waterproof protective covering for the body.

The Dermis Provides Strength and Elasticity

The dermis is the thick layer of skin beneath the epidermis (Fig. V–1). Dermis consists of dense connective tissue composed mainly of collagen fibers. Collagen is largely responsible for the mechanical strength of the skin. It also permits the skin to stretch and then return to its normal form again. Blood vessels and nerves, which are generally absent in the epidermis, are found throughout the dermis. Specialized skin structures such as hair follicles and glands are found in the dermis. They develop from cells of the epidermis that push down into the dermis.

The upper portion of the dermis has many small, fingerlike elevations that project into the epidermal tissue. Extensive networks of capillaries in these elevations deliver oxygen and nutrients to the cells of the epidermis and also function in temperature regulation. The patterns of ridges and grooves visible on the skin of the soles and palms (including the fingertips) reflect the arrangement of the dermal elevations beneath. Unique to each individual, these patterns provide the fingerprints so useful to law-enforcement officials. They also serve as friction ridges that help us hold onto the objects we grasp.

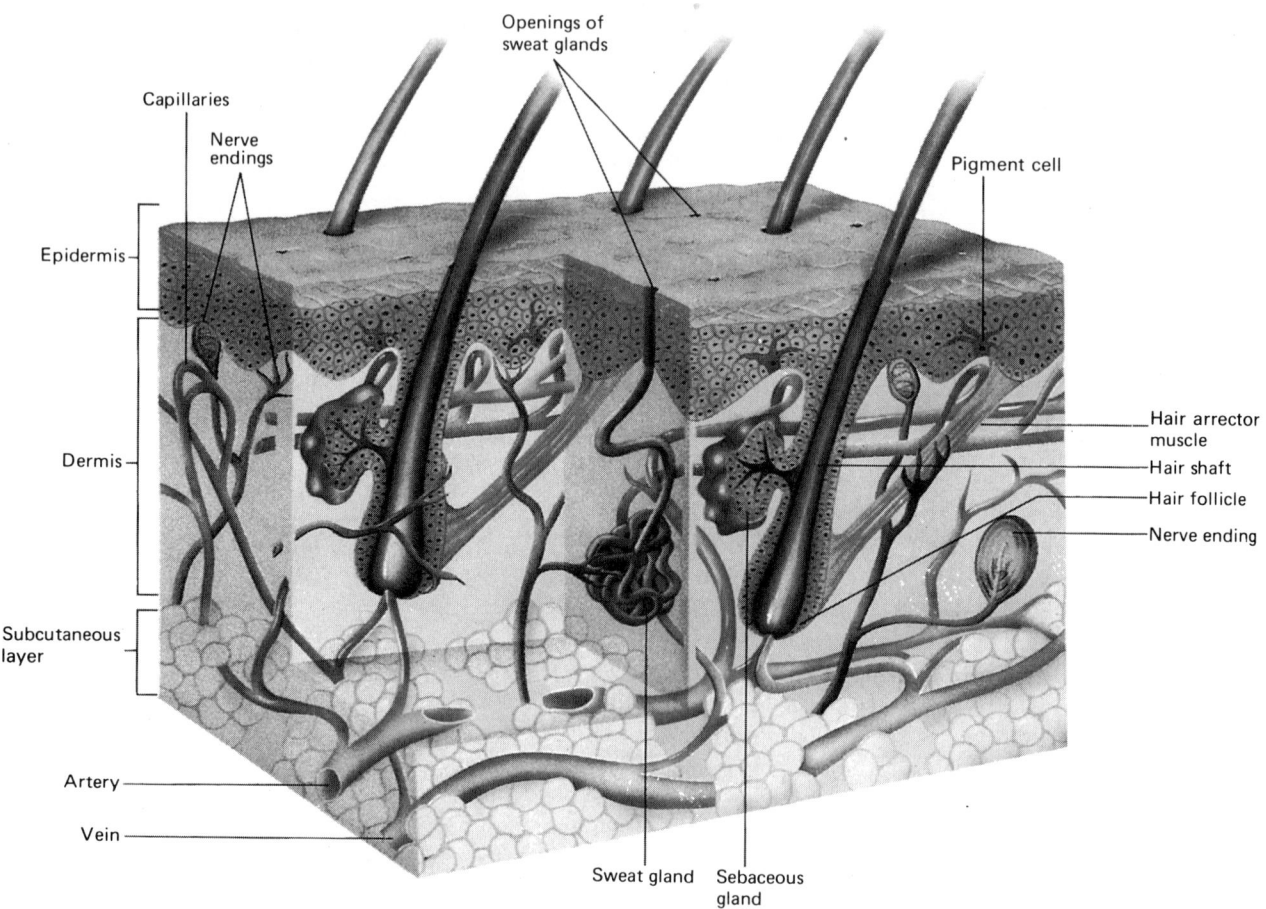

Figure V-1 Microscopic structure of skin.

The Subcutaneous Layer Attaches the Skin to Underlying Tissues

The subcutaneous layer beneath the dermis is also known as the **superficial fascia (fash'-ee-ah)**. This layer consists of loose connective tissue, usually containing a lot of adipose (fat) tissue. The subcutaneous layer attaches the skin to the muscles and other tissues beneath. This thick fatty layer helps protect underlying organs from mechanical shock. It also insulates the body, thus conserving heat. Fat stored within the adipose tissue can be mobilized and used as an energy source when adequate food is not available. Distribution of fat in the subcutaneous layer is largely responsible for characteristic male and female body shapes.

WRITING

Directions: Answer the following question based on the reading selection. Remember to use the following writing strategies:

- Organize ideas
- Write the first draft
- Revise, edit, and proofread to write the final draft

What is the overall importance of the skin for humans?

COMPREHENSION QUESTIONS

Directions: Answer the matching questions based on the selection. Use the strategies you learned for answering matching questions.

SKIN LAYER   **FUNCTION**

A. Epidermis   Attaches skin to muscle   1. ____

B. Dermis   Protects organs from mechanical shock   2. ____

C. Superficial fascia   Responsible for mechanical strength of skin   3. ____

                        Serves as a waterproof cover   4. ____

                        Allows the skin to stretch   5. ____

                        Insulates the body   6. ____

                        Conserves heat   7. ____

                        Capillaries deliver oxygen to cells   8. ____

                        Cells are pushed to outer surface by newer cells   9. ____

                        Helps with temperature regulation   10. ____

WORD PROBLEM

Directions: Use the strategies you learned for solving word problems to answer this question.

All individuals have their unique set of fingerprints, or visible ridges and grooves, on the tips of their fingers. Detective Hogwood is investigating a crime scene. Luckily, he has been able to find the fingerprints of the perpetrator. However, they are not complete. Nevertheless, he runs them through the computer looking for a partial match. Out of the 206,000 prints registered in the computer, 20% of them are potential matches. How many people does this represent?

Reading Selection 4

> **PREVIEW QUESTIONS**
> - What systems of the body does this selection discuss?
> - What do you already know about these systems?

VOCABULARY

Directions: Locate five words which are new to you in this reading. Write the meaning of each of these words in the space provided.

_____

_____

_____

_____

_____

_____

_____

_____

_____

_____

SYSTEMS NEEDED FOR MOVEMENT AND SUPPORT

The Skeletal System

The bones of the skeleton are divided into an *axial* portion, consisting of the cranium, spinal column, ribs, and sternum, and an *appendicular* portion, consisting of the shoulder girdle, the hip girdle, and the bones of the arms and legs. The skeleton gives the body structure, protects vital organs, and works with the muscular system to produce movement at the joints. Blood cells are produced within the red marrow of the bones.

From Flynn JC Jr (Ed.): Procedures in Phlebotomy. Philadelphia, W.B. Saunders, 1994, pp. 16–20.

The Muscular System

There are three types of muscle tissue: **smooth (visceral) muscle,** which makes up the walls of hollow organs and the blood vessels; **cardiac muscle,** which makes up the heart; and **skeletal (striated) muscle,** which is attached to the bones. The term *muscular system* refers to the last of these, the more than 700 muscles that move the skeleton (Fig. V–2). The main property of muscle tissue is the ability to contract in response to stimulation by the nervous system. To function, muscles need a source of energy, such as glucose; oxygen to release the energy from the nutrient; and calcium for the interactions of contractile filaments within the muscle cells. Muscles can function for a brief period without oxygen, but when they do, they accumulate **lactic acid,** which soon causes muscle fatigue. As they work, muscles generate heat. For example, shivering on a cold day boosts the energy output of the skeletal muscles to warm the body.

SYSTEMS THAT CONTROL AND COORDINATE ACTIVITIES
The Nervous System

The nervous system (Fig. V–3) is divided for study into a *central nervous system* (CNS), consisting of the brain and spinal cord, and a *peripheral nervous system* (PNS), comprising all nervous tissue outside of the CNS, including the cranial and spinal nerves that connect with the brain and spinal cord and the receptors, which respond to changes in the internal and external environments. The purpose of the nervous system is to detect such changes, known as *stimuli*, and to coordinate an appropriate response. The nervous system works by transmitting electrical signals along nerve cells, or *neurons*. It also employs chemicals, called *neurotransmitters*, to carry a stimulus across the junctions between nerve cells, contact points known as *synapses*. Information is coordinated and interpreted within the CNS, which then directs a suitable response by a muscle or a gland.

A functional subdivision of the nervous system is the *autonomic nervous system*, which controls involuntary (unconscious) behavior. It consists of two portions: the *sympathetic system*, which stimulates an alarm response ("fight-or-flight" response), and the *parasympathetic sys-*

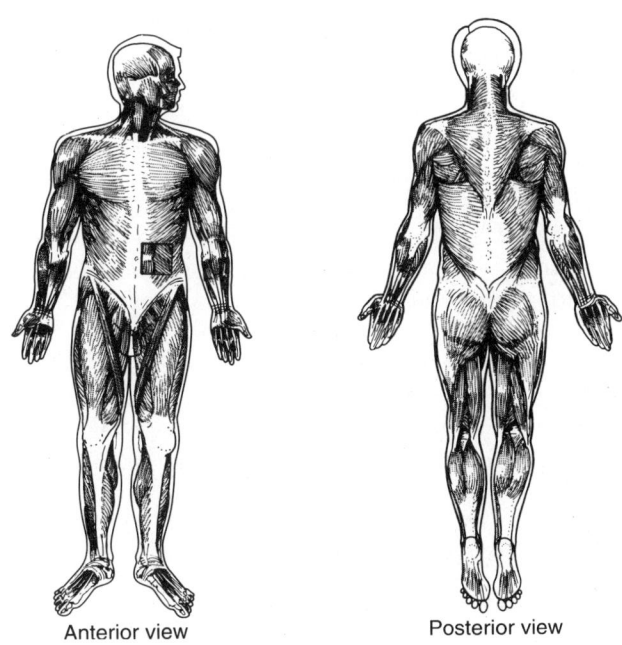

FIGURE V–2 The muscular system.

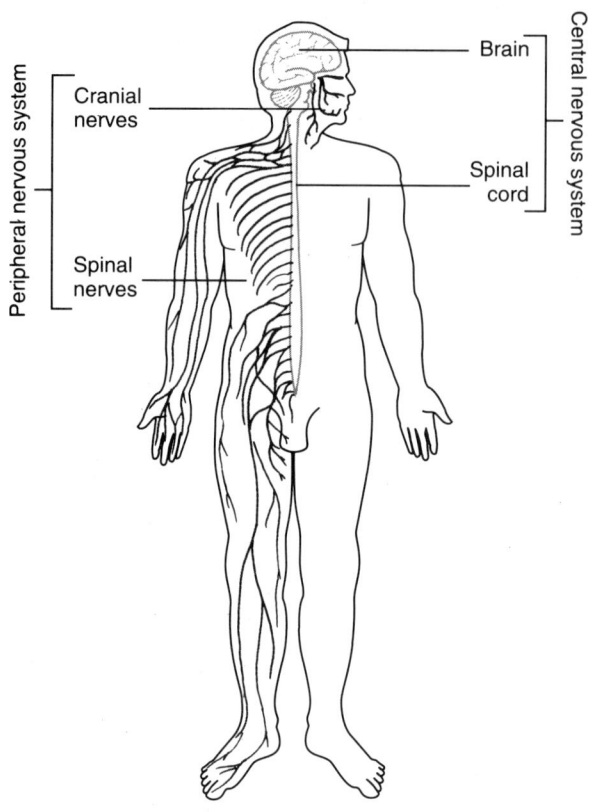

Figure V-3 The nervous system.

tem, which restores balance and stimulates maintenance systems such as the digestive and urinary systems.

The Sensory System

The sensory system is a component of the nervous system and contains specialized cells that can detect stimuli. These cells, or *receptors*, may be widely distributed throughout the body or localized in special sense organs. The latter include the ear (hearing and equilibrium), the eye (vision), the tongue (taste), and the nose (smell). General receptors detect pain, temperature, touch, pressure, and body position.

The Endocrine System

The endocrine system (Fig. V-4) consists of glands that secrete substances that affect other cells. These substances, called **hormones,** are released into the bloodstream to be carried to the target cells. They exert a wide range of effects on growth, metabolism, reproduction, and behavior. Examples of hormones include steroid hormones secreted by the adrenal glands and the sex glands, insulin secreted by the pancreas, thyroid hormone, and growth hormone secreted by the pituitary gland. The *pituitary* gland, which secretes a number of hormones that regulate other endocrine glands, is actually controlled by the hypothalamus, a region of the brain just above it. Although hormone-secreting glands are collectively referred to as the endocrine system, there are other organs that release hormones. These include the kidneys, stomach, intestine, and heart.

SYSTEMS THAT TRANSPORT MATERIALS

The Cardiovascular System

As the name suggests, the cardiovascular system (Fig. V-5) consists of the heart and blood vessels. Together these form a closed circuit for carrying blood to and from the tissues. Blood

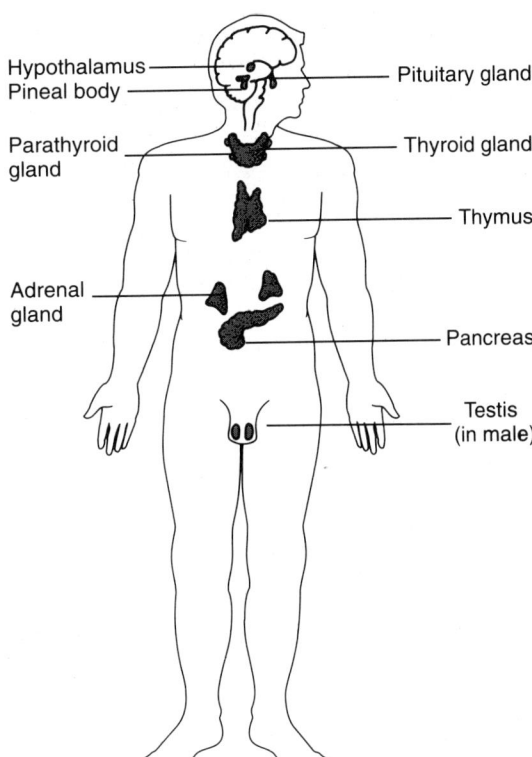

FIGURE V-4 The endocrine system.

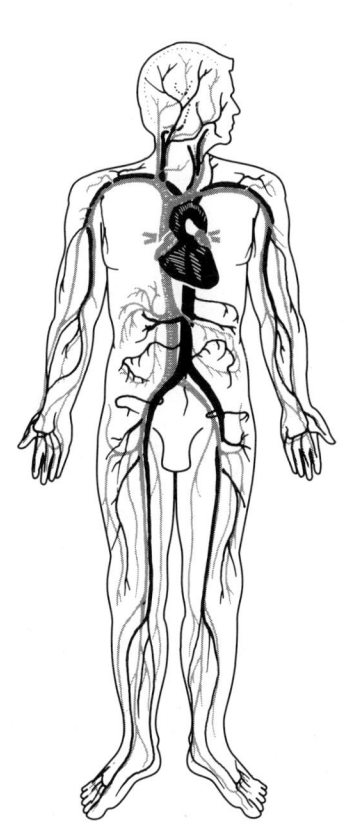

FIGURE V-5 The cardiovascular system.

brings nutrients and oxygen to the cells and carries away metabolic wastes and carbon dioxide. The blood also carries hormones, antibodies, and enzymes. As it circulates, the blood distributes body heat, which is generated largely by muscles and glands. This system is of major interest to phlebotomists and will be discussed in greater detail later.

The Lymphatic System

The lymphatic system works with the cardiovascular system to provide effective circulation. Unlike the blood vessels, which form a closed circuit, the lymphatic vessels form a one-way system that drains excess fluids and proteins from the tissues and returns them to the subclavian veins near the heart. The *thoracic duct* drains the lower portion and the upper left half of the body and empties into the left subclavian vein; the *right lymphatic duct* drains the upper right half of the body and empties into the right subclavian vein. The fluid that circulates in the lymphatic system is called **lymph.**

The lymphatic system has some other functions as well. It collects digested fats through special capillaries, called *lacteals,* in the villi of the small intestine. These nutrients are added to the general circulation when the lymph joins the blood.

Finally, the lymphatic system is considered to be part of the immune system. Lymphatic tissues help to filter blood and other body fluids, and cells active in immunity (lymphocytes) are sheltered and stimulated within organs of the lymphatic system. Lymphatic organs include the lymph nodes, which are located throughout the body; the spleen; the thymus gland; the tonsils; and the appendix.

WRITING

Directions: Answer the following question based on the reading selection. Remember to use the following writing strategies:

- Organize ideas
- Write the first draft
- Revise, edit, and proofread to write the final draft

What are the similarities and differences between the cardiovascular and lymphatic systems?

COMPREHENSION QUESTIONS

Directions: Answer the short-answer questions based on the selection. Use the strategies you learned for answering short-answer questions.

1. The three types of muscles are smooth, _____ and skeletal muscles.

2. Approximately how many muscles move the skeletal system? _____

3. CNS stands for the _____.

4. The _____ controls involuntary behavior.

5. Glands secrete _____ that affect other cells.

6. Which cells detect stimuli? _____

7. Which system consists of the heart and blood vessels? _____

8. What two ducts are part of the lymphatic system? _____

9. Blood carries away _____ and _____.

10. Body heat is generated by _____ and _____.

WORD PROBLEM

Directions: Use the strategies you learned for solving word problems to answer this question.

Red blood cells live about 120 days before they wear out and are replaced by new red blood cells. Approximately how many replacements occur in a year's time?

Reading Selection 5

> **PREVIEW QUESTION**
> - What have been your own experiences with cats?

VOCABULARY

Directions: Locate five words that are new to you in this reading. Write the meaning of each of these words in the space provided.

_____

_____

_____

_____

_____

_____

_____

_____

_____

_____

DOMESTICATION OF THE CAT

Domestication requires several generations of selective breeding to produce physiological, morphological, and behavioral changes. For *F. catus* this process has been unique. Except for the cat, breeding during domestication of most animals had been done by selection of behavioral characteristics, primarily to increase gentleness. The cat, however, was first brought into the home for religious reasons, not utilitarian ones. Because cats followed the urbanization of human populations, mating was a matter of proximity rather than of human selection. Not only was it difficult to control mating in cats, but the religious connotation prohibited selective breeding. The actual date of domestication varies from 100 B.C. to as early as 7000 B.C., and several authorities imply that even now the cat is not fully domesticated because it can

From Beaver BV: Feline Behavior. Philadelphia, W.B. Saunders, 1992, pp 4–6.

revert to total self-sufficiency. The first recorded planned feline breeding did not occur until A.D. 999, at the Japanese Imperial Palace. It soon became fashionable in that country to control cat matings and environments. But mice subsequently devastated the silkworm industry, so that by 1602, Japanese cats were released from these controls.

During the time the cat fell from favor and met with mass extermination in Europe, selective breeding was not practiced. Even with the Crusaders helping the cat return to favor, the prevailing attitude was one of tolerance rather than of full acceptance. Historically, then, it took many years before the cat achieved a position whereby the behavioral characteristics desired in a domesticated animal could be developed by selective breeding.

CURRENT STATUS OF THE FELID
Cat Population Statistics

The recent increase in the number of cats—especially registered cats—in the United States has been dramatic. This may be due in part to their adaptability to living in apartments and small homes. Figures vary greatly and are inaccurate because of the number of stray cats, but the pet cat population is between 23.1 and 56 million. Associated figures estimate 1.6 to 2.2 cats for each house that has cats, or one cat in every 3.2 single-family dwelling units. Of this cat population, only between 3 and 13 million are seen by veterinarians. Stray cats represent between 2 per cent and 28 per cent of the known population. Each year as many as 20 per cent of a city's pet population pass through its animal shelter. This large stray feline population may be reflected in another statistic: Only 38 per cent of male cats are castrated and 31 per cent of females are spayed; however, local differences have been reported.

Cat ownership is increasing worldwide, often in parallel to trends in the United States. In several European countries cat numbers now exceed those for dogs, as does the percentage of households owning cats.

Cat Owner Categorization

In addition to surviving a varied history, the cat has withstood many types of owners. Cat owners have been classified in several ways by researchers, but they tend to fall in one of two categories: those who have a weak attachment and those who have a strong one. The classification "low-involvement owner" is applied to 59 per cent of the 14,645,000 cat-owning households in one study of pet owners. These people devote little time to the care or company of the cat, and seem to enjoy having a cat around more than interacting with it. This lack of involvement with the pet is reflected in trauma statistics. Of 126 cats (89 males, 37 females) reported injured during a period of slightly more than a year, 16.3 per cent had been hit by a car, 14.7 per cent had been involved in animal interaction, and 39.5 per cent received injuries from causes unknown to the owner. The average life span for a cat is 12 years, but ages of 20 or more years are not uncommon. The current longevity record is 36 years. Although the average age for the general population is 3 years, that of the neutered cat is 3 to 5 years longer and that of the traumatized cat is only 1.3 years. One study of road kills indicated that most were kittens or young adults. Because of the low-involvement owners, cat populations, for the most part, still fulfill the criteria of random mating.

The second classification of cat owners, those with a strong attachment, has been subdivided. "Quality- or status-conscious owners" compose 21 per cent of all cat owners. The pet is an expression of how this owner views himself or herself and reflects his or her good taste, as would other material possessions. These owners believe that the cat depends on them for love, affection, and care, and as a result, the animal is well groomed and only reluctantly left alone.

"High-involvement owners," the second subdivision, constitute the remaining 20 per cent of the cat-owning population. Unlike owners in the other two categories, these people rely on the cat to supply love and affection or to serve as an emotional crutch, such as a child substitute. Attachments to the cat frequently are described as those to a human family member, friend, or child. The person believes that the cat enjoys humans, feeds it specially prepared foods, has photographs of the pet, and may celebrate the cat's birthday. Owners from this group are most likely to bury a deceased pet in a pet cemetery or mausoleum or to leave an estate to their cats. This kind of owner was responsible for bequeathing $415,000 to two cats in 1965, making them the richest cats in history.

Quality- or status-conscious owners and high-involvement owners, many of whom are in the middle or upper socioeconomic level, spend billions of dollars each year on their pets. Such people have a higher percentage of neutered cats than do low-involvement owners and a preference for lighter-colored cats.

WRITING

Directions: Answer the following question based on the reading selection. Remember to use the following writing strategies:

- Organize ideas
- Write the first draft
- Revise, edit, and proofread to write the final draft

If you were a cat owner, would you be a low-involvement owner or a high-involvement owner? Explain.

COMPREHENSION QUESTIONS

Directions: Answer the multiple-choice questions based on the selection. Use the strategies you learned for answering multiple-choice questions.

1. The cat was brought into the house from the wild for
    a. work reasons
    b. companionship reasons
    c. religious reasons
    d. utilitarian reasons

2. Some experts believe that the cat is not fully domesticated because the cat
    a. is totally self-sufficient
    b. is capable of biting
    c. it does not get along well with dogs
    d. basically does not like humans

3. In the 1600s the cat fell out of favor in
    a. Japan
    b. Europe
    c. Egypt
    d. United States

4. The population increase of cats in the United States is due to
   a. the decline of dogs
   b. the increase in the rodent population
   c. their ability to be independent
   d. their ability to live in small dwellings

5. Most cat owners are
   a. low-involvement owners
   b. high-involvement owners
   c. part high- and part low-involvement owners
   d. neither low- nor high-involvement owners

6. The majority of cats killed on the road are
   a. elderly cats
   b. partially blind cats
   c. kittens and young adults
   d. nursing mothers of young kittens

7. The type of owner who would celebrate a cat's birthday is
   a. the low-involvement owner
   b. the high-involvement cat
   c. always childless and lonely
   d. none of the above

8. The number of cats that see a veterinarian range between
   a. 3 and 13 million
   b. 15 million and 17 million
   c. 20 and 30 million
   d. undetermined

9. Cat ownership worldwide is
   a. stabilizing
   b. unknown
   c. decreasing
   d. increasing

10. You can conclude from this selection that the writer
    a. favors cats
    b. dislikes cats
    c. neither likes nor dislikes cats
    d. cannot determine

WORD PROBLEM

Directions: Use the strategies you learned for solving word problems to answer this question.

Assume that the pet cat population is 56 million and that the stray cat population represents 10% of the pet cat population. How many cats are stray cats?

Reading Selection 6

PREVIEW QUESTION
- What are the five types of dental assistants?

VOCABULARY

Directions: Locate five words that are new to you in this reading. Write the meaning of each of these words in the space provided.

___

___

___

___

___

___

___

___

___

___

THE DENTAL ASSISTANT

Educational programs for dental assistants vary considerably in length. An "accredited dental assisting program" is one that has been evaluated and approved by the Commission on Dental Accreditation of the American Dental Association.

The Generalist

Working as a generalist is a challenging but increasingly rare role. In a "one-employee" practice this dental assistant divided her time between the business office, treatment areas, dental laboratory, and darkroom.

From Ehrlich A, Torres HO: Essentials of Dental Assisting. Philadelphia, W.B. Saunders, 1992, pp 4–7.

A more common situation is one in which several assistants are employed, each of whom is a "specialist" in her own area. However, each assistant has basic knowledge of other areas and is able to substitute or help out as necessary.

The Administrative Assistant

The administrative assistant, also known as the *secretarial assistant* or *receptionist*, is primarily responsible for the smooth and efficient operation of the business office (Fig. V–6). These duties include:

- Patient reception and answering the telephone.
- Appointment control.
- Records management.
- Accounts receivable and accounts payable bookkeeping.
- Handling of all correspondence and management of the recall and inventory control systems.

The Chairside Assistant

The term **four-handed dentistry** describes the seated dentist and chairside assistant working smoothly as a team to provide quality dental care with a minimum of time, motion, and stress.

The chairside assistant is responsible for working directly with the dentist in the treatment area. Responsibilities here may include:

- Patient seating and preparation.
- Instrument and operatory care.
- Oral evacuation.
- Tongue and tissue retraction.
- Instrument exchange.

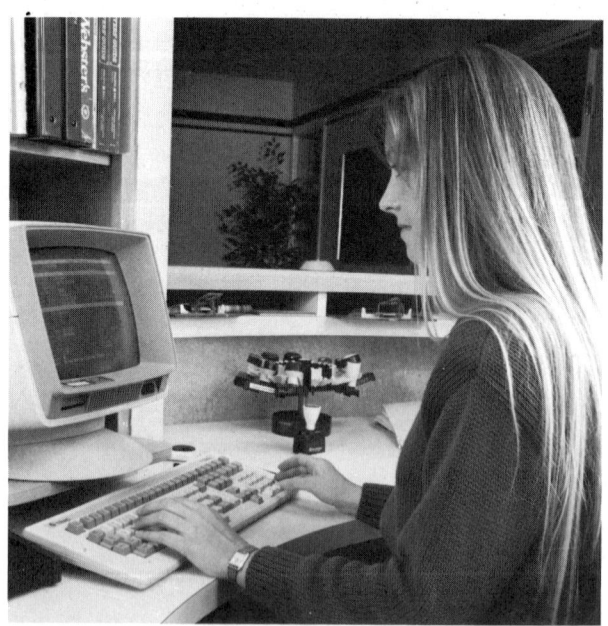

FIGURE V–6 The administrative assistant is primarily responsible for the smooth functioning of the business office. (Torres HO, Ehrlich A: Modern Dental Assisting, 4th ed. Philadelphia, W.B. Saunders, 1990, p. 904.)

- The preparation and storage of materials and supplies
- Some radiography and patient education.

In a practice where there *is* a coordinating assistant, the chairside assistant's duties are usually modified so that more time may be spent "chairside" working directly with the dentist.

The Coordinating Assistant

The term **six-handed dentistry** describes the use of an additional assistant, usually the coordinating assistant, who "serves as an extra pair of hands where needed" throughout the dental treatment (Fig. V–7).

In six-handed dentistry, the coordinating assistant also has specific responsibilities of her own. These may include:

- Exposing, processing, and mounting radiographs.
- Patient seating and dismissal.
- Mixing and passing materials to the chairside assistant or dentist.
- Operatory and instrument care and preparation.
- Patient education.
- Limited laboratory procedures and control of cases to and from the dental laboratory.

Very often a new assistant is assigned to work as a coordinating assistant until she becomes familiar with all aspects of the practice.

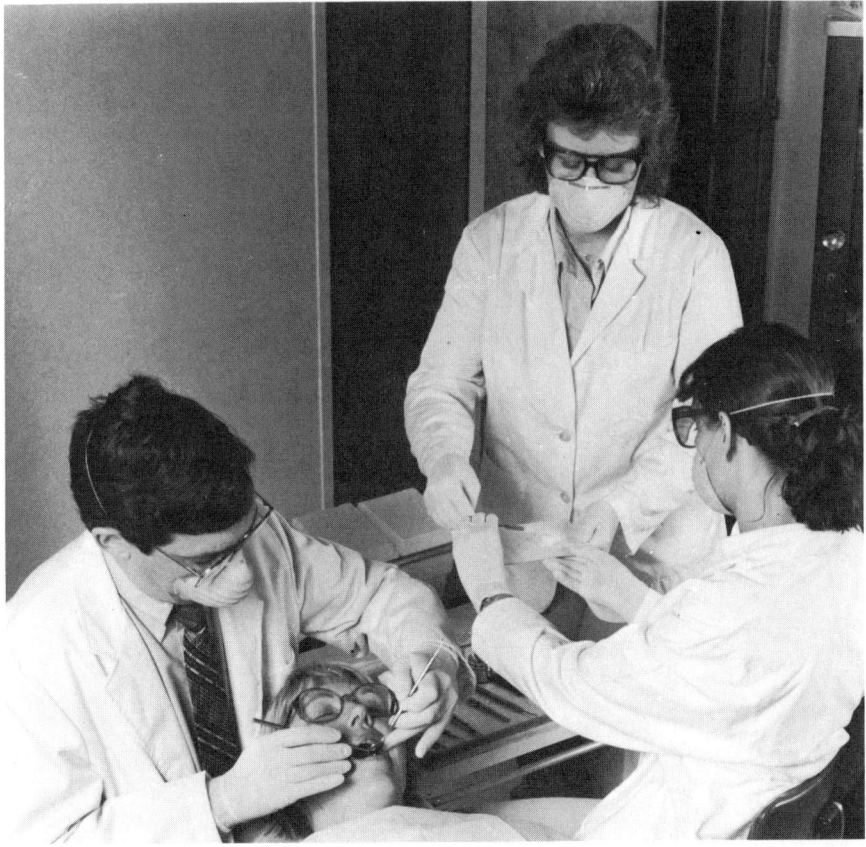

FIGURE V–7 In six-handed dentistry, the coordinating assistant serves "as an extra pair of hands where needed" throughout treatment. (Torres HO, Ehrlich A: Modern Dental Assisting, 4th ed. Philadelphia, W.B. Saunders, 1990, p. 335.)

The Extended Functions Dental Assistant (EFDA)

Under the State Dental Practice Act, "extended functions" are those duties that may legally be assigned to qualified dental auxiliaries functioning in that state (Fig. V–8).

An assistant who is qualified and registered to perform these duties is known as an extended function dental auxiliary (EFDA).

The following is a list of duties that may *potentially* be allowed for performance by an extended functions registered dental assistant:

- Making radiographic exposures.
- Taking impressions for opposing study casts.
- Taking a bite registration.
- Retracting gingivae prior to impression procedures.
- Taking impressions for cast restorations.
- Taking impressions for space maintainers, orthodontic appliances, and occlusal guards.
- Determining root length and endodontic file length.
- Fitting trial endodontic filling points.
- Placing and removing periodontal and surgical dressings.
- Removing sutures.
- Applying topical anesthetics.
- Assisting in the administration of nitrous oxide-oxygen analgesia or sedation.
- Performing preliminary oral examinations.
- Polishing coronal surfaces of teeth.
- Providing oral health instruction.

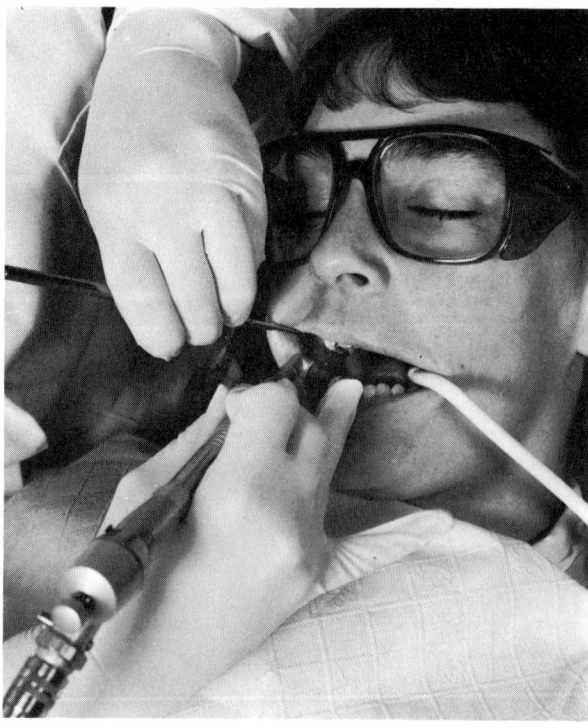

Figure V–8 The extended functions dental assistant (EFDA) performs direct patient functions in keeping with the state's dental practice act and his or her educational qualifications. (Torres HO, Ehrlich A: Modern Dental Assisting, 4th ed. Philadelphia, W.B. Saunders, 1990, p. 904.)

- Applying anticariogenic agents topically.
- Placing and removing rubber dams.
- Placing and removing wedges and matrices.
- Placing and removing sedative or temporary restorations and crowns.
- Placing, carving, and finishing amalgam restorations.
- Placing and finishing composite restorations.
- Removing excess cement from coronal surfaces of teeth.
- Preparing teeth for bonding by etching.
- Applying pit and fissure sealants.
- Applying cavity liners and bases.
- Performing additional functions that may be delegated within specialties for the state in which the auxiliary is employed.

WRITING

Directions: Answer the following question based on the reading selection. Remember to use the following writing strategies:

- Organize ideas
- Write the first draft
- Revise, edit, and proofread to write the final draft

What type of dental assistant would you choose to be? Give reasons for your choice.

COMPREHENSION QUESTIONS

Directions: Answer the true and false questions based on the selection. Use the strategies you learned for answering true and false questions.

1. The generalist role is gaining in popularity in this decade. T____ F____
2. Records management is part of an administrative assistant's duties. T____ F____
3. Handling of correspondence is done by both the dentist and the administrative assistant. T____ F____
4. The chairside assistant helps with patient seating and preparation. T____ F____
5. The coordinating assistant is described as "an extra pair of hands." T____ F____
6. The coordinating assistant is responsible for applying topical anesthetics. T____ F____
7. The coordinating assistant can do patient education. T____ F____
8. "EFDA" stands for "educated for dental assisting." T____ F____
9. The EFDA performs directly on patients according to state regulations. T____ F____
10. An EFDA can definitely make radiographic exposures. T____ F____

WORD PROBLEM

Directions: Use the strategies you learned for solving word problems to answer this question.

Ms. Happytooth worked as an administrative assistant in Dr. Fine's office. Ms. Happytooth was responsible for accounts receivable and accounts payable. At the end of the month she had to balance the books. On the accounts payable side, Ms. Happytooth noticed that Dr. Fine received $29,583 in patient fees. On the accounts payable side, she noticed that Dr. Fine paid $16,245 in salaries, $900 in rent, and $1711 in miscellaneous expenses. Did Dr. Fine make a profit for that month, or did he go further into debt? If he made a profit, what was the amount? If he went further into debt, what was the amount?

Reading Selection 7

PREVIEW QUESTION
- What are the organs of the respiratory system?

VOCABULARY

Directions: Locate five words that are new to you in this reading. Write the meaning of each of these words in the space provided.

_____

_____

_____

_____

_____

_____

_____

_____

_____

_____

_____

_____

THE RESPIRATORY SYSTEM
Organs of the Respiratory System

1. Nose
2. Pharynx
3. Larynx
4. Trachea
5. Bronchus
6. Lungs

From LaFleur-Brooks M (Ed.): Health Unit Coordinating, 3rd ed. Philadelphia, W.B. Saunders, 1993, pp. 434–436.

Functions of the Respiratory System

The function of the respiratory system is to exchange gases. Oxygen is taken into the body and carbon dioxide is removed. This process is referred to as **respiration.**

Respiration

External respiration, or breathing, is the exchange of gases between the lungs and the external environment. Oxygen is inhaled into the lungs and passes through the capillary wall into the blood to be carried to the blood cells. Carbon dioxide passes out of the capillary blood to the lungs to be exhaled to the outside environment.

The exchange of gasses also takes place within the body between the blood in the capillaries and individual body cells. This is called **internal respiration.** The body cells take on the oxygen from the blood and at the same time give off carbon dioxide to the blood to be transported back to the lungs, where it is exhaled from the body.

The Nose

Air enters the respiratory system through the nose. The nose is divided into a right and left nostril by a partition called the **nasal septum.** The nose prepares air for the body by (1) warming and moistening the air, (2) removing pathogenic microorganisms, and (3) removing foreign particles, such as dust, from the air.

The Pharynx

Both air and food travel through the **pharynx** (throat). The food passes from the pharynx to the esophagus, while the air passes from the pharynx into the larynx, which is located anterior to the esophagus.

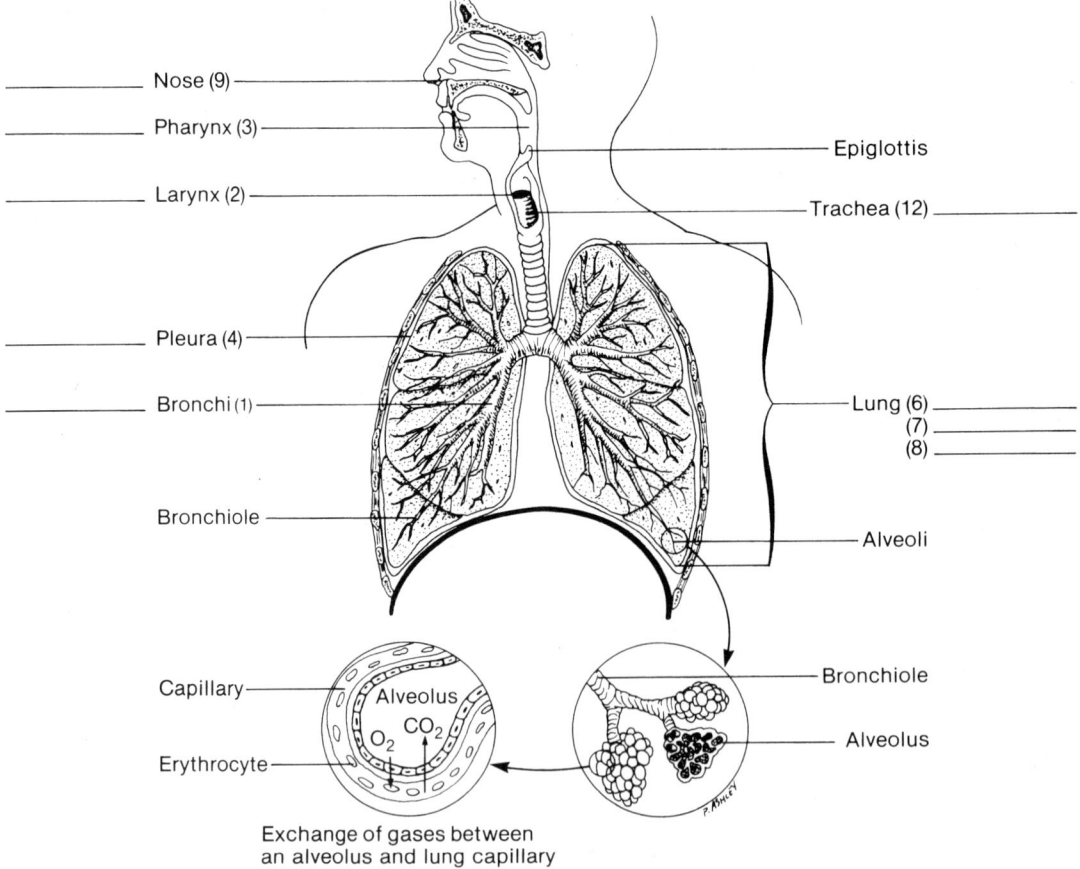

FIGURE V–9 The respiratory system.

The Larynx

The **larynx** (voice box) is a tubular structure located below the pharynx. As mentioned earlier, the pharynx is a passageway for both food and air. A flap of cartilage, called the **epiglottis,** automatically covers the larynx during the act of swallowing to prevent the food from passing from the pharynx into the larynx. The larynx contains the **vocal cords.** As the air is exhaled past the vocal cords, the vibration of the cords produces sounds.

The Trachea

The **trachea** (windpipe) is a vertical tube extending from the larynx to the bronchi (Fig. V–9). A series of C-shaped cartilage rings prevents the trachea from collapsing. The function of the trachea is the passage of air.

Bronchi

Behind the heart, close to the center of the chest, the trachea branches into two tubes: one leading to the right lung and the other leading to the left lung. These tubes are called **bronchi** (singular: *bronchus*). The function of the bronchi is the passage of air.

The Lungs

The lungs are cone-shaped organs located in the thoracic cavity. The right lung is the larger of the two and is divided into three lobes. The left lung is divided into two lobes. After the bronchus enters the lung, it divides into smaller tubes and continues to subdivide into even smaller tubes called **bronchioles.** At the end of each bronchiole is a grape-like cluster of air sacs called **alveoli** (singular: *alveolus*). The walls of the alveoli are one-celled, which allows for the exchange of gases to take place between the alveoli and the capillaries. The **pleura** is a double sac that surrounds each lung.

The Passageway of Air

The air, which carries oxygen, enters the body through (1) the nose, then travels through (2) the pharynx, (3) the larynx, (4) the trachea, and (5) the bronchi, to the lungs. In the lungs the air passes into (6) the bronchioles and then to (7) the alveoli, where the exchange of gases takes place with the surrounding capillaries.

CONDITIONS OF THE RESPIRATORY SYSTEM

Pneumothorax and Hemothorax

Pneumothorax

Pneumothorax is the collection of air or gas in the pleural cavity, resulting in a collapsed lung (Fig. V–10). It may be caused by a chest wound, or it may be a spontaneous collapse due to lung disease. The pleural cavity is airtight, with negative pressure. As air enters the pleural cavity it creates pressure against the lung, causing it to collapse.

Symptoms include sudden sharp chest pain, shortness of breath, and stopping of normal chest movements on the affected side.

Treatment consists of a thoracentesis to remove the air or gas from the cavity and a thoracotomy, with the insertion of chest tubes. The tubes are connected to an underwater drainage system and remain in place until air is no longer expelled from the pleural space.

Hemothorax

A **hemothorax** is the collection of blood in the pleural cavity; it is usually caused by trauma. Treatment includes stopping the bleeding, evacuating the blood from the pleural space, and re-expanding the lung.

Pulmonary Embolism

Pulmonary embolism is the most common complication in hospitalized patients. It strikes 6,000,000 adults a year, causing 100,000 deaths.

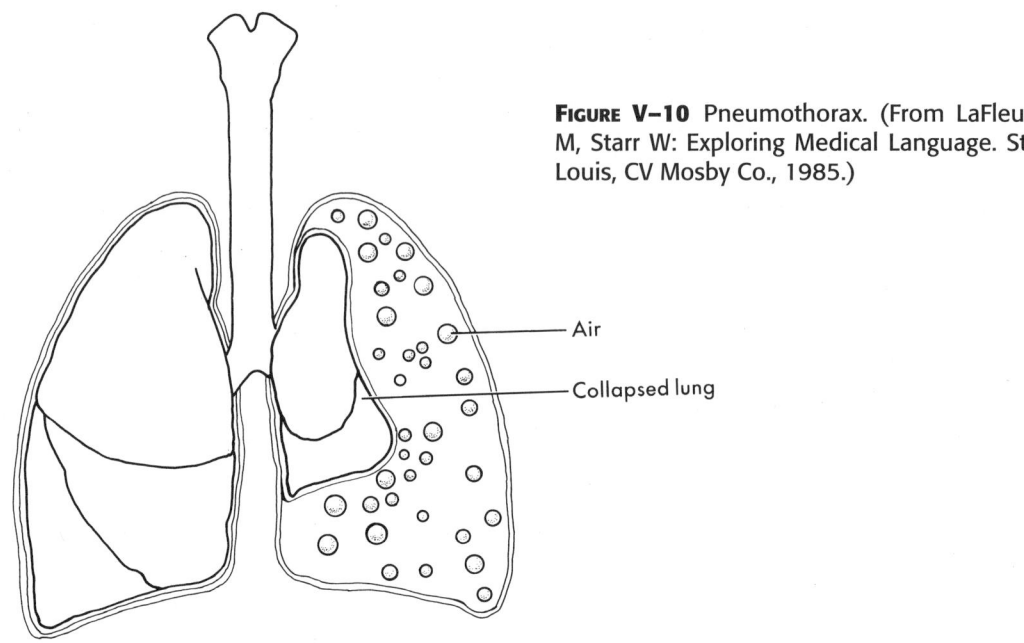

Figure V-10 Pneumothorax. (From LaFleur M, Starr W: Exploring Medical Language. St. Louis, CV Mosby Co., 1985.)

Pulmonary embolism is usually caused by a thrombus that has been dislodged from a leg vein and now blocks a pulmonary artery. Symptoms are dyspnea (difficulty in breathing), chest pain, cyanosis (blue tinge to the skin), and shock. It is difficult to distinguish from pneumonia and myocardial infarction. Chest x-ray, pulmonary angiography, and arterial blood gases are used to diagnose pulmonary embolism. Treatment includes anticoagulant and oxygen therapy.

WRITING

Directions: Answer the following question based on the reading selection. Remember to use the following writing strategies:

- Organize ideas
- Write the first draft
- Revise, edit, and proofread to write the final draft

What is the passageway of air through the respiratory system? Use sufficient details when writing your answer.

COMPREHENSION QUESTIONS

Directions: Answer the matching questions based on the selection. Use the strategies you learned for answering matching questions.

A. Nose	contains vocal cords	1. ____
B. Pharynx	located behind the heart	2. ____
C. Larynx	cone-shaped organs	3. ____

D. Trachea

E. Bronchi

F. Lungs

nasal septum divides the left and right nostrils	4. ____
passage of air	5. ____
branches into two tubes	6. ____
where the exchange of gases take place	7. ____
both air and food travel through this	8. ____
where air enters the respiratory system	9. ____
is covered by the epiglottis during swallowing	10. ____

WORD PROBLEM

Directions: Use the strategies you learned for solving word problems to answer this question.

What percentage of people die of pulmonary embolism if 6,000,000 adults are hospitalized with this condition and 100,000 patients die?

Reading Selection 8

PREVIEW QUESTION
- What does Figure V–12 describe?

VOCABULARY

Directions: Locate five words that are new to you in this reading. Write the meaning of each of these words in the space provided.

_____
_____
_____
_____
_____
_____
_____
_____
_____
_____

WRITING

Directions: Answer the following question based on the reading selection. Remember to use the following writing strategies:

- Organize ideas
- Write the first draft
- Revise, edit, and proofread to write the final draft

What is the procedure for folding a surgical gown? Write your answer in paragraph form.

Figures V–11 to V–13 are from McCurnin DM (Ed.): Clinical Textbook for Veterinary Technicians, 3rd ed. Philadelphia, W.B. Saunders, 1994, pp. 262–265.

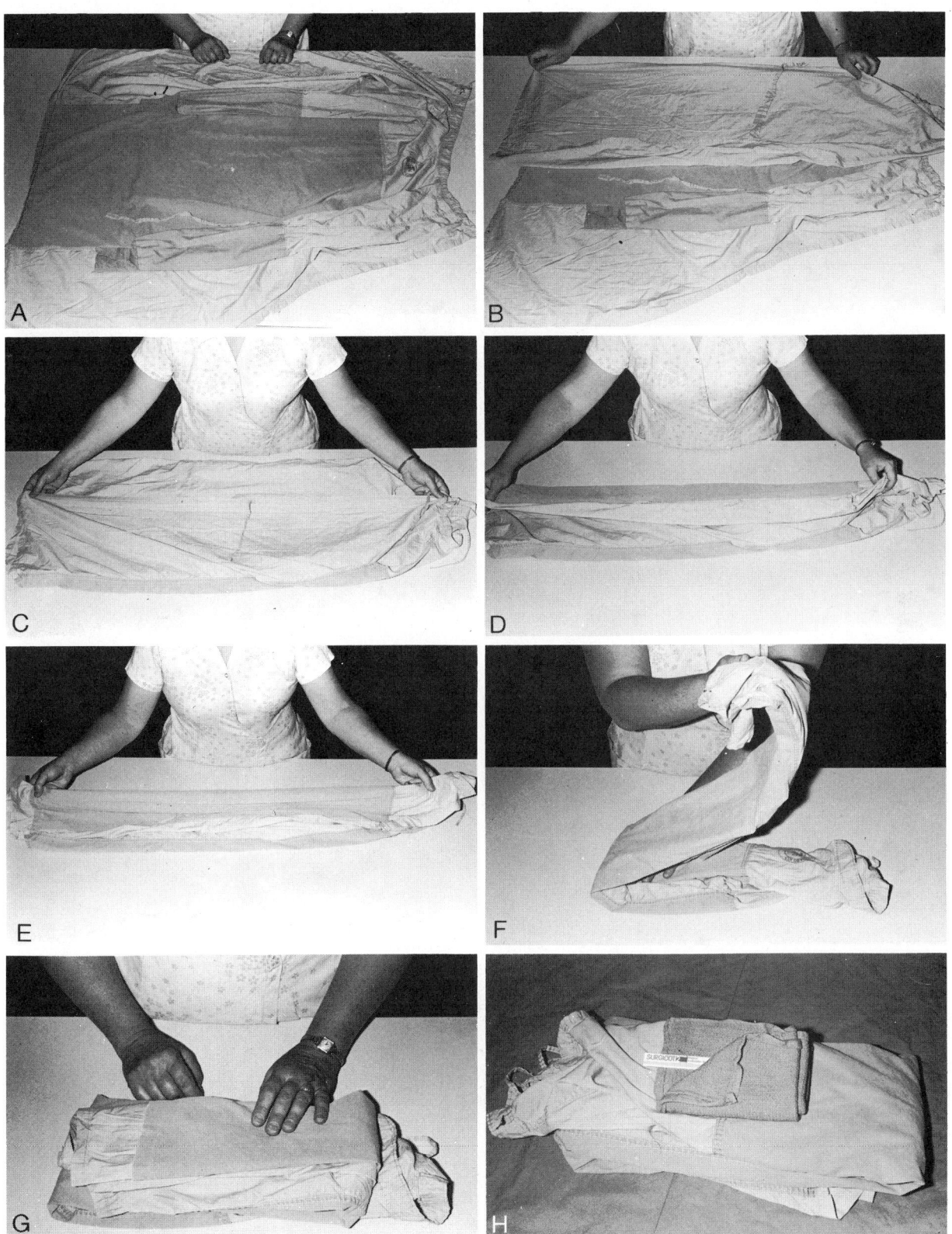

FIGURE V–11 A, Method of folding a surgical gown. The gown is spread on a countertop with the outside of the gown facing up. B, The near edge of the gown is folded to the center. C, Next, the far edge of the gown is folded toward the center to meet the near edge. D, The gown is folded in half. E, The gown is folded in half again. F and G, The gown is folded lengthwise in accordion fashion into thirds. H, A hand towel and sterilization indicator are placed on top, and the gown is ready for wrapping.

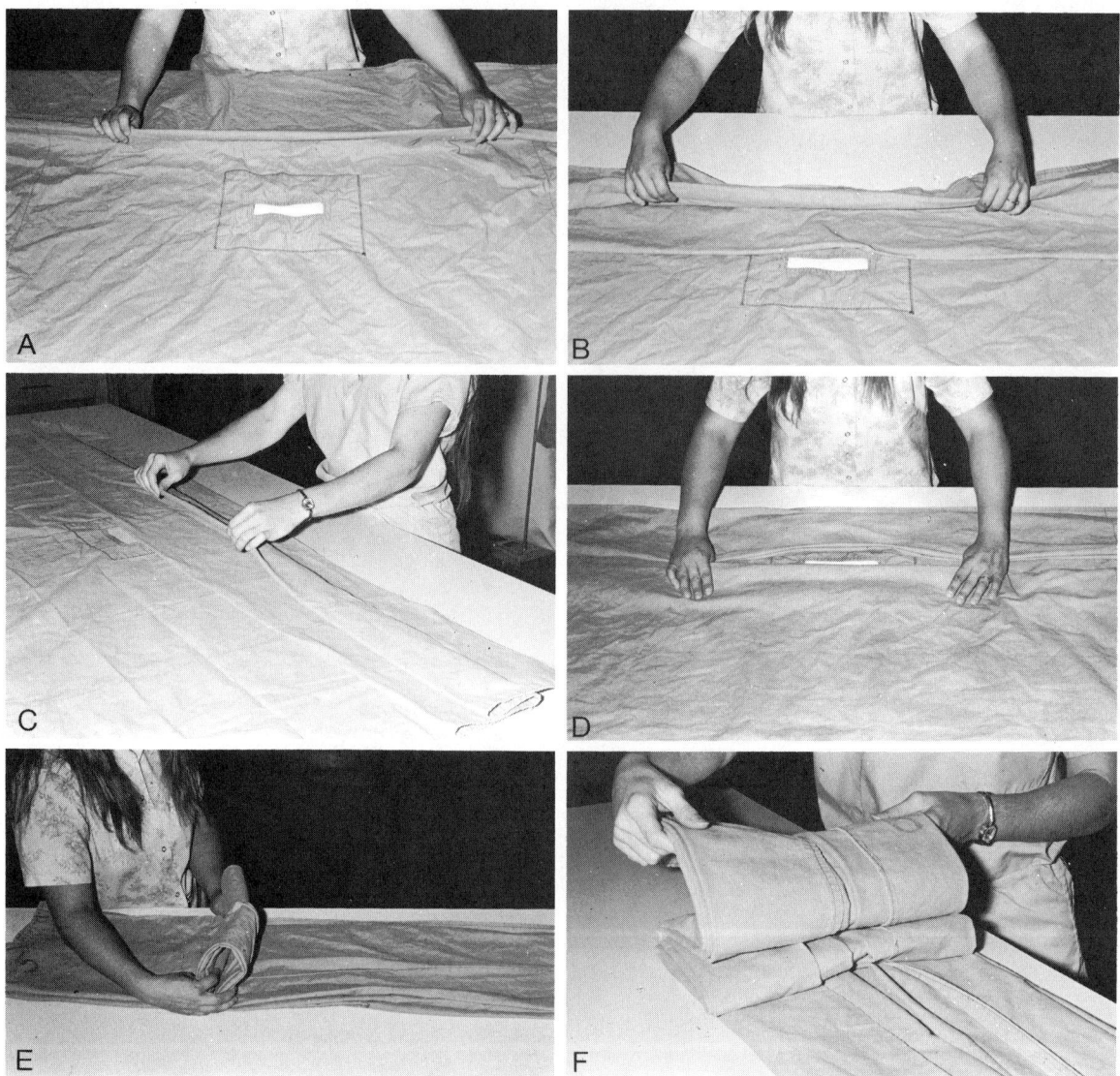

FIGURE V-12 Drapes are folded in accordion fashion so that they are easily unfolded onto the patient. A–C, One side of the drape is folded to the center in accordion fashion. Each fold is approximately 15 cm wide. D, The opposite side is folded in a similar manner. E and F, Lengthwise, the drape is again folded to the center of the fenestration in accordion fashion. These folds are also about 15 cm in width. G, The opposite side is folded in the same manner. H, The two sides are folded together, and the drape is ready for wrapping (I).

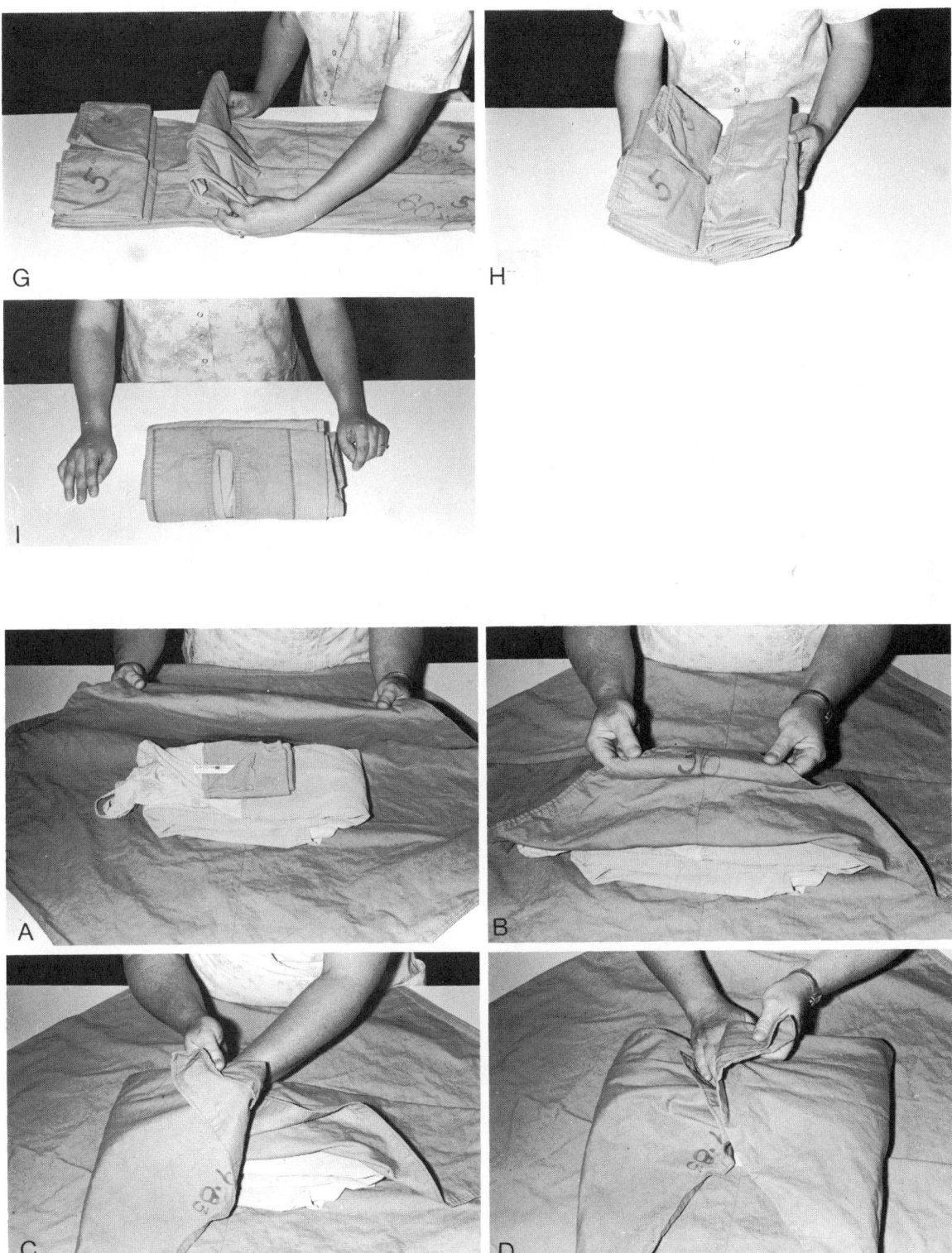

FIGURE V-13 Wrapping of fenestrated drape and gown. A, The gown, along with a hand towel and sterilization indicator, is placed diagonally onto the nonfenestrated drapes. B–E, The corners are folded over the gown. F, Three corners of the second drape are folded in a similar manner.

Continued on following page

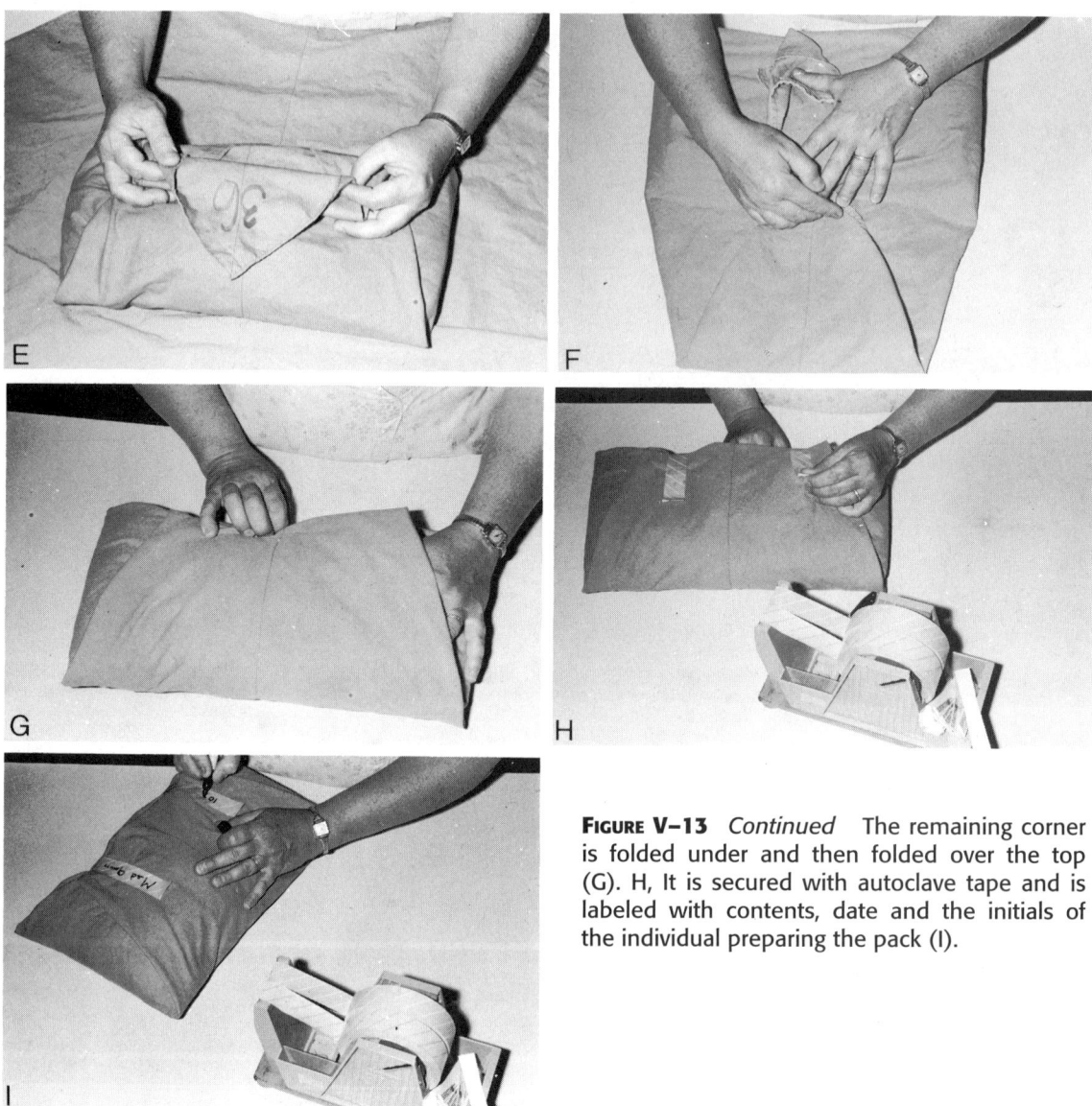

Figure V-13 *Continued* The remaining corner is folded under and then folded over the top (G). H, It is secured with autoclave tape and is labeled with contents, date and the initials of the individual preparing the pack (I).

COMPREHENSION QUESTIONS

Directions: Answer the short-answer questions based on the selection. Use the strategies you learned for answering short-answer questions.

1. When folding a surgical gown, the first step is to spread the gown on a counter top with the _____ of the gown facing _____.

2. In the final step of folding a surgical gown, what two objects are placed on top of the gown? _____

3. How many steps are there in all for folding a surgical gown? _____

4. Why are drapes folded in accordion fashion? _____
   _____

5. How wide are the folds for drapes? _____

6. How many steps are there in all for folding drapes? _____

7. What is the first step for the wrapping of a fenestrated drape and gown?
   _____
   _____

8. What is the following step for the wrapping of a fenestrated drape and gown?
   _____

9. How many steps are there in all for the wrapping of a fenestrated drape and gown? _____

10. What labeling is put on the folded drape and gown? _____
    _____

WORD PROBLEM

Directions: Use the strategies you learned for solving word problems to answer this question.

Drapes are folded in accordion pleats that are 15 cm wide. If the drape is 120 cm wide, how many folds will be made?

Reading Selection 9

PREVIEW QUESTION
- List three common diseases that affect the organs of respiration.

VOCABULARY

Directions: Locate five words that are new to you in this reading. Write the meaning of each of these words in the space provided.

_____
_____
_____
_____
_____
_____
_____
_____
_____
_____

CARE OF THE PATIENT WITH COMMON DISRUPTIONS IN RESPIRATION

Common diseases that affect the organs of respiration are

- pneumonia
- asthma
- emphysema

From Polaski A, Warner JP: Saunders Fundamentals for Nursing Assistants. Philadelphia, W.B. Saunders Co., 1994, pp. 200–201.

Each disease can affect the oxygen–carbon dioxide exchange in the lungs. Patients whose bodies lack oxygen are tired and have little energy. They breathe faster (more respirations per minute) to keep up with their body's demand for oxygen.

PNEUMONIA

Pneumonia is an acute inflammation of lung tissue. It affects the tissues of the lower respiratory tract. The inflammation interferes with the exchange of oxygen and carbon dioxide in the lungs.

Pneumonia can be caused by viruses and other harmful microorganisms. These microorganisms may be present in the form of small droplets in the air and can be breathed into the lungs. The droplets can be breathed in from spray that comes out when people talk, cough, or sneeze. An inflammation response can occur if particles of food or fluid in the stomach or esophagus are **aspirated** into the lungs; this is called aspiration pneumonia. Unusual observations you will note in a patient with pneumonia are

- fever that starts quickly
- shaking chills
- cough that may produce **purulent** sputum
- chest pain

Some patients may also become lethargic (sleepy) or weak and confused, and some may experience a loss of appetite and a loss of body fluid (dehydration).

The physician or the nurse can listen to the lungs; certain sounds indicate that oxygen and carbon dioxide are not being exchanged efficiently. The approximate location of the pneumonia can be determined from the sounds. Disease of the lungs can also be viewed and pinpointed on an x-ray if the physician orders it. The physician may order bed rest, fluids, and medications to treat the pneumonia and the fever.

ASTHMA

Asthma is a disease of the bronchi (air passages) in the lungs. The cause of asthma is not clearly understood. It is known that the lungs respond to certain stimuli (irritants). Stimuli may be

- certain foods or dust
- **pollen**
- animal **dander**
- small scales from the hair or feathers of animals
- smoke
- any number of other irritants or pollutants in the environment
- stress

Not all persons respond with asthma to these stimuli. In people who do respond, the response causes

- **spasm** of the bronchi
- swelling of the air passageways
- production of thick secretions

These responses make the air passageways more narrow, so it is difficult for enough oxygen to reach the lungs.

The major observation of a patient with asthma is dyspnea (difficulty breathing). Wheezing occurs often in asthmatic persons. Dyspnea or wheezing should be reported to the supervisor or nurse. During an asthma attack, the patient may experience the following:

PNEUMONIA
an acute inflammation or infection of lung tissue

ASPIRATION
a foreign body being drawn into the lungs; may occur in persons who are unconscious, under the effects of anesthesia, or having difficulty swallowing

PURULENT
containing pus

ASTHMA
a disease of the bronchi characterized by difficult, wheezing respiration

POLLEN
the substance that fertilizes flowering plants

DANDER
small particles from the hair or feathers of animals that may cause an allergy

SPASM
a sudden contraction (tightening) of a muscle or group of muscles

- a feeling of fullness or tightness in the chest
- shortness of breath
- coughing
- fear and irritability
- profuse sweating
- extreme anxiousness
- an inability to talk because of lack of oxygen

The physician treats asthma in a patient by ordering certain medications that dilate (open) the air passageways so that oxygen can be delivered to the lungs.

EMPHYSEMA

Emphysema results from the destruction of the alveoli and enlargement of air spaces in the lung tissue. The oxygen and the carbon dioxide cannot move in and out of the lungs as usual.

Emphysema is classified as a chronic obstructive pulmonary disease. Because an obstruction (blockage) of the air passageways causes air to become trapped in the lungs, the patient cannot empty the lungs of air. It is a chronic disease (an illness that continues over a long period of time); the patient experiences periods of remission in which the disease is quiet and does not interfere with activities of daily living. These can be followed by an **exacerbation** of the emphysema.

In the early stages of emphysema, patients may arise in the morning, cough, and produce **sputum.** As the disease progresses, the cough and amount of sputum increase. Patients also become short of breath upon exertion.

In the late stage of emphysema, patients develop a persistent cough and produce large amounts of sputum. They are too tired to perform the activities of daily living because even a small amount of movement causes them to use their oxygen reserves quickly. Observations include

- a cough that may persist
- increased amounts of sputum
- increased shortness of breath upon exertion
- decreased ability to perform activities of daily living
- fatigue

Each of these becomes more severe as the disease progresses.

The main form of treatment of emphysema is a medication to dilate the air passageways. Depending on symptoms, other medications can be ordered to make patients comfortable and help them function. Oxygen may also be ordered.

EMPHYSEMA
destruction of the alveoli (tiny air sacs in the lungs) and enlargement of air spaces so oxygen and carbon dioxide cannot move in and out of the lungs

EXACERBATION
making more severe, a flare-up

SPUTUM
a mucous secretion from the lungs, bronchi, and trachea that is ejected (brought up) through the mouth

WRITING

Directions: Answer the following question based on the reading selection. Remember to use the following writing strategies:

- Organize ideas.
- Write the first draft.
- Revise, edit, and proofread to write the final draft.

Describe the three diseases that affect the organs of respiration.

COMPREHENSION QUESTIONS

Directions: Answer the true and false questions based on the selection. Use the strategies you learned for answering true and false questions.

T F

__ __ 1. Patients whose bodies lack oxygen breathe slower to keep up with their body's demand for oxygen.
__ __ 2. Asthma is a disease of the air passages in the lungs.
__ __ 3. The cause of asthma is clearly understood.
__ __ 4. Chest pain can be a symptom of pneumonia.
__ __ 5. As emphysema progresses, the cough becomes more severe.
__ __ 6. A patient with asthma has difficulty in breathing.
__ __ 7. Another name for a cough is *sputum*.
__ __ 8. Emphysema is a chronic disease.
__ __ 9. Pneumonia causes an increase in energy.
__ __ 10. The treatment for asthma is medication which closes the air passageways.

WORD PROBLEM

Directions: Use the strategies you learned for solving word problems to answer this question.

Timothy Murray had an asthma attack. When he arrived at the hospital at 7:00 AM, the physician noticed that he was wheezing. Timothy said that the wheezing began at 5:30 AM. How long was Timothy experiencing difficulty in breathing?

Reading Selection 10

PREVIEW QUESTION
- What is a pathogen?

VOCABULARY

Directions: Locate five words that are new to you in this reading. Write the meaning of each of these words in the space provided.

___

THE IMPORTANCE OF INFECTION CONTROL

By the time a disease manifests itself, the patient is sick and the disease must be treated and cured (if cure is possible). Rather than allowing this to happen, the goal must be 100 percent **prevention** of disease transmission through the dental office.

The effects of an infection transmitted in the dental office may not be readily apparent to the dental health team for several reasons.

First, injured oral mucosal tissue usually heals rapidly and well, in spite of adverse conditions.

Second, an infection introduced into the blood stream in the mouth (the focus of infection) is often washed away in the blood stream without being localized in the mouth. As a result, the infection may be localized elsewhere in the body.

From Torres HO, Ehrlich A: Modern Dental Assisting, 4th ed. Philadelphia, W.B. Saunders, 1990, pp 147–148. For updated information see Chapter 10, Microbiology and Disease Transmission, in the 5th edition of Torres and Ehrlich, 1995, pp. 169–181.

A **focus of infection** is an infection confined to a single organ or tissue such as the periodontal tissues. From this primary site, the infection may spread through the blood stream to other sites.

Third, an infective organism that gets into the blood stream during an oral procedure may take months (or years) of incubation before the disease is manifested.

Serum hepatitis is an example of this. Although the infection may be initiated in the mouth, the liver is affected as long as five months later. It is difficult to connect previous dental treatment with the patient's liver disorder months later; however, there have been documented cases in which this has happened.

Because of these factors, which affect the appearance of infection related to dental treatment, it is particularly important at all times to maintain optimal standards of clinical control.

DISEASE TRANSMISSION

In a dental practice, there is the danger of disease transmission from the patient to the staff, from the staff to the patient, and from patient to patient through contact with the practice.

In general, diseases are transmitted when they are carried from place to place in fluids or air currents, on objects, or in waste products. In order to prevent disease transmission, it is important to understand how this transmission may take place.

Droplet Infection

This type of infection is transmitted by the numerous droplets of moisture, containing bacteria or viruses that are spread as people talk, breathe, sneeze, or cough. When someone sneezes, he sprays contaminated particles out about 8 feet and up about 4 feet.

A special droplet infection hazard for the dentist and assistant is inhaling the mist of bacteria and debris that is produced by the high-speed handpiece with water spray.

Being exposed to this mist is approximately the equivalent of having someone sneeze in your face twice per minute—at a distance of one foot!

Indirect Transmission

In the dental office, diseases may be indirectly transmitted by soiled hands and towels, dirty instruments, and even dust.

Also, anything that is touched during patient care is considered **contaminated** and potentially capable of spreading disease through indirect contact.

This includes faucet handles, switches, handpieces, instruments, drawer handles, medications, dressings, the patient's chart, and even the pen used to make the chart entry.

Self-infection

In many cases, infective microorganisms are present in the patient's mouth but will not cause infection until they enter the blood stream. However, an open wound in dental surgery may allow these microorganisms access to the blood stream, and in this way the patient may actually infect himself.

Operator Infection

Infection from the dentist's or assistant's nose, mouth, or hands may be spread to the patient via droplet infection or by indirect transmission during the operative procedure.

Also, infectious organisms sprayed from the patient's mouth can be transmitted to the dentist or assistant through his or her own nose or mouth or through a break in the skin.

Personal Contact

This mode of transmission, particularly of **sexually transmitted diseases** (STDs), also known as **venereal diseases,** requires direct person-to-person contact.

These diseases include **acquired immunodeficiency syndrome (AIDS), herpes, syphilis,** and **gonorrhea** and they may produce lesions in the oral cavity. These diseases can be transmitted through contact with contaminated blood, saliva or mucous membranes in the mouth.

Carrier Contact

A carrier is an individual who harbors in his body the specific organisms of a disease without obvious symptoms, and is capable of transmitting this disease to others.

Among carrier-transmitted diseases are **typhoid fever, tuberculosis, hepatitis B, herpes:**

- A carrier may have had the disease and recovered;
- A carrier may have been exposed to the disease and may be coming down with it but not yet have obvious symptoms; or
- A carrier may have been exposed to the disease but will never be sick with it.

Having a complete, up-to-date medical history on each patient is helpful in detecting someone who might be a carrier, but this is not 100 percent reliable. Therefore, it is always safer to assume that every patient is a potential carrier.

DISEASE-PRODUCING CAPABILITIES

There are three factors that influence the disease-producing capability of a pathogenic organism. There are (1) host resistance, (2) virulence, and (3) concentration.

Host Resistance

Host resistance is the ability of the body to resist the pathogen. The healthier you are, the better your resistance to disease. It is your responsibility to take the steps necessary to maintain your own health.

Immunization against specific diseases, such as hepatitis, is an important part of host resistance. Dental personnel should be immunized, and the immunizations should be kept up to date.

Virulence

Virulence describes the strength or disease-producing capabilities of the pathogen. A virulent pathogen is able to overcome many of the body's defenses—even in a healthy individual.

Concentration

Concentration refers to the number of pathogens that are present. The more pathogens that are present, the better their chances of overwhelming the host and producing disease.

WRITING

Directions: Answer the following question based on the reading selection. Remember to use the following writing strategies:

- Organize ideas.
- Write the first draft.
- Revise, edit, and proofread to write the final draft.

Describe six ways in which diseases can be transmitted in the dental office.

COMPREHENSION QUESTIONS

Directions: Answer the matching questions based on the selection. Use the strategies you learned for answering matching questions.

_____ A. Transmitted by droplets of moisture containing bacteria or viruses that are spread as people talk, breath, sneeze, or cough.

_____ B. Infective microorganisms are in the patient's mouth and cause infection when they enter the blood stream.

_____ C. Organisms of a disease are in an individual without obvious symptoms.

_____ D. Infections are spread from nose, hands, and mouth of dentist.

_____ E. Diseases are transmitted by soiled hands and towels.

_____ F. Sexually transmitted diseases.

_____ G. The ability of the body to resist the pathogen.

_____ H. The strength of the disease-producing capabilities of the pathogen.

_____ I. Anything touched during the patient's care.

_____ J. The number of pathogens that are present.

1. Indirect transmission
2. Personal contact
3. Droplet infection
4. Carrier contact
5. Operator infection
6. Self-infection
7. Concentration
8. Virulence
9. Contaminated
10. Host resistance

WORD PROBLEM

Directions: Use the strategies you learned for solving word problems to answer this question.

The high-speed handpiece with water spray in a dentist's office produces a mist of bacteria that is equal to having someone sneeze in your face twice per minute. Dr. Michael Peters is exposed to this mist eight hours a day, four days a week. How many sneezes does this mist equal each week?

Reading Selection 11

PREVIEW QUESTION
- Look at the figure. What is scrolling?

VOCABULARY

Directions: Locate five words that are new to you in this reading. Write the meaning of each of these words in the space provided.

_____

_____

_____

_____

_____

_____

_____

_____

_____

_____

EDITING TEXT

One of the more valuable functions of word processing is text editing. *Editing* refers to the changing or modifying of text in a document (the insertion or deletion of a word, for example), and in word processing it is accomplished through a series of commands. Although learning the editing commands of a word processing program takes time and effort, it provides a distinct advantage over the conventional method of editing with a typewriter. Specifically, the text can be edited without having to use correction paper or fluid because the corrections are made directly on the display screen rather than on paper. In addition, changes need only be made to that portion of the text requiring them. Therefore, the entire document does not

From Bonewit-West K: Computer Concepts and Applications for the Medical Office. Philadelphia, W.B. Saunders, 1993, pp. 88–91.

have to be retyped as may be required with typewriter editing, and only that portion of the document that has been changed requires proofreading because the remainder of the text remains untouched. These features greatly increase the speed and efficiency of text production.

Editing commands, in combination with cursor movement, are used to perform the editing operations of word processing. Cursor movement is used to move the cursor to the proper location on the display screen. The editing command is then activated by depressing a function key which is a special key on the computer keyboard. An example of an editing command would be the deletion of a character from a misspelled word on the display screen. The cursor is first moved to the location of the character to be deleted. The next step involves the depression of the proper function key (usually the Delete key). Depressing this key will result in the deletion of the character from the word and the movement of the remaining characters to the left to fill in the gap caused by the deleted character. The most commonly used editing operations are listed and described below.

Deletion

This is a feature in which a character, word, sentence, paragraph or larger block of text may be removed from the existing text.

Insertion

This is a feature in which a character, word, sentence, paragraph or larger block of text is added to the existing text paragraph. In insert mode, characters that are entered at the cursor location push existing text to the right.

Replacement

With this feature, characters that are entered at the cursor location replace or type over the existing character.

Centering

This is a feature which consists of a command that automatically centers a word or phrase between the margins as it is being entered. This feature eliminates the necessity of having to backspace from the center of a document.

Scrolling

Scrolling refers to the automatic movement of text up or down on the computer screen. Most documents created are too large to be seen in their entirety on the screen of the monitor. At the most, the screen can accommodate 24 to 25 lines of text. Once there is enough text to fill up a screen, the screen then acts as a "window" for viewing a portion of the document (Fig V–14). Scrolling provides the mechanism to move the window up or down to view different parts of a document that is too large to fit entirely on the screen. Scrolling the document up moves the text forward toward the beginning of the document, while scrolling the document down moves the text backwards toward the end of the document. The term scrolling is used because this function is similar to that of "rolling out a scroll." Scrolling is used to move through the document at a rapid rate when performing text editing functions to different portions of the document.

Block Action

A *block* is a group of characters such as a sentence or paragraph. Block action is a feature which allows the user to select a block of text and then perform a specific operation on the entire block. Commonly performed block actions include moving a block of text, copying a block of text, saving a block of text, and deleting a block of text from a document. With this feature, for example, a block of text can be copied and moved to a different location in the document or to an entirely different document.

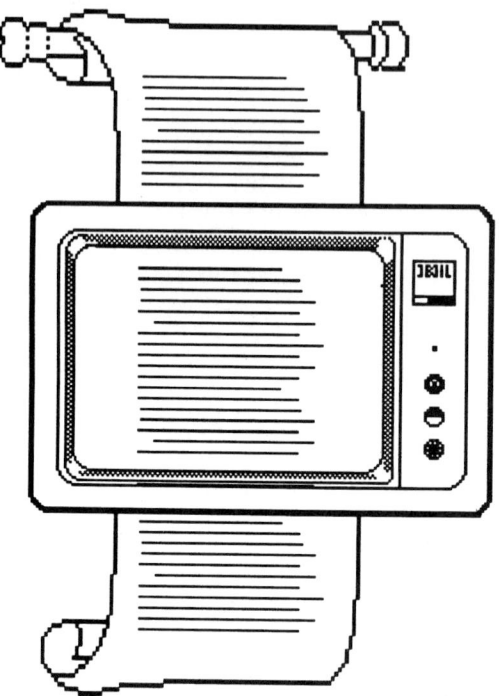

Figure V-14 Scrolling is the automatic movement of text up or down on the computer screen. Once there is enough text to fill up a screen, the screen then acts as a "window" for viewing a portion of the document.

Search and Replace

A feature which allows the user to locate a designated word or short phrase throughout an entire document and automatically change it if desired. This feature is useful when a word used frequently in a document is misspelled, when it is necessary to change a frequently used word to another word, or when a word has been used too often.

Spelling Checker

A spelling checker is used to detect possible spelling mistakes in a document by comparing each word in the document with the list of words in its dictionary. When a word is found that does not match any of the words in the dictionary, the word is highlighted. The user then decides whether or not to change the word. Most spelling checkers are able to display a list of possible suggestions to assist in locating the correct word. One disadvantage of spelling checkers is that they are unable to spot words that are used incorrectly in context. For example, if you type the word *patent* for *patient,* the spelling checker will not detect the error since *patent* is spelled correctly. In addition, a spelling checker does not include proper names in its dictionary.

FILING TEXT

Filing forms the basis of many of the unique features of word processing programs. Without this capability, it would not be possible to edit text or format text for printing. Filing functions include the storage and retrieval of documents from a secondary storage device such as a floppy disk or a hard disk. The specific procedures for saving, retrieving, and revising a document are outlined in the program user manual.

Storing or *saving* a document is the process of transferring a copy of the text that has been entered into the computer to a secondary storage device. Saving a document can be compared to placing that document in a file folder and storing it in a filing cabinet.

As previously discussed in Chapter 1, text entered into the computer is placed into the computer's memory (RAM) for temporary storage. Therefore, it is important to save a document before turning off the computer because the removal of power will result in the loss of the document. When working on a large document, it is recommended that the text be saved periodically (e.g., every 15 minutes) to prevent the loss of the entire document in the event of a power failure.

Before a document can be saved, it must be assigned a *filename*. The filename is used for later retrieval of the document from the disk. The filename should be short, but descriptive of the document that is being saved. The maximum number of characters that can be used for a filename generally ranges between eight and fifteen based on the application program being used. Each document must be assigned its own unique name. A filename that has previously been assigned to another document stored on the disk cannot be used because the computer would have difficulty in properly retrieving the documents. Therefore, if you want to store several versions of the same document, you will have to save each with a different filename. An ongoing, updated catalog of the filenames is stored along with the documents on the disk. The application program permits the display of this catalog, consisting of the list of filenames, to assist the user in retrieving a stored document.

Stored documents can later be retrieved for text editing functions and/or printing the document. When an edited document is saved again under the same filename, the revised document replaces the one previously stored on the disk.

FORMATTING TEXT

Text formatting is the arrangement or layout of the text on paper; in other words, how it will appear as printed text. Text entering and printing are two separate functions in word processing. This is in contrast to the typewriter in which these functions occur simultaneously, and the format is integrated as the document is being typed. Because of this separation in word processing, a document can be formatted a number of different ways by simply changing the formatting instructions. For example, if a document has been printed using single spacing, and the user desires the same document in a double-spaced format, the line spacing value can be changed from single- to double-spacing without having to retype the document. Formatting options included in most word processing programs are listed and described on the following page.

Line Spacing

Line spacing refers to the amount of empty space between printed lines. Word processing programs can produce single-spaced, double-spaced, and triple-spaced documents.

Margins

This feature allows you to select how much of a margin you want between your text and the edge of the paper.

Justifiction

This is a feature for making lines of text even at the left and right margins. Justification provides margin columns of even width like those of textbook print, rather than a "ragged" right edge.

Automatic Pagination

This is a feature which automatically numbers the pages of the printed document. Most word processing programs also allow the user to select the position of the number on the page (e.g., top, bottom).

Boldface

Boldface is a type in which the main strokes of the letter are thicker than normal.

Superscript

This is a feature which allows a character to be printed half a line above the usual text baseline.

Subscript

This is a feature which allows a character to be printed half a line below the usual text baseline.

WRITING

Directions: Answer the following question based on the reading selection. Remember to use the following writing strategies:

- Organize ideas.
- Write the first draft.
- Revise, edit, and proofread to write the final draft.

Which features of editing text with a word processing program would be particularly helpful to you? Explain why.

COMPREHENSION QUESTIONS

Directions: Answer the short-answer questions based on the selection. Use the strategies you learned for answering short-answer questions.

1. A _____ is a group of characters such as a sentence or paragraph.
2. A _____ is a feature in which a word or paragraph is added to the text.
3. _____ refers to the changing of text within the document.
4. Text formatting is the arrangement or _____ of text on paper.
5. The amount of empty space between printed lines is called _____.
6. A feature which automatically numbers the pages is called _____.
7. Another name for saving a document is _____.
8. _____ is a type which is thicker that normal.
9. RAM is the computer's _____.
10. Deletion _____ words or paragraphs from the text.

WORD PROBLEM

Directions: Use the strategies you learned for solving word problems to answer this question.

Julie Sands has been editing text with the word processor for 2 hours. It used to take her half of her 8-hour working day to edit the same amount of text with her typewriter. How many hours longer did editing with a typewriter take than editing with a word processor?

Reading Selection 12

PREVIEW QUESTION
- What are the three types of anesthesia discussed in this reading section?

VOCABULARY

Directions: Locate five words that are new to you in this reading. Write the meaning of each of these words in the space provided.

From Polaski A, Warner JP: Saunders Fundamentals For Nursing Assistants. Philadelphia, W.B. Saunders, 1994, pp. 702–704.

ANESTHESIA

When patients arrive in the operating room, they are given a medication to cause a loss of sensation in one part of the body or in the entire body. This loss of sensation is called *anesthesia*. The anesthetic (the medication that produces anesthesia) is given by a physician who specializes in giving such medication. The physician is called an *anesthesiologist*. An *anesthetist* is a registered nurse who is certified to administer anesthetics under the direction of the physician. The patient receives one of the following types of anesthesia:

> General anesthesia
> Local anesthesia
> Spinal anesthesia

General Anesthesia

During a lengthy or complex surgery, the patient receives an anesthetic that blocks sensation in the entire body.

General anesthesia is a deep sleep. A general anesthetic causes this effect because it is introduced into the blood. A general anesthetic is used for patients who have surgery on body organs such as the heart, liver, or kidney. It is also used in joint (for example, hip or knee) replacement or special tests. A general anesthetic affects many body functions (see chart on The Effects of General Anesthesia on Body Functions).

Local Anesthesia

When a patient undergoes **local anesthesia,** an anesthetic is injected directly into the surgical area where the loss of sensation is needed. For example, when a wound needs sutures (stitches), local anesthesia blocks the pain that would be caused by the needle going through the skin. As the local anesthetic wears off, sensation returns to the affected area.

A local anesthetic may also be applied directly to the skin or mucous membrane. For example, an anesthetic ointment can be applied to gums in the mouth to relieve the feeling of soreness.

The patient remains awake when a local anesthetic is used. During some surgical procedures in which a local anesthetic is used, the surgeon may order a medication to help the patient relax. This medication does not produce the deep sleep that a general anesthetic does.

Spinal Anesthesia

For **spinal anesthesia,** the anesthetic is injected into the spinal canal and produces a loss of sensation from the point of injection down to the toes of both feet. The impulses from the nerves in the spinal cord are blocked so that the brain no longer receives a message of pain from the areas served by the nerves. The patient remains awake and alert during the surgical procedure but cannot move the lower extremities or feel anything below the area of the injection. A medication that relaxes the patient and decreases anxiety may also be ordered. As the spinal anesthetic wears off, sensation returns to the lower extremities.

Spinal anesthesia is commonly used in surgeries performed on the male genital organs. For the mother who is about to give birth, spinal anesthesia helps decrease the pain caused by contractions of the uterus. Spinal anesthesia is also used for surgical procedures on the lower back.

GENERAL ANESTHESIA
loss of feeling or sensation in the entire body caused by an anesthetic medication introduced into the blood

LOCAL ANESTHESIA
loss of feeling or sensation in the part of the body in which an anesthetic medication has been injected or applied on the skin

SPINAL ANESTHESIA
loss of feeling or sensation in the body parts below the area of the back where anesthetic medication was injected

The Effects of General Anesthesia on Body Functions

Thinking Function
- The patient may experience mental confusion, sleepiness, or agitation because the anesthesia affects the brain. The patient may also be slow to respond to questions.

Respiratory Function
- The patient's respiration rate may slow down because the anesthetic affects the brain's breathing control center.
- Respiratory complications can occur if
  - the surgery involves the chest or upper abdominal area
  - a disease of the lungs was present before surgery
  - the patient is overweight
  - the patient is elderly
  - postoperative activities such as coughing and deep breathing are not done

Circulatory Function
- The patient's inactivity and slower blood flow may cause circulatory problems such as the formation of blood clots.
- Changes in blood pressure after surgery may cause dizziness.

Protective Function of the Skin
- The patient's skin may become dry in the hospital environment. Dry skin breaks down easily.
- The patient may discover that lying in one position decreases pain or discomfort. By lying in one position, however, the patient can develop decubitus ulcers over bony areas of the body.
- Patients who are at risk for skin complications after surgery are those
  - with nutritional problems
  - with circulation problems
  - who do not turn in bed
  - who have had skin problems in the past

Gastrointestinal Function
- General anesthesia slows down the movement of food through the gastrointestinal tract. This can cause constipation.
- The general anesthetic used may cause nausea and vomiting.

Urinary Function
- When anesthesia affects the bladder, the bladder may not empty completely. Urinary retention can result in urinary infection.
- Insertion of an indwelling catheter as part of preoperative preparation also increases patients' risk for bladder infection.

Activity Function
- The patient may be weak and move slowly after surgery. The patient may not move the part of the body on which the surgery was performed. The lack of movement causes the muscles to atrophy (shrink).

Fluids
- The patient's fluid balance may change after surgery. Patients who experience nausea and vomiting after surgery lose fluids. They will receive fluids intravenously (through the vein) until they are able to take fluids by mouth.

WRITING

Directions: Answer the following question based on the reading selection. Remember to use the following writing strategies:

- Organize ideas.
- Write the first draft.
- Revise, edit, and proofread to write the final draft.

What are the differences in the three types of anesthesia?

COMPREHENSION QUESTIONS

Directions: Answer the multiple-choice questions based on the selection. Use the strategies you learned for answering multiple-choice questions.

1. An anesthesiologist is a
   a. registered nurse
   b. a physician
   c. a medication
   d. an illness

2. General anesthesia is a
   a. body organ
   b. spinal tap
   c. deep sleep
   d. deep wound

3. Local anesthesia is often used for
   a. stitches
   b. complex surgery
   c. changing blood pressure
   d. surgery on body organs

4. Intravenous feeding is through the
   a. mouth
   b. veins
   c. joints
   d. skin

5. The anesthesia which is injected directly into the surgical area is
   a. local
   b. spinal
   c. general
   d. ineffective

6. After surgery, the patient's fluid balance
   a. always changes
   b. never changes
   c. stays the same
   d. may change

7. Loss of feeling in the entire body is caused by
   a. a relaxing medication
   b. general anesthesia
   c. local anesthesia
   d. spinal anesthesia

8. A loss of sensation is called
   a. anesthesia
   b. anesthesiologist
   c. anesthetist
   d. sutures

9. Muscles which atrophy
   a. grow
   b. stiffen
   c. shrink
   d. disappear

10. When spinal anesthesia is administered, the patient
    a. can move all extremities
    b. cannot move the upper extremities
    c. cannot move the lower extremities
    d. can move only the upper extremities

WORD PROBLEM

Directions: Use the strategies you learned for solving word problems to answer this question.

The anesthetist planned to administer anesthesia to the patient 70 minutes before surgery. The surgery was scheduled for 3:00 PM. What time was the anesthesia administered?

Reading Selection 13

> **PREVIEW QUESTION**
> - What specific injuries can be caused by electrical burns?

VOCABULARY

Directions: Locate five words that are new to you in this reading. Write the meaning of each of these words in the space provided.

_____
_____
_____
_____
_____
_____
_____
_____
_____
_____

ELECTRICAL BURNS

Electricity is a fundamental entity of nature consisting of negative and positive forces. It is observable in the attractions and repulsions of bodies electrified by friction and in natural phenomena such as lightning or the aurora borealis.

In the United States, about 1,000 people die each year from electrical injuries. At high risk are workers involved in industrial accidents and children. Electrical accidents occur due to downed power lines, the malfunctioning of home appliances, children chewing through electrical lines, accidental contact with TV antennae by unskilled individuals, and contact with high-tension power lines (often by adolescent boys).

From Henry MC, Stapleton ER (Eds.): EMT Prehospital Care. Philadelphia, W.B. Saunders, 1992, pp. 508–509.

When electricity traverses the body, it is converted to heat that burns the tissues in its path. High-voltage arcs generate intense amounts of heat and can burn a person nearby. Death can result from the passage of current through vital organs, which causes respiratory or cardiac arrest.

The EMT must take due precautions to protect himself or herself and the victim from further injury. Knowing some basic properties of electricity may help guide you to take correct actions. Electricity is the movement of electrons from a point of higher concentration to a point of lower concentration. Electricity is often described in terms of three variables: amperage, voltage, and resistance. Amperage is the number or volume of electrons flowing. Voltage is the force with which movement occurs. Resistance is the degree of hindrance to electron flow. These three concepts are interrelated by the formula

$$A \text{ (amperage)} = V \text{ (voltage)}/R \text{ (resistance)}$$

Current can be direct or unidirectional in flow or it can alternate or switch the direction of electron flow at a given number of cycles per second. Flow from a battery is direct current, whereas household current is usually alternating current.

Generally, exposure to low voltage is less serious than to high voltage. However, fatalities have occurred with voltage as low as 45 to 60 cycles per second. Household current is capable of causing tetanic contraction of human muscle, preventing release of the electrified object by the victim. Amperage, which is not usually known, also does more damage as the milliamperes increase: from tingling, to tetanic contraction, to fatal organ damage. If current passes through the brain, it may cause respiratory arrest. If it passes through the heart, it may cause cardiac arrest.

Resistance is defined as a measure of the hindrance to electron flow through a given material. Materials vary tremendously in their resistance. For example, copper wires offer relatively low resistance and conduct electricity readily; they serve as good conductors. Rubber has a very high resistance to electrical flow; rubber serves as an insulator. Good conductors offer low resistance. Poor conductors offer high resistance. Lightning rods illustrate some of these properties. Lightning rods, made of metal, which is a good conductor, are used to direct electricity from the roof of a house along insulated wires to the ground. Since electricity seeks to flow along the path of least resistance from a higher to a lower potential, lightning rods prevent electricity from traveling through a highly resistant wooden roof, which would generate heat and fire. Instead the electricity is directed to the earth, which can absorb the current. In fact, *Webster's* Dictionary defines the term "ground" as a large conducting body, as the earth, used as a common return for an electrical circuit and an arbitrary zero of potential.

Cars are insulated from the ground by their rubber tires. Thus, a downed power line in contact with a car may leave the occupants unharmed as long as they avoid direct contact with the ground. However, if they step out of the car while holding onto the door, they will be part of the circuit consisting of the wire, the car, their bodies, and the ground, and they will suffer electrical injury.

When electrical current passes through the body as part of its circuit (usually to the ground), it follows an internal path of least resistance. Skin and bone offer high resistance to electrical current, muscle offers less, and the vessels and nerves offer the lease resistance to electrical flow. Therefore, current passing from arm to arm tends to pass along the vessels and nerves in the arms and thorax. Even high current can enter and exit at relatively small surface areas and one cannot gauge the extent of internal injury from the external appearance.

Wet skin, offering less resistance, is more easily penetrated by electricity than dry skin. For example, even household current that penetrates wet skin can cause fatal ventricular fibrillation.

Electrical Burns to Skin

Burns to the soft tissues, because of the heat generated from electric current, can extend from first-degree to fourth-degree burns. Third-degree and fourth-degree burns can vary from those that look gray-white to those that appear charred. Thermal burns can also be caused by the intense heat generated by electric arcs that are nearby but not in direct contact with the body. The longer the duration of contact, the greater the burn. Remember that electrical burns tend to be more extensive than can be judged from their external marks.

Types of Electrical Burns

Arc Burns

A high-voltage current traveling through the air can cause temperatures to reach 2,000 to 3,000°F, an intense heat (flash) that causes thermal injury. For example, clothing may ignite, adding to the burns.

Specific Injuries

The most immediate life-threatening effects of electrical injuries are respiratory and cardiac arrest. Early resuscitation can salvage some victims. For example, respiratory arrest following a lightning injury can be prolonged, but victims who have received early respiratory support have recovered. Associated falls may cause fractures and other injuries.

Assessment and Treatment

The first priority is to assess whether hazards continue to exist. Are there fallen wires? Any downed wire should be considered as charged until the appropriate authorities such as power company personnel confirm that the power is off. When encountering victims entrapped in a vehicle in contact with a downed wire, have them remain in the vehicle. Do not touch the vehicle yourself, since that will place you in a circuit from the vehicle to the ground. If there is a fire in the car, victims should jump out or throw small children to rescue personnel (making sure there is never a circuit from the car to the ground). After ensuring rescuer safety, perform the ABCs of life support with appropriate concern for the cervical spine if falls or violent contractions have occurred. Look closely for any fractures and splint appropriately. When assessing the skin, look for both entrance and exit wounds. Cover the wounds with sterile dressings and transport the patient to the hospital.

WRITING

Directions: Answer the following question based on the reading selection. Remember to use the following writing strategies:

- Organize ideas.
- Write the first draft.
- Revise, edit, and proofread to write the final draft.

What should the EMT know about electricity to protect the burn victim from further injury?

COMPREHENSION QUESTIONS

Directions: Answer the true and false questions based on the selection. Use the strategies you learned for answering true and false questions.

T F

___ ___ 1. Electricity consists of only negative forces.

___ ___ 2. In the United States, 10,000 people die each year from electrical injuries.

___ ___ 3. Death can result from the passage of current through vital organs.

___ ___ 4. A = V/R

___ ___ 5. Exposure to low voltage is more serious than exposure to high voltage.

___ ___ 6. Burns to the soft tissue extend from the third to the fourth degree.

___ ___ 7. Amperage is the number or volumes of electrons flowing.

___ ___ 8. Downed wire should be considered as charged.

___ ___ 9. Cars are insulated from the ground by their rubber tires.

___ ___ 10. If a current passes through the heart, it will always cause cardiac arrest.

WORD PROBLEM

Directions: Use the strategies you learned for solving word problems to answer this question.

Fatalities can occur with voltage as low as 45 to 60 cycles per second. If the voltage is 90 to 180 cycles per second, how much greater is the risk?

Reading Selection 14

PREVIEW QUESTION
- What is another name for amyotrophic lateral sclerosis?

VOCABULARY

Directions: Locate five words that are new to you in this reading. Write the meaning of each of these words in the space provided.

___

DEGENERATIVE, MOVEMENT, AND SEIZURE DISORDERS

Alzheimer's disease
    Brain disorder marked by deterioration of mental capacity (**dementia**) beginning in middle age.
    The disorder develops gradually, and early signs are loss of memory for recent events, persons, and places, followed by impairment of judgment, comprehension, and intellect. Anxiety, depression, and emotional disturbances can occur as well. On autopsy of the brain there is cerebral cortex atrophy and widening of the cerebral sulci, especially in the frontal and temporal regions. Microscopic examination shows senile plaques resulting from degeneration of neurons and neurofibrillary tangles (bundles of fibrils in the cytoplasm of a neuron) in the cerebral cortex. There is as yet no effective treatment.

amyotrophic lateral sclerosis (ALS)
    Progressive disorder characterized by degeneration of motor neurons in the spinal cord and brain stem; also called **Lou Gehrig's disease.**

From Chabner DE: The Language of Medicine, 5th ed. Philadelphia, W.B. Saunders, in press.

Named for a famous baseball player, Lou Gehrig, who became a victim of the disease, ALS presents in adulthood and affects men more often than women. Symptoms are weakness in skeletal muscles, difficulty in swallowing and talking, and dyspnea as the respiratory muscles become affected. Eventually muscles atrophy, and the patient becomes quadriplegic. Etiology (cause) and cure for ALS are both unknown.

epilepsy

Chronic disorder characterized by recurrent seizure activity.

A seizure is an abnormal, sudden excessive discharge of electrical activity within the brain. Seizures are often symptoms of underlying brain pathological conditions, such as brain tumors, meningitis, vascular disease, or scar tissue from a head injury. **Tonic-clonic seizures (grand mal seizures)** are characterized by a sudden loss of consciousness, falling down, and then tonic contractions (stiffening of muscles) followed by clonic contractions (twitching and jerking movements of the limbs). Often, these convulsions are preceded by an **aura**, which is a peculiar sensation appearing before more definite symptoms. Dizziness, numbness, or visual disturbances are examples of an aura. **Absence seizures (petit mal seizures)** are a minor form of seizure consisting of momentary clouding of consciousness and loss of contact with the environment. Drug therapy (anticonvulsants) is used for control of epileptic seizures. The term comes from the Greek *epilepsis* meaning a laying hold of. The Greeks thought a victim of a seizure was laid hold of by some mysterious force.

Huntington's chorea

Hereditary nervous disorder due to degenerative changes in the cerebrum and involving bizarre, abrupt, involuntary, dance-like movements.

This condition begins between the ages of 30 and 45 and results in mental decline with choreic (meaning dance) movements (uncontrollable, irregular, jerking movements of the arms, legs, and face). The recent discovery that the genetic defect in patients with Huntington's disease is located on chromosome 4 has made it possible to test and identify those who will eventually develop the disease. Inheritance is a dominant trait (the disorder appears when only one of a pair of chromosomes carries the defective gene) and the offspring of a parent with the disease has a 50 per cent chance of eventually manifesting the condition. There is no cure; management is symptomatic.

multiple sclerosis (MS)

Destruction of the myelin sheath on neurons in the CNS and its replacement by plaques of sclerotic (hard) tissue.

One of the leading causes of neurologic diability in persons 20–40 years of age, MS is a chronic disease marked by periods of remission and then relapse. **Demyelination** prevents the conduction of nerve impulses through the axon and causes paresthesias, muscle weakness, unsteady **gait** (manner of walking), and paralysis. Etiology is unknown, and there is no effective treatment, although immunosuppressive agents are often given with some benefit.

myasthenia gravis

Neuromuscular disorder characterized by relapsing weakness (-asthenia) of skeletal muscles (attached to bones).

Myasthenia gravis means grave muscle weakness and is a chronic autoimmune disorder. Antibodies block the ability of *acetylcholine* (a neurotransmitter) to transmit the nervous impulse from nerve to muscle cell, and normal muscle contraction fails to occur. Muscles on the outside of the eye (extraocular) are affected (causing ptosis of the eyelid) as well as those of the face, tongue, and extremities. Therapy to reverse symptoms includes anticholinesterase drugs, which inhibit the enzyme that breaks down acetylcholine. Corticosteroids (prednisone), and immunosuppressive drugs (azathioprine, methotrexate, and cyclophosphamide) are also used in treatment. Thymectomy (removal of the thymus gland, the source of antibody-producing white blood cells) is an alternative method of treatment and is beneficial to many patients.

palsy

Paralysis (partial or complete loss of motor function).

Cerebral palsy is partial paralysis and lack of muscular coordination caused by damage to the cerebrum during gestation or in the perinatal period. **Bell's palsy** involves unilateral facial paralysis, which is due to a disorder of the facial nerve. Etiology is unknown, but complete recovery is possible.

Parkinson's disease

Degeneration of nerves in the brain, occurring in later life, leading to tremors, weakness of muscles, and slowness of movement.

This slowly progressive condition is caused by a deficiency of **dopamine** (a neurotransmitter) that is made by cells in the midbrain (below the cerebrum and above the pons and medulla). Motor disturbances include stooped posture, shuffling gait, muscle stiffness (rigidity), and often a tremor of the hands. Drugs (such as levodopa) that increase dopamine levels in the brain are useful **palliative** (relieving but not curative) measures to control symptoms. Implantation of fetal brain tissue containing dopamine-producing cells is currently being used as an experimental treatment with uncertain results.

WRITING

Directions: Answer the following questions based on the reading selection. Remember to use the following writing strategies:

- Organize ideas.
- Write the first draft.
- Revise, edit, and proofread to write the final draft.

What are the signs of Alzheimer's disease? How do these signs differ from Parkinson's disease?

COMPREHENSION QUESTIONS

Directions: Answer the short-answer questions based on the selection. Use the strategies you learned for answering short-answer questions.

1. Dementia is the _____ of mental capacity.
2. Lou Gehrig was a famous _____.
3. _____ is marked by abnormal, recurrent firing of nerve impulses within the brain.
4. Bell's palsy is due to a disorder of the _____ nerve.
5. Extraocular muscles are on the _____ of the eye.
6. The genetic defect in patients with Huntington's disease is located on chromosome _____.
7. The removal of the thymus gland is called a _____.
8. Parkinson's disease is a _____ of nerves in the brain.
9. _____ is partial or complete loss of motor function.
10. Drugs that relieve but do not cure are called _____.

WORD PROBLEM

Directions: Use the strategies you learned for solving word problems to answer this question.

A class training to become nursing assistants was taught the signs of MS. Two-thirds of the students were able to recognize those patients who had this disease. If there are 30 students, how many still have to learn to recognize the signs of MS?

Reading Selection 15

PREVIEW QUESTION
- How many generations of antihistaminic drugs are available?

VOCABULARY

Directions: Locate five words that are new to you in this reading. Write the meaning of each of these words in the space provided.

_____
_____
_____
_____
_____
_____
_____
_____
_____
_____
_____

ASTHMA

The mast cells of the airway contain most of the histamine that is found in the lungs. Physical (e.g., exercise, cold air) as well as chemical (e.g., allergens) insults stimulate its release. An increase in the plasma level of histamine has been associated with both allergen-induced and spontaneous bronchoconstriction.

Among the classic actions of histamine is bronchoconstriction, which can occur directly by the stimulation of H_1-receptors or indirectly by the stimulation of vagal reflexes. The inhalation of histamine may be used in a test to quantify airway hyperresponsiveness. Other actions of histamine that may contribute to asthma include an increase in the permeability of the pul-

From Witek TJ Jr, Schachter EN: Pharmacology and Therapeutics in Respiratory Care. Philadelphia, W.B. Saunders, 1994, pp. 266–271.

monary epithelium of the airway, an enhancement of the release of other mediators and, possibly, a change in immunoregulatory functions.

Studies of first-generation H_1-receptor antagonists used to treat asthma found them to be somewhat effective in producing bronchodilation, but their use has been limited by their side effects, especially when they are given at high dosages. The second-generation H_1-receptor antagonists are more potent agents and devoid of sedative side effects. These newer agents have been shown to be protective against provocation from a variety of insults and have been shown to provide benefits in the treatment of asthma. The efficacy of some of these drugs may extend beyond their function as antagonists of H_1-receptors and may be due to the inhibition of some of the cellular events that occur in patients who have chronic asthma.

INDIVIDUAL AGENTS

Two generations of antihistaminic drugs are available.

First-Generation Compounds

H_1-receptor antagonists have been used for more than five decades in the treatment of respiratory disease. Current United States federal regulations governing the clinical development of pharmaceuticals were not in place when these agents were first introduced, and the safety and efficacy of many of the older drugs have not been extensively evaluated. Nevertheless, many of the first-generation compounds have been reviewed for safety and efficacy in the over-the-counter (OTC) monograph process of the federal Food and Drug Administration (FDA), and Table V–1 lists drugs that have been approved by the FDA in a Final Monograph. Clinical data for some of these and other first-generation compounds are provided as follows.

Brompheniramine

Brompheniramine is a commonly used H_1-receptor antagonist that is available in several preparations (e.g., Dimetane). Pharmacokinetic studies of its use by healthy adults have documented a mean serum half-life of 24.9 ± 9.3 hours.

Brompheniramine has been shown to have a prolonged antihistaminic effect on the skin. Its beneficial effects on nasal breathing have been demonstrated both by provocative challenge and by trials of its use against seasonal allergic rhinitis. Subjective observations of sleepiness and alterations in **psychomotor performance** have been reported by subjects after single doses of 4 mg and 12 mg.

Chlorpheniramine

Chlorpheniramine is available in many products, either alone or in combination with other drugs. Its mean half-life in adults exceeds 20 hours; a shorter half-life (13.1 hr) has been observed in children who have allergic rhinitis.

As previously noted, chlorpheniramine has been reported to be effective in reducing the symptoms that are associated with acute infections of the upper respiratory tract. A relief of symptoms and better nasal clearance after the use of chlorpheniramine were also reported in trials of this drug against induced rhinovirus colds; nasal patency, measured by rhinomanometry, or the response of the middle ear and the eustachian canal proved to be the same, however, in a comparison of chlorpheniramine and a placebo.

Relief from the symptoms of seasonal allergic rhinitis has been observed in subjects whose symptoms were treated with chlorpheniramine; head-to-head trials of chlorpheniramine and the second-generation drug terfenadine found them to be comparable in relieving these symptoms. In another trial, 4.0 mg of chlorpheniramine provided a relief of symptoms similar to that of 0.5 mg of azelastine. In an eight-week trial during ragweed season, both chlorpheniramine (24 mg/day) and hydroxyzine (150 mg/day) provided significantly more relief than a placebo; hydroxyzine ranked best in this study. Protection against bronchospasm induced by exercise and against isocapneic hyperventilation has also been demonstrated after subjects inhaled chlorpheniramine.

TABLE V-1 Adult Dosages for Antihistamines Available Without a Prescription

Antihistamine	Adult Dose (mg) (Maximum per 24 hr)	Administration Interval (hr)
Brompheniramine	4 (24)	4–6
Chlorcyclizine	25 (75)	6–8
Chlopheniramine	4 (24)	4–6
Clemastine*	1.34 (2.68)	12
Dexbrompheniramine	2 (12)	4–6
Dexchlorpheniramine	2 (12)	4–6
Diphenhydramine	25–50 (300)	4–6
Phenindamine	25 (150)	4–6
Pheniramine	12.5–25 (150)	4–6
Pyrilamine	25–50 (200)	6–8
Thonzylamine	50–100 (600)	4–6
Triprolidine	2.5 (10)	4–6

*Clemastine was granted over-the-counter status in 1992.

Sedation after the use of chlorpheniramine was reported to be greater than after taking a placebo in clinical trials of patients who suffered from seasonal allergic rhinitis. For example, in the trial reported by Kemp and co-workers, the incidence of the sedation that followed the use of chlorpheniramine, terfenadine, and placebo was 19%, 7.6% and 2.4% of the group studied, respectively. Alterations in psychomotor performance have been observed in studies of the effect of single doses of 4 mg, 8 mg, and 10 mg. In a trial of 10 mg chlorpheniramine, the addition of 15 mg ephedrine hydrochloride reduced the impairment in tasks that require sustained attention and discrimination that had been observed after the administration of 10 mg of chlorpheniramine alone.

Diphenhydramine

Diphenhydramine (e.g., Benadryl) is one of the few H_1-receptor antagonists that is available for intravenous administration. It is widely prescribed for the treatment of the symptoms of urticaria and anaphylaxis. It is also used for the treatment of the symptoms of allergies and infections of the upper respiratory tract. In a trial of the drug with patients who had perennial allergic rhinitis, diphenhydramine was found to be as effective as cetirizine in providing relief from symptoms. Diphenhydramine is an antitussive agent as well.

Studies have shown that the mean serum half-life of diphenhydramine differs significantly in the elderly (13.5 ± 4.2 hr), in young adults (9.2 ± 2.5 hr), and in children (5.4 ± 1.8 hr). In the elderly and in young adults, diphenhydramine inhibited the eruption of histamine-induced wheals and areas of flare significantly for approximately 1 to 12 hours as compared with their appearance without the use of the drug. In children, the significant suppression lasted only from one to eight hours. In a trial of diphenhydramine with young adults, the administration of a dose at bedtime of a formula that contained diphenhydramine was found to inhibit the sneezing associated with morning nasal antigen challenge. Diphenhydramine causes marked drowsiness, which can limit its use in the daytime. It has been shown that the use of 25–50 mg of diphenhydramine significantly shortens latency to daytime sleep and alters psychomotor performance in comparison with a placebo.

Phenindamine

Phenindamine was introduced in the late 1940s and is available in a limited number of products (e.g., Novahist). Early reports of the efficacy of this drug have been published, and a trial of its use in the treatment of seasonal allergic rhinitis confirmed its usefulness. Although the use of phenindamine does not shorten latency to daytime sleep more than a placebo does or differ from a placebo in tests of psychomotor performance, the incidence of both sedation and insomnia is significantly greater after therapy with phenindamine than after the administration of a placebo.

Triprolidine

Triprolidine is an H_1-receptor antagonist of the alkylamine class; it is found in several preparations, primarily in the Actifed line of products. Triprolidine has a short half-life; studies of its effect on healthy subjects show a mean serum half-life of 2.1 ± 0.8 hours. The mean peak serum concentration occurs approximately two hours after its ingestion orally.

The efficacy of triprolidine in the treatment of allergic rhinitis has been demonstrated both when used alone and when combined with pseudoephedrine. The combination of the two drugs is often prescribed to reduce the size of swollen, congested nasal vessels and to inhibit the histamine-driven symptoms of sneeze and rhinorrhea. For example, Diamond and coworkers reported that although the use of triprolidine elicited the greatest reduction in the symptoms of rhinitis, the combination of triprolidine and pseudoephedrine was more effective than pseudoephedrine or a placebo taken alone. As expected, the combination was more effective than triprolidine or a placebo in reducing nasal congestion.

Triprolidine is associated with sedation. Decrements in psychomotor performance have been observed after the ingestion of a single dose.

Hydroxyzine

Hydroxyzine (e.g., Atarax, Vistaril) is widely used for the relief of pruritus. Its efficacy in the treatment of allergic rhinitis has also been demonstrated. The mean half-life of hydroxyzine has been reported to be 2.0 hours in healthy adults; a longer half-life has been reported for the drug when used by the elderly. One trial found that 50 mg of hydroxyzine given at bedtime maintained skin H_1-receptor antagonism the following morning and alleviated the decline in psychomotor performance.

The side effects of hydroxyzine include sedation, impairment of cognitive function, and confusion as well as anticholinergic responses such as dry mouth, blurred vision, and urinary retention, particularly troublesome in the elderly. Hydroxyzine's effects on the CNS have been demonstrated in studies that use several sleep latency tests and tests of psychomotor performance.

Second-Generation Compounds

All of the second generation of antihistaminic compounds are available in the United States by prescription only (Table V–2). Some of these agents have been available without prescription in Canada and Europe.

TABLE V–2 H_1-receptor Antagonists Available by Prescription Only

Generic (Proprietary)	U.S.A. Regulatory Status	Adult Dosage*
Astemizole (Hismanal)	NDA approved 12/29/88	10 mg q.d.
Azatadine (Optimine)	NDA approved 3/20/77	1–2 mg q. 12 hr
Cyproheptadine HCl (Periactin)	NDA approved 10/17/61	4 mg q. 8 hr
Promethazine (Phenergan)	Classification changed from OTC Category 1 to Rx only	12.5–25 mg q. 6–24 hr
Terfenadine (Seldane)	NDA approved 5/8/85	60 mg b.i.d.
Loratadine (Claritin)	NDA approved 4/12/93	10 mg q.d.
Cetirizine (Reactine)	NDA pending	—

*Usual single oral adult dose for conventional dosage forms.
KEY: NDA = new drug application to the federal Food and Drug Administration, OTC = over-the-counter, Rx = by prescription.

Acrivastine

Acrivastine is related structurally to its parent triprolidine. It is a short-acting H_1-receptor antagonist under development in the United States. Its half-life is between 1.5 and 2.0 hours, and its recommended dosage is three times per day.

Acrivastine is effective in relieving the symptoms of allergic rhinitis. The studies of the drug available suggest that acrivastine has a low potential for sedation.

Astemizole

Astemizole (Hismanal), the second nonsedating H_1-receptor antagonist to be introduced in the United States, has a long duration of action and is administered once a day. Desmethylastemizole is the metabolite that is principally active in humans; the mean serum half-life of a single 30-mg dose of astemizole plus demethylastemizole metabolite is 9.5 days.

Several clinical studies have established the effectiveness of astemizole in the treatment of seasonal and perennial rhinitis. Astemizole is as effective or slightly more effective in providing relief from rhinitis than is either chlorpheniramine or terfenadine.

The incidence of sedation after therapy with astemizole is comparable to that of a placebo. In one trial of psychomotor performance, no changes were observed after the ingestion of astemizole (10 mg and 20 mg) or of terfenadine (60 mg). Astemizole may increase a patient's appetite and weight after its prolonged use. Like terfenadine, astemizole has been associated with cardiac tachyarrhythmias.

Azatadine

Azatadine (Optimine) is a tricyclic H_1-receptor antagonist that also possesses anticholinergic and antiserotonin properties. It is available in combination with pseudoephedrine (Trinalin). Azatadine's half-life is approximately nine hours; it is recommended for use twice a day.

Azatadine has been shown to be effective in the relief of the symptoms of allergic rhinitis when taken either alone or in combination with pseudoephedrine. The alleviation of the symptoms associated with an infection of the upper respiratory tract have been reported for formulas that contain azatadine.

The administration of azatadine topically inhibits both the symptoms and the release of histamine (and of other mediators associated with mast cells) into nasal secretions after a challenge by an antigen. After a provocation by histamine, the use of azatadine inhibits the onset of symptoms and reduces the level of albumin in nasal secretions. Azatadine has no effect on either symptoms or the release of histamine after a nasal challenge by cold or dry air, which suggests that mast cells release histamine by different mechanisms when stimulated by an antigen than when stimulated by the physical characteristics of the air inhaled.

Azatadine causes drowsiness, but little effect on psychomotor performance has been observed in clinical studies.

Azelastine

In addition to its H_1-receptor antagonism, azelastine also inhibits the release of histamine from mast cells; it has negligible anticholinergic activity. Its half-life is 25.0 hours after a single dose administered orally and 35.5 hours after several doses. For the treatment of allergic rhinitis, 2 mg taken twice a day is recommended; higher dosages are recommended for the treatment of asthma.

Administered either orally or intranasally, azelastine provides relief from the symptoms of allergic rhinitis. Azelastine may offer some benefits in the treatment of asthma, as evidenced by an alleviation of symptoms, by bronchodilation, and by a reduction in the number of attacks. The most common side effects of azelastine are an altered perception of taste and drowsiness; the soporific effect of azalastine is not clearly established.

Cetirizine

Cetirizine is an H_1-receptor antagonist to be administered once a day that is expected to be available in the United States in the near future. It is the active carboxylic acid metabolite of its parent drug hydroxyzine. It is highly selective for the H_1-receptor.

A mean serum half-life of approximately seven hours has been established for this drug in both children and adults; a longer half-life has been found in the elderly and in adults who have mild to moderate renal insufficiency.

Clinical trials have documented the effectiveness of 5–20 mg cetirizine in the treatment of seasonal and perennial allergic rhinitis and of urticaria. Cetirizine has been shown to block the infiltration of eosinophils at the site of cutaneous reactions induced by allergens. Preliminary trials have demonstrated that the drug offers some benefit in the treatment of pollen-associated asthma.

Compared with its parent drug hydroxyzine, the carboxyl group of cetirizine is negatively charged at physiologic pH, which results in a decrease in its penetration into the CNS across the blood-brain barrier. Studies of psychomotor performance and latency to daytime sleep have generally shown that cetirizine causes minimal impairment.

Loratadine

Loratadine (Claritin), related structurally to azatadine, has a neutral carbamate group in the place of azatadine's basic tertiary amino group and an additional chloro group on the benzocycloheptapyridine ring. The administration of this drug in single dosages results in an elimination half-life of 8 and 11 hours for 20 mg and 40 mg, respectively. The recommended adult dose is 10 mg taken once a day.

The efficacy of loratadine has been established in several clinical trials. In one trial, 10 mg of loratadine provided relief comparable to 60 mg of terfenadine from the symptoms of allergic rhinitis. The effectiveness of loratadine (5 mg) with pseudoephedrine (120 mg) administered as an immediate and slow-release core (Claritin-D) has been demonstrated in trials of its effectiveness against seasonal allergic rhinitis. In one trial that evaluated the ingredients both individually and in combination, pseudoephedrine alone was found to be more effective than loratadine in relieving nasal stuffiness, and the combination was more effective than either a placebo or loratadine.

Loratadine is relatively free from the soporific effects common to first-generation H_1-receptor antagonists. In tests of psychomotor performance and latency to daytime sleep, 10 mg of loratadine produced effects comparable to those produced by a placebo.

Terfenadine

Terfenadine is an H_1-receptor antagonist that has little or no activity at H_2-, cholinergic, or serotoninergic receptors. Terfenadine is absorbed rapidly and metabolized extensively after a single dose administered orally. Terfenadine's principal metabolite, metabolite I, has antihistaminic activity and reaches its peak level two to three hours after a single dose of terfenadine was administered to healthy subjects. The elimination half-life of metabolite I is approximately 17 hours. Terfenadine is recommended at a dosage of 60 mg taken twice a day, although an equivalent relief from the symptoms of allergic rhinitis has been reported after the use of 120 mg taken once a day.

Several trials have demonstrated the effectiveness of terfenadine in the treatment of perennial or seasonal rhinitis. Terfenadine has been shown to reduce the symptoms of asthma and the need for bronchodilators. The role of terfenadine and other second-generation H_1-receptor antagonists in the treatment of asthma needs further study. Terfenadine does not appear to provide significant relief from the symptoms of infections of the upper respiratory tract, and it is not indicated for this purpose.

Terfenadine was the first H_1-receptor antagonist to be introduced in the United States as nonsedating. Although sedation is the most frequently reported adverse effect of terfenadine therapy, its incidence does not differ significantly from the incidence of sedation that is reported by patients who have received a placebo and is less than that reported by patients who received first-generation agents. In addition, several studies have shown that psychomotor performance is not altered significantly by the use of terfenadine and that terfenadine does not shorten latency to daytime sleep.

Terfenadine, like astemizole, has been associated with **torsades de pointes,** a serious ventricular arrhythmia associated with prolongation of the **QT interval.** Factors that predispose a patient to this side effect include preexisting cardiac disease, overdose of the drug, cirrhosis of the liver, the antifungal agent ketoconazole, and the antibiotic erythromycin.

WRITING

Directions: Answer the following question based on the reading selection. Remember to use the following writing strategies:

- Organize ideas.
- Write the first draft.
- Revise, edit, and proofread to write the final draft.

Compare the advantages and disadvantages of the two generations of antihistaminic drugs.

COMPREHENSION QUESTIONS

Directions: Answer the multiple choice questions based on the selection. Use the strategies you learned for answering multiple choice questions.

1. Benadryl is an example of
   a. Triprolidine
   b. Diphenhydramine
   c. Clemastine
   d. Chlorcyclizine

2. Clemastine was granted over-the-counter status in
   a. 1990
   b. 1991
   c. 1992
   d. 1993

3. The administration interval for taking the adult dose of pyrilamine is
   a. 4-6 hours
   b. 6-8 hours
   c. 2-6 hours
   d. 12 hours

4. H_1-receptor antagonists have been used in the treatment of respiratory disease for
   a. two decades
   b. five decades
   c. less than five decades
   d. more than five decades

5. The side effects of hydroxyzine include all of the following except
   a. increase of cognitive function
   b. dry mouth
   c. blurred vision
   d. urinary retention

6. The second generation of antihistaminic compounds is available
   a. only by prescription world wide
   b. only in the United States
   c. in the United States only by prescription
   d. only by prescription in Canada and Europe.

7. NDA means
   a. National Drug Application
   b. New Drug Application
   c. New Drugs Available by prescription only.
   d. New Drugs Available only in Canada

8. Hismanal was NDA approved on
   a. December 29, 1988
   b. March 20, 1977
   c. October 17, 1961
   d. May 8, 1985

9. The symbol for "by prescription" is
   a. OTC
   b. NDA
   c. FDA
   d. R_x

10. The first H_1-receptor antagonist to be introduced to the United States as nonsedating was
   a. Claritin
   b. Cetirizine
   c. Terfenadine
   d. Loratadine

WORD PROBLEM

Directions: Use the strategies you learned for solving word problems to answer the following question.

Steven Everfore is taking triprolidine once every four hours. If his first dose was taken at 10:00 AM, when should he take his third dose?

References

Beaver BV: Feline Behavior: A Guide for Veterinarians. Philadelphia, W.B. Saunders, 1992.

Bonewit-West K: Computer Concepts and Applications for the Medical Office. Philadelphia, W.B. Saunders, 1993.

Chabner D-E: The Language of Medicine, 4th ed. Philadelphia, W.B. Saunders, 1991.

Diehl MO, Fordney MT: Medical Typing and Transcribing: Techniques and Procedures, 3rd ed. Philadelphia, W.B. Saunders, 1991.

Ehrlich A, Torres HO: Essentials of Dental Assisting. Philadelphia, W.B. Saunders, 1992.

Flynn JC Jr (Ed.): Procedures in Phlebotomy. Philadelphia, W.B. Saunders, 1994.

Henry MC, Stapleton ER (Eds.): EMT Prehospital Care. Philadelphia, W.B. Saunders, 1992.

Kinn ME, Woods MA, Derge EF: The Medical Assistant: Administrative and Clinical, 7th ed. Philadelphia, W.B. Saunders, 1993.

LaFleur-Brooks M (Ed.): Health Unit Coordinating, 3rd ed. Philadelphia, W.B. Saunders, 1993.

Lewis N (Ed.): Roget's New Pocket Thesaurus in Dictionary Form. New York, Washington Square Press, 1978.

McCurnin DM (Ed.): Clinical Textbook for Veterinary Technicians, 3rd ed. Philadelphia, W.B. Saunders, 1994.

Miller-Keane Encyclopedia & Dictionary of Medicine, Nursing, & Allied Health, 5th ed. Philadelphia, W.B. Saunders, 1992.

Polaski A, Warner JP: Saunders Fundamentals for Nursing Assistants. Philadelphia, W.B. Saunders, 1994.

Purtilo R: Ethical Dimensions in the Health Professions, 2nd ed. Philadelphia, W.B. Saunders, 1993.

Solomon EP: Introduction to Human Anatomy and Physiology. Philadelphia, W.B. Saunders, 1992.

Torres HO, Ehrlich A: Modern Dental Assisting, 4th ed. Philadelphia, W.B. Saunders, 1990.

Witek TJ Jr, Schachter EN: Pharmacology and Therapeutics in Respiratory Care. Philadelphia, W.B. Saunders, 1994.

Glossary

abuse harmful treatment.
academic having to do with school or learning.
accredited credentialed.
analyzing breaking down a whole into its parts.
aneurysm a sac formed by the localized dilation of the wall of an artery, vein, or the heart.
aneurysmectomy surgical removal of an aneurysm.
anxiety emotional pain.
apprenticeship the practical experience of training under skilled workers.
approximate nearly the same or nearly correct.
asepsis freedom from infection (Miller-Keane, p. 141).
associate closely connected.
attending physician a doctor who works in a teaching hospital.
audience the people who will read your writing.
autocratic pertaining to one who has total power.
battered bruised.
beneficence kindness.
brainstorming spontaneously forming ideas.
cardiac pertaining to the heart (Miller-Keane, p. 250).
caret a punctuation mark that shows in what place something must be inserted.
chaotic pertaining to being in a state of utter confusion.
choppy short sentence.
chronological arranged in order of time.
common belonging to or shared by two or more mathematical entities.
comparison showing similarities of two or more items.
complement to complete or make perfect.
concentrate focus.
concepts ideas.
conclusions outcomes or results.
condensing making something more compact.
confidence self-assurance.
content the material to be learned in a course.
context the words around an unknown word that are used to figure out the meaning of the unknown word.
conventional traditional.
conversion the act of changing or transforming.
coworkers fellow employees.

credentials diplomas or certificates.
data factual information, usually in number form.
delete remove.
denominator the part of a fraction below the line that signifies division.
detect to see.
diabetes mellitus a disturbance in the oxidation and utilization of glucose (Miller-Keane, p. 142).
diagonal passing from the upper left to the lower right or the upper right to the lower left.
disclosure something made known.
discombobulated confused or upset.
distracted to have attention taken away.
document informational paper.
draft a rough version of written work.
E-mail electronic mail, a message sent on a computer.
efficiently pertaining to being productive without any waste.
emphasis stresses the importance of something.
endangered subject to being destroyed.
equation a mathematical expression of similarity.
ethicist a person who studies morality.
expanded expressed in greater detail.
exponent a mathematical number written to the right and above a number to show the raising of a power.
extends stretch forward.
external outside the body.
focused directed.
form the medium for the written message.
formulate devise.
function keys special control keys on the computer keyboard.
gastrointestinal pertaining to the stomach and intestine.
goals aims, intentions.
hemostasis stopping blood flow by natural or artificial means.
highlight emphasize.
hormones chemical transmitter substance produced by cells of the body and transported by the bloodstream to the cells and organs on which it has a specific regulatory effect (Miller-Keane, p. 702).
host an animal or plant that harbors and provides sustenance for another organism.
hypertrophy increase in volume of a tissue or organ produced entirely by enlargement of existing cells.
hypotension lowered blood pressure.
identical the same.
imperative essential.
inadequate not good enough.
indentation the division of a document to create sections.

indicate demonstrate.
ingested taken in.
interfere to get in the way of.
internal inside the body.
intimidated made timid or fearful.
inverse opposite.
invoice a list showing items purchased and how much money is owed.
ions charged particles
journal an account of daily events.
juggling dealing with several things at one time.
logically relating to the ability to use reason.
lymph a transparent, usually slightly yellow, often opalescent liquid found within the lymphatic vessels (Miller-Keane, p. 867).
mechanics punctuation, sentence style, word choice, capitalization, grammar.
microcapillary minute vessels connecting arterioles and venules (Miller-Keane, p. 245).
microorganisms an organism that is too small to be seen with the unaided eye.
mobilize to put into action.
molecules the smallest amount of a substance that possesses its characteristic properties (Miller-Keane, p. 929).
monitoring asking yourself if you are understanding what you are reading; watching; observing.
narrating telling a story.
neurologist a specialist in that branch of health science that deals with the nervous system (Miller-Keane, p. 1021).
numerator the part of a fraction above the line that signifies division.
objective lack of feeling toward or against.
obligation a commitment to acting in certain ways.
opponents those who disagree.
ovum egg.
pancreas a large gland located behind the stomach.
passive not active.
pathogenic having the ability to cause disease.
plaque food debris on tooth that fosters bacteria.
portable able to carry easily.
presentation the appearance.
prewriting plan for writing.
prioritize in order of importance.
procedure steps taken in a logical manner to accomplish something.
process the several steps involved in doing something.
procrastination delaying what needs to be done.
product the answer in a multiplication problem.
product the end result of the creative effort of writing.
protein any large organic compound made from one or more polypeptides (Miller-Keane, p. 1228).

pulse rate the pressure on the arteries used for the counting of heart beats.
purpose why the author is writing.
quadrants one of four parts.
quadrupled made four times greater.
quantity total amount.
quotient the answer in a division problem.
radiation energy carried by waves or a stream of particles.
recreational having to do with activities designed for relaxation and fun.
reference a book containing information, like an encyclopedia or dictionary.
resistant tending to oppose.
respectively in the given order.
reverse to go in an opposite direction.
revision rewriting.
rote use of memory mechanically.
secrete to synthesize and release a substance.
sequence the order of events.
slanted biased.
sodium salt.
statistic numerical data.
subject the topic.
subject area to be learned.
sum the answer in an addition problem.
supine lying with the face up (Miller-Keane, p. 1438).
syllables parts of a word that contain at least one consonant and one vowel.
tedious boring.
tendency leaning toward.
topical pertaining to a particular area (Miller-Keane, p. 1506).
transmission passage or transfer of a disease from one individual to another.
typical having the nature or being part of a type.
utility usefulness.
vague not clearly stated.
values numerical quantities.
variable a symbol representing a number that may have any value.
venipuncture surgical puncture of a vein (Miller-Keane, p. 1597).
veracity truthfulness.
veterinary relating to the diagnosis and cure of disease in animals.
visualize to make a mental picture.
welts a lump on the body caused by a heavy blow.

Answer Key

CHAPTER 1

Vocabulary Check
1. efficiently
2. asepsis
3. lymph
4. topical
5. neurologist
6. supine
7. autocratic
8. hemostasis
9. document
10. conclusions

Exercise 1–1
1. L
2. A
3. I
4. I
5. L
6. A
7. A
8. L
9. L
10. I

Exercise 1–2
1. confidentiality
2. hemostasis
3. checking references
4. cats and psychotherapy
5. appointment scheduling

Exercise 1–3
1. Topic = The cell.
   Main idea = The cell is the basic unit of all life.
2. Topic = Connective tissue fibers.
   Main idea = Collagen fibers are the most numerous.
3. Topic = Liquid topical anesthetics.
   Main idea = (unstated). Answers may vary, but they should contain the following ideas: Liquid topical anesthetics can be used for numbing and relieving pain in the mouth.
4. Topic = Computer service.
   Main idea = It is important to choose a service that will explain what can be expected from the computer and that will provide all the instruction and supervision necessary to ensure success in using it.
5. Topic = Preparing surgical site.
   Main idea = (unstated). Answers may vary, but they should contain the following ideas: Before surgery and after the animal is anesthetized, the hair should be clipped and the skin in and around the surgical site should be scrubbed with a special skin preparation.

Exercise 1–4
1. b
2. a
3. d
4. a
5. c

Exercise 1–5
Answers may vary, but they should include the following ideas:
- "Will you wait, or should I have the doctor call you back?"

329

- "I am sorry, but the doctor is still busy."
- "I am sorry that you are waiting so long. Would you like me to have the doctor call you back when he is free?"
- "Thank you for waiting. The doctor should be free in a few minutes."
- "Will you please wait while I get the information?"

Exercise 1–6

I
G
D
A
C
E
H
B
F
K
J

CHAPTER 2

Vocabulary Check
1. apprenticeship
2. beneficence
3. accredited
4. veracity
5. disclosure
6. sodium
7. quadrants
8. aneurysm
9. aneurysmectomy
10. pancreas

Exercise 2–1
See below

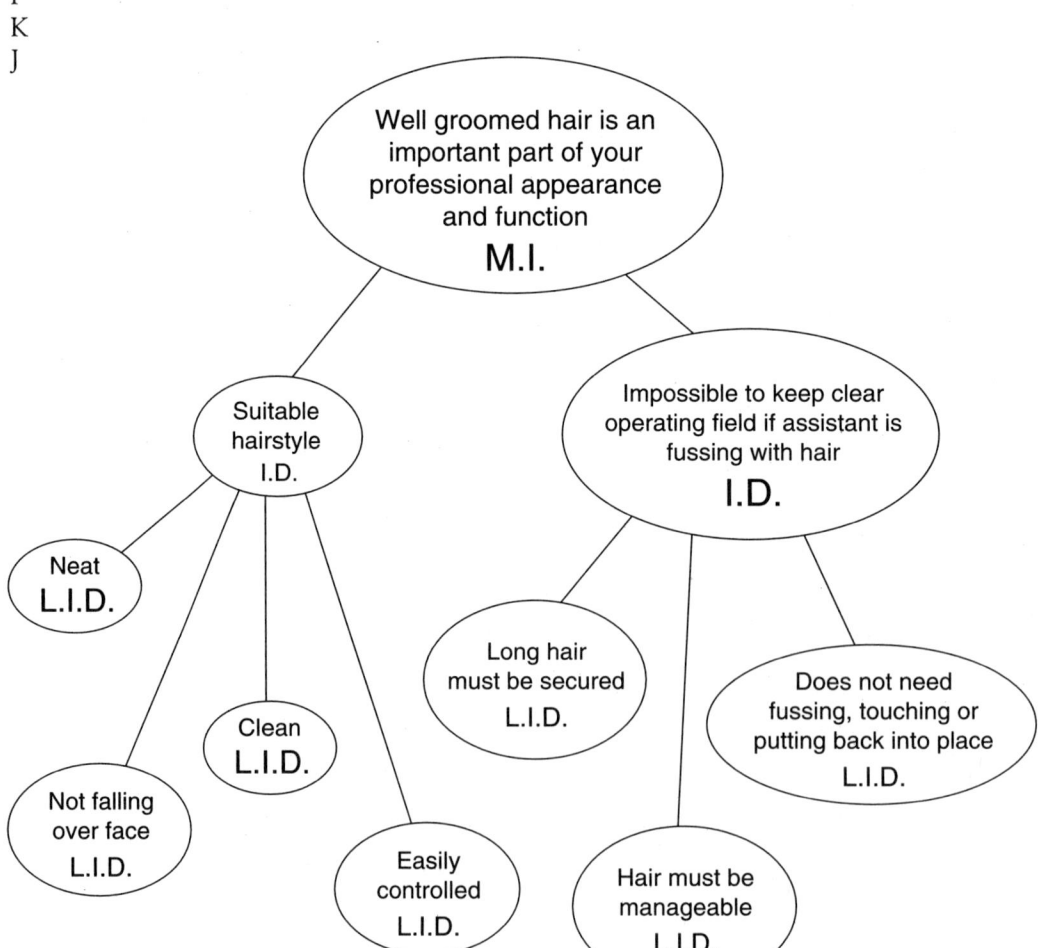

Exercise 2–2
1. b   par #3
        line 4-5
2. d   par #5
        line 3
3. c   par #4
        line 5
4. d   par #2
        line 5-6
5. a   par #1
        line 4

Exercise 2–3
1. Additional precautions in handling 5.25 floppy disks.
2. 5
3. before, immediately, after, when
4. 1, 4, 5, 3, 2

Exercise 2–4
1. Sequence
2. Mixing polysulfide impression materials
3. 5
4. 3, 1, 5, 2, 4

Exercise 2–5
1. Classification
2. Yes
3. Quadrants of the abdominopelvic area or quadrants of the abdomen
4. 4
5. Right upper quadrant
   Right lower quadrant
   Left upper quadrant
   Left lower quadrant
6. Right upper quadrant

Exercise 2–6
1. Classification
2. Yes
3. Divisions of the back (spinal column)
4. 1
5. 2

Exercise 2–7
1. Examples and illustration
2. High blood pressure in arteries
3. 140/90 mm Hg
4. Diuretics, beta-blockers, losing weight, limiting salt intake, stopping smoking, reducing fat in diet.
5. essential, secondary

Exercise 2–8
1. Comparison-contrast
2. An argument against disclosure vs. arguments favoring disclosure
3. Honesty
   Death not taboo
   Caring entails sharing information
4. Maintain hope of patient
   Patient passive
   Benevolence
5. Answers will vary

Exercise 2–9
1. Cause-effect
2. The cause of congestive heart failure
3. Heart cannot pump required amount of blood, and blood accumulates in the lungs
4. Fluid
5. Right-sided heart failure

CHAPTER 3

Vocabulary Check
1. context
2. vague
3. analyzing
4. hormones
5. syllable
6. inadequate
7. veterinary
8. ovum
9. pathogenic
10. microorganisms

Exercise 3–2
1. (a catheter coated with a substance that does not permit the passage of x-rays)
2. also known as oil glands
3. ("tail vein")
4. (those that are used only once)
5. a portable file

Exercise 3–3
Answers will vary.

Exercise 3–4
Discrimination that is not entirely defined by law may be just as harmful as the discrimination that is defined. This type of discrimination is often referred to as *subtle discrimination*. Subtle discrimination is <u>not obvious</u> and is <u>seldom expressed openly</u>. It includes <u>discrimination based on a person's appearance, values, or lifestyle or on some other personal factor</u>.

    Much of the discrimination that occurs in medical facilities falls into this category. Examples include <u>discrimination against overweight people, divorced people, gay people, people receiving public assistance, and people with sexually transmitted diseases</u>. Often you may not even be aware that your words or actions reflect subtle discrimination against another.

Exercises 3–5 and 3–6
See table on page 333.

Exercise 3–7
Answers will vary.

Exercise 3–8
1. metastasis
2. boldface
3. four
4. Germany
5. One
6. adjective
7. cancer

Exercise 3–9
1. two
2. testosterone
3. heel bone
4. acquired immune deficiency syndrome
5. abdomen

Exercises 3–10
Answers will vary.

Exercise 3–11
Answers will vary.

CHAPTER 4

Vocabulary Check
1. glossary
2. pulse rate
3. reference
4. monitoring
5. diabetes mellitus
6. invoice
7. approximate
8. function keys
9. attending physician
10. visualize

Exercise 4–1
Answers will vary.

Exercise 4–2
Answers will vary.

Exercise 4–3
Answers will vary.

Exercise 4–4
Some of the main points that can be included in the summary are
- Not all information from a medical record should be released to a third party.
- The attending physician should be consulted if there is a question about what information is to be released.
- Summaries, abstracts, or standardized forms can be used to release information.
- Attending physicians can receive medical information on their patients without the patients' written approval.

Exercise 4–5
Answers will vary.

Exercise 4–6
C
B
A
C
B
A

Exercise 4–7
Answers will vary.

Exercise 3-5 and 3-6

	DEFINITION	EXAMPLE	DEFINITION OF EXAMPLE	YOUR EXAMPLE
Prefix				
anti	against	anti-inflammatory	something that stops inflammation	answers will vary
*dys	bad, difficult	dyslexia	difficulty with the printed word	answers will vary
*exo	outside	exoskeleton	external skeleton, shell	answers will vary
*hem, hemato	relating to the blood	hemodiagnosis	blood used for diagnostic purposes	answers will vary
*hyper	over, above, beyond	hyperkinesia	above normal motor activity	answers will vary
inter	between	intersession	Time between academic semesters	answers will vary
mal	poor, bad	maladjusted	poorly adjusted	answers will vary
*peri	around, near	perigastric	near the stomach	answers will vary
semi	half	semiretired	working only half-time	answers will vary
tele	distant, far	telescope	instrument for seeing objects at a distance	answers will vary
Root				
*arthro, arthr	joint	arthritis	inflammation on the joint	answers will vary
bio	life	biology	study of life forms	answers will vary
*cardi, cardio	heart	cardiopathy	disease of the heart	answers will vary
*derm, dermo	skin	dermatitis	inflammation of the skin	answers will vary
fac, fact	make, do	factory	place where objects are made	answers will vary
*path	disease	pathologist	a person who studies the disease process	answers will vary
port	carry	portable	able to be carried	answers will vary
*psych	mind	psychiatry	field of medicine concerned with mental disorders	answers will vary
spec, spect	to look at	spectator	one who looks at something	answers will vary
vers	turn	reversible	able to be turned around	answers will vary
Suffix				
able, ible	capable of	trainable	able to be trained	answers will vary
ation	act of	sanitation	act of making sanitary	answers will vary
*ectomy	excision	hysterectomy	removal of the uterus	answers will vary
ful	full of	hateful	full of hate	answers will vary
*itis	inflammation of	bursitis	inflammation of the bursa	answers will vary
ology	study	psychology	study of the mind	answers will vary
*oma	tumor	hematoma	collection of clotted blood	answers will vary
*osis	disease	nephrosis	disease of the kidneys	answers will vary
*phobia	fear	xenophobia	fear of strangers	answers will vary
scope	see	periscope	instrument for seeing around obstacles	answers will vary

*Word parts with a medical use.

CHAPTER 5

Vocabulary Check
1. plaque
2. ingested
3. secrete
4. ions
5. hypertrophy
6. credentials
7. discombobulated
8. statistics
9. chaotic
10. protein

Exercise 5-1
1. *Clinical Textbook for Veterinary Technicians*
2. Dennis M. McCurnin
3. two degrees
4. Louisiana State University
5. W.B. Saunders Company
6. Philadelphia, London, Toronto, Montreal, Sydney, Tokyo
7. Third edition

Exercise 5-2
1. new students of phlebotomy and those collecting blood for many years
2. topics directly related to blood collection
3. professional topics
4. glossary
5. review questions and answers, 100-item review examination, quick reference chart

Exercise 5-3
1. ten chapters
2. Feline Social Behavior
3. page 174
4. Feline Locomotive Behavior
5. seven major headings

Exercise 5-4
1. abdomen
2. adventitia
3. actin
4. alphabetical
5. acid

Exercise 5-5
1. *The Language of Medicine*
2. 1986
3. third edition
4. *Understanding Medical Terminology*
5. alphabetical

Exercise 5-6
1. audition
2. olfaction
3. gustation
4. touch
5. vision

Exercise 5-7
1. Letters I through L
2. page 747
3. six subtopics
4. yes
5. 86, 87, 88, 89, 90, 91

Exercise 5-8
Answers will vary.

Exercise 5-9
1. The characteristics of x-rays that are useful to physicians in the diagnosis and treatment of disease.
2. Six.
3. Charged particles.
4. Answers will vary.
5. Answers will vary.

Exercise 5-10
1. Answers will vary.
2. Answers will vary.

Exercise 5-11
1. DNA.
2. DNA controls not only the production of new cells but also the cell's ability to grow.
3. When a cell reproduces itself.
4. DNA is located in the nucleus of a cell.
5. By directing the making of new proteins, DNA copies itself.

Exercise 5-12
1. Muscle separating the chest and abdomen
2. Breathing in
3. Breathing out
4. How the diaphragm helps the breathing process

Exercise 5–13
1. Fat-soluble Vitamins
2. Vitamin A
   Vitamin D
   Vitamin E
   Vitamin K
3. K
4. The functions, sources, and deficiency symptoms of fat-soluble vitamins
5. a. Answers will vary.
   b. Answers will vary.

Exercise 5–14
1. The Role of Nutrition in Preventive Dentistry.
2. No written answer required.
3. a. The desire to learn.
   b. The development of knowledge or skill.
4. Four.
5. Answers will vary.
6. Answers will vary.
7. No written answer required.
8. Nutritionally sound snacks.
9. Sugar content of popular food.
10. It shows the sugar content of foods that are to be avoided as snacks because they are damaging to dental health.
11. Answers will vary.
12. Answers will vary.
13. Answers will vary.
14. Answers will vary.

CHAPTER 6

Vocabulary Check
1. prewriting
2. process
3. form
4. purpose
5. narrating
6. E-mail
7. subject
8. audience
9. brainstorming
10. abuse

Exercise 6–1
Answers will vary.

Exercise 6–2
Answers will vary.

Exercise 6–3
Answers will vary.

Exercise 6–4
Answers will vary.

Exercise 6–5
Answers will vary.

Exercise 6–6
Answers will vary.

Exercise 6–7
Answers will vary.

Exercise 6–8
Subject   *Unconscious patient*
Main Idea   *Patient unconscious because of large laceration and temperature of 31°C.*
Purpose   *Description*
Form   *Case history*
Audience   *Hospital emergency staff*

Subject   *Printer paper*
Main Idea   *To describe the types of paper used with a printer*
Purpose   *Describing*
Form   *Description*
Audience   *Person learning how to use computers*

Subject   *When to start CPR*
Main Idea   *Factor to consider when starting CPR*
Purpose   *Explanation*
Form   *Directions*
Audience   *EMTs*

CHAPTER 7

Vocabulary Check
1. product
2. draft
3. confidence
4. revision
5. expanded
6. endangered
7. slanted
8. sequence
9. detect
10. emphasis

Exercise 7–1
Answers will vary.

Exercise 7–2
Answers will vary.

Exercise 7–3
Answers will vary.

Exercise 7–4
Answers will vary.

Exercise 7–5
Answers will vary.

Exercise 7–6
Answers will vary.

Exercise 7–7
Answers will vary.

Exercise 7–8
Answers will vary.

CHAPTER 8

Vocabulary Check
1. focused
2. delete
3. mechanics
4. imperative
5. resistant
6. tedious
7. choppy
8. presentation
9. battered
10. welts

Exercise 8–1
Answers will vary.

Exercise 8–2
Both children had been battered. In the last month, two of the seven reported cases of child abuse were from middle class homes with both parents. Therefore it is imperative that you report all cases of suspected child abuse. No.
Answers will vary.

Exercise 8–3
Answers will vary.

Exercise 8–4
Answers will vary.

Exercise 8–5
1. copied
2. poked
3. neighbor
4. guardian
5. handkerchief
6. easier
7. hopeless
8. judgment
9. temperature
10. dried

Exercise 8–6
1. Who's
2. stationery
3. principal
4. chose
5. except
6. They're
7. allowed
8. too
9. dessert
10. lose

Exercise 8–7
1. fragment
2. correct sentence
3. fragment
4. run-on
5. run-on
6. correct sentence
7. fragment
8. correct sentence
9. run-on
10. fragment

Exercise 8–8
1. noun
2. preposition
3. pronoun
4. adjective
5. verb
6. interjection
7. adverb
8. interjection

Exercise 8–9
1. live
2. were
3. is
4. his
5. they
6. it
7. expects
8. her

9. his
10. follows

Exercise 8–10

Rosa is taking **E**nglish lessons so that she will be able to get a better job. She is hoping to improve her skills in reading**,** writing, and conversation. **W**hen she finishes this course**,** she will be able to enter a community college. Will this course give her skills she needs to succeed**?** She will have to meet the following requirements**:** taking notes, understanding lectures, and comprehending her textbooks. **R**osa hopes to become a technician when she moves to **P**hiladelphia in two years**.**

CHAPTER 9

Exercise 9–2
1. $\frac{1}{4}$
2. $\frac{24}{36}$
3. $\frac{128}{14}$ or $\frac{64}{7}$
4. $\frac{2}{11}$
5. $\frac{27}{28}$
6. $\frac{1}{6}$
7. $\frac{2}{3}$
8. $\frac{1}{10}$
9. 6
10. $3\frac{1}{8}$

Exercise 9–3
1. 14.326
2. 8.805
3. 15.889
4. 41.35
5. 471.635
6. 0.7524404
7. 280
8. 400
9. $\frac{1}{50}, \frac{4}{5}, \frac{9}{20}$
10. 0.8, 0.075, 0.2

Exercise 9–4
1. $\frac{1}{2}$, 0.5
2. $12\frac{1}{2}\%$, $\frac{1}{8}$
3. $16\frac{2}{3}\%$, $0.16\frac{2}{3}$
4. 70%, $\frac{7}{10}$
5. $\frac{3}{5}$, 0.6
6. 40%, 0.4
7. $66\frac{2}{3}\%$, $\frac{2}{3}$
8. $37\frac{1}{2}\%$, 0.375
9. $\frac{4}{5}$, 0.8
10. 25%, 0.25
11. 6
12. $112\frac{1}{2}\%$
13. 120
14. $37\frac{1}{2}\%$
15. 18.75

Exercise 9–5
1. 10:400 = 1:40, $\frac{1}{40}$, 1 to 40
2. 5:20 = 1:4, $\frac{1}{4}$, 1 to 4
3. 48:6 = 8:1, 8, 8 to 1
4. 19.209 = $\frac{19}{209}$, 19 to 209
5. 15:35 = 3:7, $\frac{3}{7}$, 3 to 7

Exercise 9–6
1. 4:12 = 1:3 $\frac{4}{12} = \frac{1}{3}$
2. 16:40 = 2:5 $\frac{16}{40} = \frac{2}{5}$
3. 35:30 = 7:6 $\frac{35}{30} = \frac{7}{6}$
4. 108:24 = 9:2 $\frac{108}{24} = \frac{9}{2}$
5. 77:99 = 7:9 $\frac{77}{99} = \frac{7}{9}$

Exercise 9–7
1. 8
2. 7
3. 81
4. 3
5. 63
6. 120
7. 210

8. 2040
9. 22
10. 124

CHAPTER 10

Vocabulary Check
1. exponent
2. extends
3. procedure
4. inverse
5. concentrate
6. equation
7. concepts
8. indicate
9. variable
10. identical

Exercise 10–1
1. +5
2. −12
3. +3
4. +35
5. −106
6. +555
7. +1
8. −32
9. +418
10. −1835

Exercise 10–2
1. −3
2. +15
3. +26
4. 0
5. −983
6. 579
7. +34,304
8. 64,108
9. 2,000,000
10. −1,000,000

Exercise 10–3
1. +8
2. −21
3. 448
4. +8775
5. −2020
6. +88,000
7. +24
8. −100
9. +1008
10. −8,400,000

Exercise 10–4
1. $+\frac{1}{3}$
2. $-\frac{1}{5}$
3. $\frac{1}{10}$
4. -0.125 or $-\frac{1}{8}$
5. +12
6. +2
7. −5
8. +4.5
9. −5
10. +2

Exercise 10–5
1. $c = 16$
2. $p = 6$
3. $k = 16$
4. $m = 30$
5. $k = \frac{1}{4}$
6. $v = 10$
7. $b = 968$
8. $k = 448$
9. $n = 31$
10. $= 5$

Exercise 10–6
1. 10 inches
2. $\frac{1}{2}$ inch
3. 4.75 inches
4. 14 inches
5. 50 inches
6. 1.5 inches
7. 78.5 square inches
8. 379.94 square inches
9. 1962.5 square inches
10. 0.0314 square inches

Exercise 10–7

TYPE OF TRIANGLE	ANGLE A	ANGLE B	ANGLE C
equilateral	60	60	60
scalene	23	55	102
right (isosceles)	45	45	90
isosceles	35.5	109	35.5
scalene	18.2	66	95.8
isosceles	15	15	150
scalene	99.4	3.6	77
right	answers will vary but one angle must = 90°		
scalene	answers will vary		
isosceles	answers will vary		

Exercise 10–8
1. 20 inches
2. 42 inches
3. 37 feet
4. 51 miles
5. 400 kilometers

Exercise 10–9
1. 49 square inches
2. 4096 square feet
3. 20.25 square miles
4. 36,000,000 square kilometers
5. 7,840,000 square yards

Exercise 10–10
1. 26
2. 60 inches or 5 feet
3. 34 yards
4. 132 kilometers
5. 556 centimeters

Exercise 10–11
1. 40 square units
2. 4.75 square inches
3. 12.5 square feet
4. 378 square centimeters
5. 12 square miles

Exercise 10–12
1. 3.18 quarts
2. 19.08 quarts
3. 1.395 square inches
4. 1.55 square inches
5. 2.48 miles
6. 18.6 miles
7. 6.42 meters
8. 41.28 meters
9. 8.1 kilograms
10. 22.7 kilograms

CHAPTER 11

Vocabulary Check
1. quadrupled
2. quantity
3. quotient
4. data
5. intimidated
6. product
7. respectively
8. sum
9. logically
10. formulate

Exercise 11–1
Strategies: answers will vary
Solutions: 934 kilowatt hour; 1,553 hundred cubic feet

Exercise 11–2
1. 1088 feet per second
   186,324 miles per second
   2 hours
2. How far does sound travel in 2 hours?
   How far does light travel in 2 hours?
3. 7,833,600 feet per 2 hours
   1,341,532,800 miles per 2 hours
4. Answers will vary.

Exercise 11–3
A. 1. 6 Bunsen burners, 5 Bunsen burners, 11 Bunsen burners
   2. How many Bunsen burners are in the veterinary school altogether?
   3. How many
   4. altogether
   5. addition
   6. 22 Bunsen burners
   7. Answers will vary.
B. 1. 322 persons in Chicago, 403 persons in Boston, 659 persons in Atlanta
   2. What is the total number of persons applying to dental school?
   3. What
   4. total
   5. add
   6. 1384 persons
   7. Answers will vary.

Exercise 11–4
A. 1. 5 feet 8 inches, 4 inches
   2. How tall is Mrs. Francis?
   3. How
   4. smaller than
   5. subtraction
   6. 5 feet, 4 inches
   7. Answers will vary.
B. 1. 8 hours, 24 hours
   2. How many study hours remain for Benny?
   3. How many
   4. remain or decrease by

5. subtraction
   6. 16 hours
   7. Answers will vary.

Exercise 11–5
   A. 1. 250 words, per minute
      2. How many words can he read in an hour?
      3. how many "more"
      4. time for 1 minute, time for many minutes
      5. multiplication
      6. 15,000 words
      7. Answers will vary.
   B. 1. $1000, quadrupled
      2. How much is she earning now?
      3. how much
      4. quadrupled
      5. multiplication
      6. $4000
      7. Answers will vary.

Exercise 11–6
   A. 1. 9 years and 10 months, half of that
      2. How old is Lauren?
      3. how old
      4. half of
      5. division
      6. 4 years and 11 months
      7. Answers will vary.
   B. 1. 12 videos for $250
      2. What was the cost of one video?
      3. cost of one
      4. cost of many, cost of one
      5. division
      6. $20.83
      7. Answers will vary.

Exercise 11–7
   1. 43 trays
   2. 559 trays
   3. $3000
   4. $30.03
   5. $6.25
   6. $24\frac{1}{4}$ hours
   7. 2%
   8. 59.5 hours
   9. $18\frac{1}{4}$ flasks
   10. 33,983.9 miles
   11. 2.1 seconds
   12. $2.50
   13. $0.77
   14. $\frac{5}{8}$
   15. $\frac{11}{16}$ ounce
   16. $\frac{1}{3}$ yard
   17. 66,500
   18. 5,000
   19. $168\frac{3}{4}$ pages
   20. $75.50

CHAPTER 12

Vocabulary Check
   1. anxiety
   2. recreational
   3. prioritize
   4. juggling
   5. tendency
   6. goals
   7. procrastination
   8. external
   9. internal
   10. academic

Exercise 12–1
Answers will vary.

Exercise 12–2
Answers will vary.

Exercise 12–3
Answers will vary.

Exercise 12–4
Answers will vary.

Exercise 12–5
Answers will vary.

CHAPTER 13

Vocabulary Check
   1. highlight
   2. coworkers
   3. subject
   4. distracted
   5. journal
   6. rote
   7. content
   8. interfere
   9. objective
   10. passive

Exercise 13–1
Answers will vary.

Exercise 13–2
Answers will vary.

CHAPTER 14

Vocabulary Check
1. complement
2. venipuncture
3. cardiac
4. microcapillary
5. molecules
6. portable
7. chronological
8. molecules
9. indentation
10. conventional

Exercise 14–1
Answers will vary.

Exercise 14–2
Answers will vary.

Exercise 14–3
Answers will vary.

Exercise 14–4
Answers will vary but should resemble the sample below.

BLOOD LANCETS

What are blood lancets?
 For difficult patients, including situations that normally call for microcapillary techniques, a blood lancet may be used. This is a small sterile, disposable instrument used for skin puncture.... Lancets are available with a variety of point lengths to help control the depth of puncture, which is especially important in children and infants. A variety of semiautomated devices are commercially available, but the manual lancet is the most commonly used device for microcapillary puncture.

Exercise 14–5
Answers will vary.

Exercise 14–6
Answers will vary but should look something like this:

 Two medical emergencies that require quick action are cardiac arrest and respiratory arrest.
 These are referred to as code arrests. Cardiac arrest: there are no heart contractions, pulse, or blood pressure. Respiratory arrests: patient does not breathe, and body cells die.
 In both conditions, treatment must be immediate because brain cells die in 3 to 4 minutes.
All nursing units have an emergency cart and fully equipped code arrest carts. It is important for the health unit coordinator to know the location of these carts.
Hospitals have personnel who report code arrests.
 They are employed in various hospital departments.

Exercise 14–7
Results and timing will vary.

Exercise 14–8
Answers will vary.

Exercise 14–9

Proofreading marks = Topic = Heading
What are proofreading marks? = Heading question
When copy is prepared for printing, it is corrected and marked, with correction symbols placed either in the margin or between the lines to indicate the changes to be made. If more than one marginal note is necessary, a slash mark (/) divides the notes. Either or both margins are used.
 In proofreading your own copy, you may be more informal, using marginal notes only when there is no room on the single-spaced copy to indicate the change.
 While you are a student, your instructor will proofread your work and may mark the copy and use marginal notes in a variety of ways. Therefore let us examine the proofreading marks as they are used formally and see how we may modify them for our own use. Your instructor may wish to add his or her marking symbols as well.

CHAPTER 15

Vocabulary Check
1. hypotension
2. obligation
3. utility
4. mobilize
5. radiation
6. transmission
7. ethicist
8. host
9. opponents
10. gastrointestinal

Exercise 15–1
1. a
2. b
3. d
4. a
5. d
6. b
7. c
8. d
9. c
10. d

Exercise 15–2
1. consequences
2. utilitarianism
3. Jeremy Bentham and John Stuart Mill
4. utilitarian
5. usefulness
6. consequences
7. a. to restore Mr. Harvey to maximum health within the limits of his impairment
   b. to treat him in such a way that everyone else will be able to have the same treatment as he received
   c. to live within my own conscience
8. Jeremy Bentham and John Stuart Mill
9. the most important consequence
10. duties, rights, and responsibilities

Exercise 15–3
1. d
2. i
3. f
4. j
5. a
6. b
7. h
8. c
9. k
10. g

Exercise 15–4
1. T
2. F
3. T
4. F
5. F
6. T
7. F
8. T
9. T
10. F

Exercise 15–5
Part I
1. host
2. reservoir
3. typhoid fever
4. incubation period
5. exposure

Part II
1. e
2. d
3. a
4. b
5. c

Part III
1. d
2. a
3. b
4. d
5. c

Part IV
1. F
2. F
3. T
4. F
5. F

Exercise 15–6
Answers will vary.

Exercise 15–7
Answers will vary.

READING SELECTION 1

Preview Question
Answers will vary.

ANSWER KEY

Vocabulary
Answers will vary.

Writing
Answers will vary.

Comprehension Questions
1. c
2. d
3. a
4. c
5. b
6. a
7. d
8. a
9. b
10. d

Word problem
$2916.67
$26,000
$2166.67

READING SELECTION 2

Preview Question
Answers will vary.

Vocabulary
Answers will vary.

Writing
Answers will vary.

Comprehension Questions
1. F
2. T
3. F
4. T
5. F
6. T
7. F
8. F
9. F
10. T

Word Problem
270 cassettes
30 cassettes

READING SELECTION 3

Preview Question
Epidermis: constantly renewing itself; waterproofing
Dermis: provides strength and elasticity
Superficial fascia: attaches skin to underlying tissue

Vocabulary
Answers will vary.

Writing
Answers will vary.

Comprehension Questions
1. C
2. C
3. B
4. A
5. B
6. C
7. C
8. B
9. A
10. B

Word Problem
41,200 people

READING SELECTION 4

Preview Question
Skeletal, muscular, nervous, sensory, endocrine, cardiovascular, and lymphatic systems
Answers will vary.

Vocabulary
Answers will vary.

Writing
Answers will vary.

Comprehension Questions
1. cardiac
2. 700 muscles
3. central nervous system
4. autonomic nervous system
5. hormones
6. receptors
7. cardiovascular system
8. thoracic and right lymphatic ducts
9. metabolic waste and carbon dioxide
10. muscle and glands

Word Problem
approximately 3 replacements

READING SELECTION 5

Preview Question
Answers will vary.

Vocabulary
Answers will vary.

Writing
Answers will vary.

Comprehension Questions
1. c
2. a
3. b
4. d
5. a
6. c
7. b
8. a
9. d
10. d

Word Problem
5,600,000 stray cats

READING SELECTION 6

Preview Question
generalist, administrative assistant, chairside assistant, coordinating assistant, the extended functions dental assistant

Vocabulary
Answers will vary.

Writing
Answers will vary.

Comprehension Questions
1. F
2. T
3. F
4. T
5. T
6. F
7. T
8. F
9. T
10. F

Word Problem
Profit; $10,727

READING SELECTION 7

Preview Question
nose, pharynx, larynx, trachea, bronchi, lungs

Vocabulary
Answers will vary.

Writing
Answers will vary.

Comprehension Questions
1. C
2. E
3. F
4. A
5. D
6. E
7. F
8. B
9. A
10. C

Word Problem
1.6%

READING SELECTION 8

Preview Question
Drapes are folded in accordion fashion so that they are easily unfolded onto the patient.

Vocabulary
Answers will vary.

Writing
Answers will vary.

Comprehension Questions
1. outside, up
2. hand towel, sterilization indicator
3. 8 steps
4. so they are easily unfolded unto the patient
5. 15 cm in width
6. 9 steps
7. The gown, along with a hand towel and sterilization indicator, is placed diagonally onto the nonfenestrated drapes.
8. The corners are folded over the gown.

9. 6 steps
10. contents, date, initials of the individual preparing the pack

Word Problem
8 accordion folds

READING SELECTION 9

Preview Question
1. pneumonia
2. asthma
3. emphysema

Vocabulary
Answers will vary.

Writing
Answers will vary.

Comprehension
1. F
2. T
3. F
4. T
5. T
6. T
7. F
8. T
9. F
10. F

Word Problem
$1\frac{1}{2}$ hours

READING SELECTION 10

Preview Question
A pathogen is a microorganism that is capable of causing disease.

Vocabulary
Answers will vary.

Writing
Answers will vary.

Comprehension
A. 3
B. 6
C. 4
D. 5
E. 1
F. 2
G. 10
H. 8
I. 9
J. 7

Word Problem
3,840

READING SELECTION 11

Preview Question
Scrolling is the automatic movement of text up or down on the computer screen.

Vocabulary
Answers will vary.

Writing
Answers will vary.

Comprehension
1. block
2. insertion
3. editing
4. layout
5. line spacing
6. automatic pagination
7. storing
8. boldface
9. memory
10. removes

Word Problem
2 hours

READING SELECTION 12

Preview Question
General anesthesia, local anesthesia, and spinal anesthesia

Vocabulary
Answers will vary.

Writing
Answers will vary.

Comprehension
1. b
2. c
3. a
4. b
5. a
6. d

7. b
8. a
9. c
10. c

Word Problem
1:50 PM

READING SELECTION 13

Preview Question
respiratory and cardiac arrest

Vocabulary
Answers will vary.

Writing
Answers will vary.

Comprehension
1. F
2. F
3. T
4. T
5. F
6. F
7. T
8. T
9. T
10. F

Word Problem
two times the risk

READING SELECTION 14

Preview Question
Lou Gehrig's disease

Vocabulary
Answers will vary.

Writing
Answers will vary.

Comprehension
1. deterioration
2. baseball player
3. epilepsy
4. facial
5. outside
6. four
7. thymectomy
8. degeneration
9. paralysis
10. palliative

Word Problem
10 students

READING SELECTION 15

Preview Question
two generations

Vocabulary
Answers will vary.

Writing
Answers will vary.

Comprehension
1. b
2. c
3. b
4. d
5. a
6. c
7. b
8. a
9. d
10. c

Word Problem
6:00 PM

Index

Note: Page numbers in *italics* refer to illustrations; page numbers followed by t refer to tables.

A

Abbreviations, for note-taking, 219
Abdomen, quadrants of, 29, *29*
Acrivastine, 319
Acronyms, in test-taking, 226
Agreement, grammatical, 128
Algebra, 152–160
   addition in, 152–153
   division in, 156–157
   equations in, 157–159
   multiplication in, 154–156
   subtraction in, 153–154
Anesthesia, 304–307
Aneurysm, aortic, *32*
Angle, in geometry, 160
Antihistamines, 316–321, 317t, 319t
Aorta, aneurysm of, *32*
Appendix, of textbook, 74–75
Area, metric, 169t
   of circle, 163
   of rectangle, 168
   of square, 166–167
Astemizole, 319
Asthma, 291–292, 315–323
Attention, pretending to, 200
Audience, in writing process, 102
Audiotape, of lecture, 220
Azatadine, 319–320
Azelastine, 319–320

B

Back, divisions of, 30–31, *30*
Bibliography, of textbook, 74
Brompheniramine, 316
Burns, electrical, 308–311

C

Calendar, daily, 195, *195*
   monthly, 192, *193*
   weekly, 193–194, *194*
Capitalization, 129

Cardiovascular system, 264, *265*, *266*
Cat, 268–272
Cause-effect, as pattern of organization, 36
Cements, dental, 31, *31*
Cetirizine, 320
Chlorpheniramine, 316–317
Circle, 161–164
   area of, 163
   circumference of, 162–163
   diameter of, 161, 162
   radius of, 162
Circumference, of circle, 162–163
Classification, as pattern of organization, 27–31
Comparison and contrast, as pattern of organization, 33–35
Comprehension, 53–64
   in textbook reading, 61–64
   making connections for, 57–58
   monitoring of, 55
   rereading for, 55
   researching for, 60–61
   summarizing for, 58–59
   visualizing for, 59–60
   vocabulary development for, 56
Computer, 253–257
   in revision process, 119–120
   word processing on, 298–302
Computer software, 253–254
Connections, for comprehension, 57–58
Context clues, for vocabulary, 40–43
   location of, 41–43
Conversion chart, 169t

D

Daydreaming, 200
Decimals, 141–144
   addition of, 142
   division of, 142–143
   multiplication of, 142
   subtraction of, 142
   to fractions, 143
   to percentages, 145

Degenerative disorders, 312–314
Dental assistant, 273–278, *274–276*
Dental cements, 31, *31*
Dermis, 259, *260*
Description, in writing process, 101, 111
Details, in interpretive understanding, 10–11
   mapping of, 18–19
   order of, 23–25
   supporting, 17
   vs. main idea, 17
Diameter, of circle, 161, *162*
Diaphragm, 86
Dictionary, 45–46
Dictionary entry, 45–46
Diphenhydramine, 317–318
Disclosure, argument against, 34
   argument for, 35
Disk, computer, 23–24, 254
Distraction, 200
   elimination of, 196
Division, 136–137, 137t

E

Editing, in writing process, 120
Electrical burns, 308–311
Embolism, pulmonary, 281–282
Emphysema, 292
Endocrine system, 264, *265*
Epidermis, 259, *260*
Equation(s), algebraic, 157–159
   addition in, 157–158
   checking answer to, 159
   division in, 159
   multiplication in, 158
   solution of, 157
   subtraction in, 158
Equilateral triangle, 164
Essay test, 240–243
Explanation, in writing process, 101, 111

F

Facial bones, 27–28, *28*
Facts, verification of, 20–22
Fascia, superficial, 260
Final draft, in writing process, 114–130
First draft, in writing process, 106–113
Floppy disk, 23–24, 254
Form, in writing process, 102, 102t
Fraction(s), 137–141
   addition of, 138–139
   division of, 140–141
   higher term of, 138
   lowest term of, 137–138
   multiplication of, 139–140
   subtraction of, 138–139

Fraction(s) (*Continued*)
   to decimals, 143
   to percentages, 144

G

Geometry, 160–168
   basic terms of, 160–161
Glands, 78–80, *79*
Glossary, 46–47
   of textbook, 70, 73
Goal setting, in time management, 190–191
Graphic aids, in reading, 85–88, *86*, 87t

H

Handwriting, for note-taking, 218
Hearing, vs. listening, 199
Heart, high blood pressure effects on, 36
Hemothorax, 281
Highlighting, for note-taking, 211–212
Hydroxyzine, 318
Hypertension, 32

I

Index, of textbook, 76–77
Infection, 294–297
Integumentary system, 258–261, *260*
Isosceles triangle, 164

L

Lecture, note-taking from, 214–216, *215*
   taping of, 220
Length, metric, 169t
Line, in geometry, 160
Liquid measure, metric, 169t
Listening, vs. hearing, 199
Listening skills, 198–203
   application of, 203
   evaluation of, 199–200
   monitoring of, 201, 202
   5W questions in, 201
Listing, in writing process, 98–99
Logical relationships, 23
Loratadine, 320–321
Lymphatic system, 266

M

Main idea, in writing process, 100, 109
   of passage, 8–10
   vs. supporting details, 17
Mapping, 18–19
   in reading, 18–19
   in writing process, 98–99

Margin writing, for note-taking, 212–214
Matching tests, 232–233
Medical assistant, 247–252
Metric system, 168–170, 169t
Misspelled words, 123–124
Misused words, 125
Modem, computer, 254–255
Movement disorders, 312–314
Multiple-choice tests, 227–228
Multiplication, 135–136, 135t
Muscles, 263, *263*

N

Narration, in writing process, 101, 111
Nervous system, 263–264, *264*
   disorders of, 312–314
Notebook, for note-taking, 207–208
Note-taking, 204–222
   abbreviations for, 219
   from lecture, 214–216, *215*
   from textbook, 210–211, *211*
   handwriting for, 218
   headings for, 220–221
   highlighting for, 211–212
   importance of, 205–206
   instructors' cues in, 217
   margin writing for, 212–214
   notebook for, 207–208
   notepaper organization for, 208–210, *209*
   quantity of, 217
   rote, 200
   speed of, 217–220
   studying from, 220–222
   symbols for, 219
   time management and, 207
   use of, 207
Nutrition, in preventive dentistry, 89–91, 90t

O

Objective tests, 227–240
Organization, in writing process, 98–99, 111–112

P

Parts of speech, 127
Patterns of organization, 22
   cause-effect, 36
   classification, 27–31
   comparison and contrast, 33–35
   sequence, 25–27
Percentages, 144–147, 145t
   problems with, 145–146
   to decimals, 144
   to fractions, 144
Perimeter, of rectangle, 167–168
   of square, 166

Persuasion, in writing process, 101, 111
Phenindamine, 318
Pheumothorax, 281, *282*
Pneumonia, 291
Point, in geometry, 160
Polysulfide syringe material, 25–27, *26*
Preface, of textbook, 68–69
Prefix, 43, 44t
Previewing, 78–82
Prewriting, 97
Printer ribbon, 254
Prioritization, in time management, 191–192
Procrastination, avoidance of, 197
Pronoun agreement, 128
Proofreading, in writing process, 120
   symbols for, 121–122
Proportions, 148–149
Pulmonary embolism, 281–282
Punctuation, 129
Purpose, in writing process, 100

Q

5W Questions, in active listening, 201
   in reading, 82–84
   in writing process, 98, 113

R

Radiology, 80–82, *81*
Radius, of circle, 161, *162*
Ratios, 147–148
Reading, applied understanding in, 5, 13–14
   cause-effect in, 36
   classification in, 27–31
   comparison and contrast in, 33–35
   comprehension of, 53–64. See also *Comprehension.*
   difficult, 88
   examples in, 31–32
   fact verification in, 30
   facts in, 20–22
   graphic aids in, 85–88, *86*, 87t
   illustrations in, 31–32
   interpretative understanding in, 5, 10–13
   literal understanding in, 5, 6–10
   logical relationships in, 23
   main idea in, 17
   mapping details in, 18–19
   order of details in, 23–25
   organizational patterns in, 23–36
   previewing of, 78–82
   purpose for, 4–5
   purpose in, 4–5
   questioning in, 82
   review of, 88
   sequence in, 25–27
   supporting details in, 17

Reading, applied understanding in (*Continued*)
  texbook, 65–92. See also *Textbook, reading of.*
  vocabulary in, 38–52. See also *Vocabulary.*
  5W questions in, 82–84
Reading selections, anesthesia, 303–307
  asthma, 315–323, 317t, 319t
  body systems, 262–267, *263–265*
  cat, 268–272
  computers, 253–257
  dental assistant, 273–278, *274–276*
  electrical burns, 308–311
  infection control, 294–297
  medical assistant, 247–252
  nervous system disorders, 312–314
  respiratory diseases, 290–293
  respiratory system, 279–283, *280, 282*
  skin, 258–261
  surgical gown folding, 284–289, *285–288*
  text editing, 298–300, *300*
  word processing, 298–302
Rectangle, 167–168
  area of, 168
  in geometry, 161
  perimeter of, 167–168
Rereading, for comprehension, 55
Researching, for comprehension, 60–61
Respiratory system, 279–283, *280*
Revision, computer in, 119–120
  in writing process, 116–119
Revision checklist, 116
Rhymes, in test-taking, 226
Right triangle, 165
Root, of word, 43, 44t

S

Scalene triangle, 165
Scheduling, in time management, 192–196
Sebaceous glands, 78–80, *79*
Seizures, 312–314
Sentence errors, in writing process, 126–127
Sequence, as pattern of organization, 25
Short-answer tests, 230–231
Signal words, in word problems, 176–183, 176t, 179t, 181t, 182t
Skeleton, 262–263
Skin, 258–261, *260*
Spelling, in writing process, 122–124
  rules for, 123
Spine, divisions of, 30–31, *30*
Square, 166–167
  area of, 166–167
  in geometry, 161
  perimeter of, 166
Subject-verb agreement, 128
Suffix, of word, 43, 44t
Summarizing, for comprehension, 58–59

Surgical gown, 284–289, *285–288*
Sweat glands, 79
Symbols, for note-taking, 219

T

Table of contents, of textbook, 70, *71–72*
Terfenadine, 321
Test-taking, 223–244
  acronyms in, 226
  evaluation of, 243
  for essay test, 240–243
  for matching questions, 232–233
  for multiple-choice questions, 227–228
  for objective tests, 227–240
  for short-answer questions, 230–231
  for true-false questions, 234–235
  planning for, 225
  rhymes in, 226
  schedule for, 225
  strategies for, 224–227
  study for, 225–227
Text editing, 298–300
Text filing, 300–301
Text formatting, 301–302
Textbook, appendix of, 74–75
  bibliography of, 74
  glossary of, 70, 73
  index of, 76–77
  note-taking from, 210–211, *211*
  preface of, 68–69
  reading of, 65–92
    comprehension in, 61–64
    difficult, 88
    graphic aids in, 85–88, *86*, 87t
    health care literacy in, 84–85
    previewing of, 78–82
    questioning in, 82
    review of, 88
    5W questions in, 82–84
  survey of, 67–77
  table of contents of, 70, *71–72*
  title page of, 67–68
Thesaurus, 47–49
Time management, 189–197
  daily calendar in, 195, *195*
  goal setting in, 191
  monitoring of, 197
  monthly calendar in, 192, *193*
  note-taking and, 207
  prioritization in, 191–192
  scheduling in, 192–196
  to-do list in, 195, 196t
  weekly calendar in, 193–194, *194*
Title page, of textbook, 67–68
To-do list, in time management, 195, 196t
Topic, of passage, 6–7

Topic outline, in writing process, 98–99
Transcription equipment, 255–256
Triangle, 164–165
   equilateral, 164
   in geometry, 161
   isosceles, 164
   right, 165
   scalene, 165
Triprolidine, 318
True-false tests, 234–235

U

Understanding, 3–15
   applied, 5, 13–14
   interpretive, 5, 10–13
   literal, 5, 6–10

V

Vitamin, fat-soluble, 87
Vitamin A, 87
Vitamin D, 87
Vitamin E, 87
Vitamin K, 87
Vocabulary, 38–52, 40
   context clues for, 40–43
   dictionary for, 45–46
   for comprehension, 56
   glossary for, 46–47
   thesaurus for, 47–49
   word cards for, 50–51
   words parts of, 43–45, 44t

W

Weight, metric, 169t
Word(s), in dictionary, 45–46
   memorization of, 49–51
   misspelled, 123–124
   misused, 125
Word cards, memorization of, 50–51
Word problems, 172–186
   careful reading for, 173–174
   in addition, 176–178, 176t

Word problems (*Continued*)
   in division, 182–183, 182t
   in multiplication, 180–181, 181t
   in subtraction, 178–180, 179t
   question formulation for, 174–176
   signal words in, 176–183, 176t, 179t, 181t, 182t
Word processing, 298–302
Writing plan, in writing process, 108–109
Writing process, 96–97
   audience in, 102
   beginning in, 112
   computer in, 119–120
   description in, 101, 111
   editing in, 120
   ending in, 112
   explanation in, 101, 111
   final draft in, 114–130
   first draft in, 106–113
   form in, 101–102
   listing in, 98–99
   main idea in, 100, 109
   mapping in, 98–99
   middle in, 112
   misused words in, 125
   narration in, 101, 111
   organization in, 98–99, 111–112
   persuasion in, 101, 111
   presentation in, 122
   prewriting strategies in, 97
   proofreading in, 120
      symbols for, 121–122
   purpose in, 100
   revision in, 116–119
   sentence errors in, 126–127
   spelling in, 122–124
   subject selection in, 98
   topic outline in, 98–99
   5W questions in, 98, 113
   writing plan in, 108–109

X

X-rays, 80–81, 81